Essentials of Surgery

Essentials of Surgery

Edited by **Valerie Kent**

hayle medical

New York

Published by Hayle Medical,
30 West, 37th Street, Suite 612,
New York, NY 10018, USA
www.haylemedical.com

Essentials of Surgery
Edited by Valerie Kent

International Standard Book Number: 978-1-63241-384-0 (Hardback)

Printed in the United States of America.

Contents

Preface   IX

Chapter 1   **Comparison of Subcuticular Suture Materials in Cesarean Skin Closure**   1
Pınar Solmaz Hasdemir, Tevfik Guvenal, Hasan Tayfun Ozcakir,
Faik Mumtaz Koyuncu, Gonul Dinc Horasan, Mustafa Erkan and Semra Oruc Koltan

Chapter 2   **Negative Pressure Incision Management System in the Prevention of Groin
Wound Infection in Vascular Surgery Patients**   6
Jan H. Koetje, Karsten D. Ottink, Iris Feenstra and Wilbert M. Fritschy

Chapter 3   **Evaluation of Early versus Delayed Laparoscopic Cholecystectomy in
Acute Cholecystitis**   10
Rati Agrawal, K. C. Sood and Bhupender Agarwal

Chapter 4   **Guidelines for Perioperative Management of the Diabetic Patient**   17
Sivakumar Sudhakaran and Salim R. Surani

Chapter 5   **Biomechanical Evaluation of a Mandibular Spanning Plate Technique
Compared to Standard Plating Techniques to Treat Mandibular
Symphyseal Fractures**   25
Matthew Richardson, Jonathan Hayes, J. Randall Jordan, Aaron Puckett and
Matthew Fort

Chapter 6   **Will Septal Correction Surgery for Deviated Nasal Septum Improve the Sense of
Smell? A Prospective Study**   31
Neelima Gupta, P. P. Singh and Rahul Kumar Bagla

Chapter 7   **Pharyngoesophageal Suturing Technique May Decrease the Incidence of
Pharyngocutaneous Fistula following Total Laryngectomy**   36
Mahmut Deniz, Zafer Ciftci and Erdogan Gultekin

Chapter 8   **Surgical Audit of Patients with Ileal Perforations Requiring Ileostomy in
a Tertiary Care Hospital in India**   41
Hemkant Verma, Siddharth Pandey, Kapil Dev Sheoran and Sanjay Marwah

Chapter 9   **Superior Mesenteric Artery Syndrome: Clinical and Radiological Considerations**   45
M. Ezzedien Rabie, Olajide Ogunbiyi, Abdullah Saad Al Qahtani, Sherif B. M. Taha,
Ahmad El Hadad and Ismail El Hakeem

Chapter 10   **Perioperative Evaluation of Patient Outcomes After Severe Acid Corrosive Injury**   50
Ming-Ho Wu and Han-Yun Wu

Chapter 11   **Local Anaesthetic Infiltration and Indwelling Postoperative Wound Catheters for Patients with Hip Fracture Reduce Death Rates and Length of Stay**   56
William D. Harrison, Deborah Lees, Jamie A'Court, Thomas Ankers, Ian Harper, Dominic Inman and Mike R. Reed

Chapter 12   **Factors Associated with Perforated Appendicitis in Elderly Patients in a Tertiary Care Hospital**   64
Siripong Sirikurnpiboon and Suparat Amornpornchareon

Chapter 13   **An Assessment of the Clinical and Economic Impact of Establishing Ileocolic Anastomoses in Right-Colon Resection Surgeries Using Mechanical Staplers Compared to Hand-Sewn Technique**   70
S. Roy, S. Ghosh and A. Yoo

Chapter 14   **Knowledge, Practice and Associated Factors towards Prevention of Surgical Site Infection among Nurses Working in Amhara Regional State Referral Hospitals, Northwest Ethiopia**   77
Freahiywot Aklew Teshager, Eshetu Haileselassie Engeda and Workie Zemene Worku

Chapter 15   **Audit of Orthopaedic Surgical Documentation**   83
Fionn Coughlan, Prasad Ellanti, Cliodhna Ní Fhoghlu, Andrew Moriarity and Niall Hogan

Chapter 16   **Panniculectomy Combined with Bariatric Surgery by Laparotomy: An Analysis of 325 Cases**   87
Vincenzo Colabianchi, Giancarlo de Bernardinis, Matteo Giovannini and Marika Langella

Chapter 17   **The Use of Tutomesh for a Tension-Free and Tridimensional Repair of Uterovaginal and Vaginal Vault Prolapse: Preliminary Report**   97
Danilo Dodero and Luca Bernardini

Chapter 18   **To Investigate the Effect of Colchicine in Prevention of Adhesions Caused by Serosal Damage in Rats**   105
Ehsan Yıldız and Yavuz Savas Koca

Chapter 19   **Long-Term Outcomes of Sacrococcygeal Germ Cell Tumors in Infancy and Childhood**   109
Rangsan Niramis, Maitree Anuntkosol, Veera Buranakitjaroen, Achariya Tongsin, Varaporn Mahatharadol, Wannisa Poocharoen, Suranetr La-orwong and Kulsiri Tiansri

Chapter 20   **Evaluation of Factor VIII as a Risk Factor in Indian Patients with DVT**   117
Darpanarayan Hazra, Indrani Sen, Edwin Stephen, Sunil Agarwal, Sukesh Chandran Nair and Joy Mammen

Chapter 21   **Operative Exposure of a Surgical Trainee at a Tertiary Hospital in Kenya**   121
Daniel Kinyuru Ojuka, Jana Macleod and Catherine Kwamboka Nyabuto

Chapter 22   **Hiatus Hernia Repair with Bilateral Oesophageal Fixation**   126
Rajith Mendis, Caran Cheung and David Martin

Chapter 23   **Teamwork Assessment Tools in Modern Surgical Practice: A Systematic Review**   131
George Whittaker, Hamid Abboudi, Muhammed Shamim Khan, Prokar Dasgupta
and Kamran Ahmed

Chapter 24   **Patient Satisfaction and Quality of Life in DIEAP Flap versus Implant Breast
Reconstruction**   142
Rossella Sgarzani, Luca Negosanti, Paolo Giovanni Morselli,
Veronica Vietti Michelina, Luigi Maria Lapalorcia and Riccardo Cipriani

Chapter 25   **A EWTD Compliant Rotation Schedule Which Protects Elective Training
Opportunities is Safe and Provides Sufficient Exposure to Emergency
General Surgery: A Prospective Study**   149
Andrew Emmanuel, Ezzat Chohda, Carolyn Sands, Joseph Ellul and
Hamid Khawaja

Chapter 26   **Review of Subcutaneous Wound Drainage in Reducing Surgical Site Infections
after Laparotomy**   154
B. Manzoor, N. Heywood and A. Sharma

Chapter 27   **Leakage After Surgery for Rectum Cancer: Inconsistency in Reporting to the
Danish Colorectal Cancer Group**   160
L. Borly, M. B. Ellebæk and N. Qvist

Chapter 28   **Comparing Supervised Exercise Therapy to Invasive Measures in the
Management of Symptomatic Peripheral Arterial Disease**   165
Thomas Aherne, Seamus McHugh, Elrasheid A. Kheirelseid, Michael J. Lee,
Noel McCaffrey, Daragh Moneley, Austin L. Leahy and Peter Naughton

Chapter 29   **Delorme's Procedure for Complete Rectal Prolapse: A Study of Recurrence
Patterns in the Long Term**   175
Carlos Placer, Jose M. Enriquez-Navascués, Ander Timoteo, Garazi Elorza,
Nerea Borda, Lander Gallego and Yolanda Saralegui

Chapter 30   **Surgical Management of Endometrial Polyps in Infertile Women: A
Comprehensive Review**   181
Nigel Pereira, Allison C. Petrini, Jovana P. Lekovich, Rony T. Elias and
Steven D. Spandorfer

Permissions

List of Contributors

Preface

Surgery is inevitable in extreme cases like that of severe accident, organ failure or gangrene and even in the complicated cases of child birth. In some cases it helps in relieving pain and in other cases it optimizes body function. Different kinds of surgeries are available depending upon the body parts such as breast surgery, colon and rectal surgery, endocrine surgery, general surgery, gynecological surgery, hand surgery, head and neck surgery, neurosurgery, orthopedic surgery, etc. Use of precision instruments in surgeries has made it further advanced and accurate. The various sub-fields of surgery along with technological progress that have future implications are glanced at in this book. The aim of this text is to present researches that have transformed this discipline and aided its advancement. It will help the readers in keeping pace with the rapid changes in this field. This book is appropriate for students seeking detailed information in this area as well as for experts.

The researches compiled throughout the book are authentic and of high quality, combining several disciplines and from very diverse regions from around the world. Drawing on the contributions of many researchers from diverse countries, the book's objective is to provide the readers with the latest achievements in the area of research. This book will surely be a source of knowledge to all interested and researching the field.

In the end, I would like to express my deep sense of gratitude to all the authors for meeting the set deadlines in completing and submitting their research chapters. I would also like to thank the publisher for the support offered to us throughout the course of the book. Finally, I extend my sincere thanks to my family for being a constant source of inspiration and encouragement.

Editor

Comparison of Subcuticular Suture Materials in Cesarean Skin Closure

Pınar Solmaz Hasdemir,[1] Tevfik Guvenal,[1] Hasan Tayfun Ozcakir,[1]
Faik Mumtaz Koyuncu,[1] Gonul Dinc Horasan,[2] Mustafa Erkan,[1] and Semra Oruc Koltan[1]

[1]Department of Obstetrics and Gynecology, Celal Bayar University Medical School, 45000 Manisa, Turkey
[2]Department of Statistics, Celal Bayar University Medical School, Manisa, Turkey

Correspondence should be addressed to Pınar Solmaz Hasdemir; solmazyildiz@yahoo.com

Academic Editor: Antonio Boccaccio

Aim. Comparison of the rate of wound complications, pain, and patient satisfaction based on used subcuticular suture material. *Methods.* A total of 250 consecutive women undergoing primary and repeat cesarean section with low transverse incision were prospectively included. The primary outcome was wound complication rate including infection, dehiscence, hematoma, and hypertrophic scar formation within a 6-week period after operation. Secondary outcomes were skin closure time, the need for use of additional analgesic agent, pain score on numeric rating scale, cosmetic score, and patient scar satisfaction scale. *Results.* Absorbable polyglactin was used in 108 patients and nonabsorbable polypropylene was used in 142 patients. Wound complication rates were similar in primary and repeat cesarean groups based on the type of suture material. Skin closure time is longer in nonabsorbable suture material group in both primary and repeat cesarean groups. There was no difference between groups in terms of postoperative pain, need for additional analgesic use, late phase pain, and itching at the scar. Although the cosmetic results tended to be better in the nonabsorbable group in primary surgery patients, there was no significant difference in the visual satisfaction of the patients. *Conclusions.* Absorbable and nonabsorbable suture materials are comparable in cesarean section operation skin closure.

1. Introduction

Cesarean sections are one of the most commonly performed abdominal operations in women worldwide [1]. Wound healing is an important factor for lower complication rate and patient satisfaction in patients undergoing cesarean section.

Tully et al. showed that 73.9% of the obstetricians preferred to close skin with subcuticular sutures using Prolene (41.1%), Vicryl (17.5%) followed by dexon (13.5%), and staples (10.4%) [2]. The subcuticular absorbable sutures and surgical staples in cesarean wound closure were compared in the literature. Although there are conflicting results, closure with subcuticular suture materials were reported to be more advantageous in terms of wound healing, better cosmetic results and more patient satisfaction rates [3, 4].

The outcome of wound healing and patient satisfaction based on the use of subcuticular suture material (absorbable versus nonabsorbable) is unknown. The aim of this study is to compare the rate of wound complications, pain, and patient satisfaction based on used subcuticular suture material.

2. Materials and Methods

A total of 250 consecutive patients with viable pregnancies greater than 24 gestational weeks undergoing scheduled or unscheduled first or repeat cesarean delivery with low transverse incision were prospectively included between July 2014 and January 2015 at Celal Bayar University Hospital, Manisa, Turkey. The randomization of the patients to the groups was made by weekly alternating the type of suture (absorbable or nonabsorbable) used in cesarean operations. Obstetricians performing the operation were blind for the procedure characteristics including type of suture material, time needed for skin closure, and length of the wound. An inquiry form was filled by a resident from the study team the day after the operation and at the 6th weeks of follow-up. Wound infection was defined as any discharge, mild to severe requiring dressing and antibiotic use. Wound dehiscence was defined as separation of skin edges more than 1 cm in length. Hematoma was defined as wound swelling more than 1 cm in diameter accompanied by changing in colour of the skin. Hypertrophic scar was defined as pink-red coloured, hard, itchy, visible, and raised from the normal tissue level scar. Body mass index (BMI) was calculated at the time of delivery.

2.1. *Exclusion Criteria.* Patients with inability to obtain informed consent (emergent cases in which there was no time to get informed consent and patients who did not prefer to be in such a study protocol), fetal death, history of nonobstetric abdominal operation, known diabetes or gestational diabetes (except from abnormal glucose tolerance test values under control with diet only), any known immunological disorder, history of allergy for antibiotics and analgesics, and steroid drug usage were excluded. Patients implemented a nonroutine procedure (midline skin incision, postpartum hysterectomy or relaparotomy) because of an unexpected complication and patients who did not come for a second visit were also excluded.

The total number of the cesarean operations during the study period was 453 in our hospital. The main reasons for exclusion were lack of follow-up in 91 (20%), inability to obtain informed consent in 52 (11.8%), and presence of diabetes in 16 (3.5%) patients.

2.2. *Ethical Consent.* The study was approved by the Institutional Review Board of the Celal Bayar University with the number of 20.478.486-137, on March 26, 2014. Informed patient consent was obtained from the cases.

2.3. *Operative Technique.* Skin of the patients was cleaned with povidone iodine 3 to 4 minutes before the operation started. Prophylactic antibiotic (2nd generation cephalosporin) was administered in all patients right after cord clamping. The same operation technique (Pfannenstiel technique) was used for all patients. Subcutaneous tissues were closed with interrupted sutures (3.0 Vicryl Rapide [polyglactin 910]) in case of more than 1 cm subcutaneous tissue thickness. Polyglactin-910 (3.0 Vicryl) was used as absorbable and polypropylene (3.0 Prolen) was used as nonabsorbable suture material for skin closure. Continuous suturing with curved needle was used in all patients regardless of the suture type. Closure of the skin was performed by the attending physician who performed the operation and did not have information about the study protocol. Nonabsorbable suture materials were removed at postoperative 7 to 10 days. All patients included in the study were advised not to use any medication that would potentially affect wound healing.

Wound evaluations were initially performed at hospital discharge at postoperative day 2 or 3 and at 6th week of follow-up. The primary outcomes were complications related to wound healing (infection, dehiscence, hematoma, and hypertrophic scar formation) at 6th week of follow-up. Secondary outcomes were operative time, pain score on numeric rating scale (NRS) (0 = no pain; 2 = mild; 5 = moderate; 7 = severe; 10 = excruciating), itching at the scar site, cosmetic score (no scar or just a line, mild ridge with minimal change in colour, and presence of severe scar [>0,5 cm ridge and red in colour]), and patient scar assessment scale (1 = minimum and 10 = maximum). NRS, cosmetic score, and patient scar assessment scale were evaluated by asking the patient verbally to grade the extent and severity of the scar or pain on a scale of zero to ten for NRS and one to ten for patient scar assessment scale [5–8].

2.4. *Statistical Analysis.* Statistical analysis was performed with IBM SPSS Statistics 15.0 (SPSS Inc., Chicago, IL). A stratified analysis was made for patients with primary and repeat cesarean delivery. The Shapiro-Wilk test was used to calculate whether the numeric variables were normally distributed. For normally distributed variables, differences in the distributions of the patient characteristics were analyzed with Student's t test. The Mann-Whitney U test was used for abnormally distributed variables. Cross-tables and chi square analysis were employed in the evaluation of the categorical data. P value <0.05 was considered statistically significant.

3. Results

A total of 250 patients underwent cesarean section. Absorbable polyglactin-910 (3.0 Vicryl) was used in 108 (43.2%) and nonabsorbable polypropylene (3.0 Prolen) was used in 142 (56.8%) patients. Of the 250 patients, 167 underwent primary and 83 underwent repeat cesarean deliveries. Baseline characteristic including age, BMI, type, and length of skin incisions was similar in absorbable and nonabsorbable suture material groups for both primary and repeat cesarean patients (Table 1). Wound complication rates were similar in primary and repeat cesarean groups based on the type of suture material (Table 2). Skin closure time was longer in nonabsorbable suture material group in both primary and repeat cesarean patients ($P = 0.016$ and $P = 0.035$, resp.). There was no statistical difference between absorbable and nonabsorbable suture groups in terms of postoperative pain, need for additional analgesic use, itching, and pain at the scar tissue at 6th weeks follow-up (Table 3). Although the cosmetic results tended to be better in nonabsorbable group in primary surgery patients ($P = 0.089$), there were no significant differences in the visual satisfaction of the patients ($P = 0.717$) (Table 3).

4. Discussion

Functional and cosmetic aspects of cesarean surgeries gain increasing importance in recent years. There is still a lack of data in terms of the best method for skin closure in cesarean operations [9, 10]. There are several studies in the literature comparing staples with suture in closure of cesarean

TABLE 1: Descriptive statistics of study groups.

	Primary Cesarean			Repeat Cesarean		
	Absorbable (n = 80)	Nonabsorbable (n = 87)	P value	Absorbable (n = 28)	Nonabsorbable (n = 55)	P value
Age (years) (mean ± SD)	26.78 ± 4.83	27.11 ± 5.35	0.678*	30.71 ± 5.36	29.16 ± 4.92	0.192*
BMI (mean ± SD)	27.24 ± 4.48	28.38 ± 4.88	0.130*	30.12 ± 5.25	29.29 ± 4.92	0.487*
Wound length (mm)						
mean ± SD	11.00 ± 1.36	11.27 ± 1.70		11.03 ± 1.29	11.20 ± 1.67	
Median (25th–75th)	11 (10–12)	11 (10–12)	0.813**	11 (10–12)	11 (10–12)	0.775**

*Student's t test, **Mann-Whitney U test.

TABLE 2: Comparison of the groups in terms of the primary outcomes (complication rates).

Complication	Primary Cesarean			Repeat Cesarean		
	Absorbable (n = 80)	Nonabsorbable (n = 87)	P value	Absorbable (n = 28)	Nonabsorbable (n = 55)	P value
Wound infection (%)	22.5%	14.9%	0.210*	14.3%	12.7%	1.000**
Hematoma	6.3%	3.4%	0.480**	0.0	5.5%	0.546**
Dehiscence	5.0	5.7	1.000**	10.7	10.9	1.000**
Hypertrophic scar	3.8%	2.3%	0.668**	3.6%	0.0	0.352**

*Chi square test, **Fisher's exact test.

incisions [3, 7, 10–13]. A meta-analysis which included 877 women from 5 studies compared the use of staples and subcuticular sutures. Study results showed that wound dehiscence and complication rates increased with staples, although the operation time was shortened only by a mean of 5.05 minutes. The authors recommended that subcuticular closure of the skin should be preferred [12]. Similar results were found by Mackeen et al. in 2015 [13]. Frishman et al. compared the staples with absorbable subcuticular suture in 66 women undergoing cesarean section and reported that operation time was significantly shorter with the use of staples. But the use of absorbable subcuticular suture resulted in less pain and use of lower dose of analgesics [11, 14]. A 2012 Cochrane review reported that staples and subcuticular absorbable sutures were similar in terms of wound infection and wound complication rates except that the incidence of wound dehiscence was increased with early (<4 days) removal of staples in women with Pfannenstiel incisions [9].

According to a recent prospective, randomized study closing cesarean incisions with suture is associated with 57% decrease in wound complications compared to closure with staples [13] along with better patient satisfaction rates [15]. Gaertner et al. compared subcuticular sutures with staples in both subcuticular layer closure and nonclosure group of patients and found no significant difference among the groups in terms of wound complications and patient satisfaction at 4th month of follow-up [16].

Based on the results of the abovementioned studies, subcuticular sutures seem to be more advantageous compared to staples [3, 12, 13]. But there is a lack of data comparing the outcome of different types of subcuticular suture materials. Tan et al. conducted a study comparing the suture materials and reported that absorbable and nonabsorbable

sutures have similar short-term outcomes but nonabsorbable sutures have a disadvantage of requirement of removal. Additionally, late-term itching at the scar site was seen more frequently in absorbable suture material group possibly due to the late absorption of this kind of suture material [17]. This study was a randomized, controlled study comparing absorbable (poliglecaprone 25) and nonabsorbable (polypropylene) suture materials in low-transverse incisions. Inclusion of obstetric and nonobstetric cases as well as diabetic cases was the downside of this study. In our study, we compared the most commonly used suture materials (Vicryl and Prolen) [2] just in cesarean sections and performed a stratified analysis for first and repeat cesarean patients. In addition, we excluded patients with diabetes which is an important confounder in wound healing.

4.1. Study Limitations. The major limitation of this study was the difference in the number of the patient population in the study groups despite the fact that we expected them to be similar when making the sample size calculations. However this was due to the weekly randomization process and was not expected to have confounder effect on the results of our study because patient characteristics such as age, BMI, and wound length were found similar.

5. Conclusion

Our results showed that there was no significant difference in terms of wound complications. There is a tendency to get better wound healing with nonabsorbable suture materials, although this difference did not affect the patient's satisfaction rate.

TABLE 3: Comparison of the groups in terms of the secondary outcomes.

| | Primary Cesarean | | | Repeat Cesarean | | |
	Absorbable (n = 80)	Nonabsorbable (n = 87)	P value	Absorbable (n = 28)	Nonabsorbable (n = 55)	P value
Skin closure time						
Mean ± SD	6.77 ± 1.12	7.31 ± 1.23		7.3 ± 0.97	7.83 ± 1.04	
Median (25th–75th)	7 (6–8)	7 (7–8)	0.016**	7 (7–8)	8 (7–9)	0.035**
Analgesic use	12.5%	30.2%	0.006*	21.4%	29.1%	0.455*
Postoperative pain (VAS)						
Mean ± SD	3.40 ± 2.74	4.02 ± 2.66		4.0 ± 3.30	4.11 ± 2.69	
Median (25th–75th)	3 (1–5)	3 (2–6)	0.099**	4 (1–6.75)	4 (2–6)	0.652**
Pain at 6th week	11.3%	21.8%	0.067*	28.6%	27.3%	0.901*
Itching	3.8%	3.4%	1.000***	0.00	0.00	NA
Cosmetic results			0.089*			0.723*
No scar or just a line	41.3%	56.3%		57.1%	63.6%	
Mild ridge with minimal change in colour	52.5%	35.6%		35.7%	27.3%	
Severe scar (>0,5 cm ridge and red in colour)	6.3%	8.0%		7.1%	9.1%	
Satisfaction						
Mean ± SD	6.70 ± 2.62	6.56 ± 2.61		7.28 ± 2.44	7.05 ± 2.79	
Median (25th–75th)	8 (5–9)	7 (5–9)	0.717**	8 (5.25–9.75)	8 (5–10)	0.879**

*Chi square, **Mann-Whitney U test, ***Fisher's exact test, and NA: not applicable.

Conflict of Interests

The authors declare that there is no conflict of interests regarding the publication of this paper.

References

[1] L. Gibbons, J. M. Belizán, J. A. Lauer, A. P. Betrán, M. Merialdi, and F. Althabe, "The global numbers and costs of additionally needed and unnecessary caesarean sections performed per year: overuse as a barrier to universal coverage," World Health Report, World Health Organization, Geneva, Switzerland, 2010.

[2] L. Tully, S. Gates, P. Brocklehurst, K. McKenzie-McHarg, and S. Ayers, "Surgical techniques used during caesarean section operations: results of a national survey of practice in the UK," European Journal of Obstetrics Gynecology and Reproductive Biology, vol. 102, no. 2, pp. 120–126, 2002.

[3] D. Figueroa, V. C. Jauk, J. M. Szychowski, R. Garner, J. R. Biggio, and W. W. Andrews, "Surgical staples compared with subcuticular suture for skin closure after cesarean delivery: a randomized controlled trial," Obstetrics & Gynecology, vol. 121, no. 5, pp. 33–38, 2013.

[4] A. D. MacKeen, T. Devaraj, and J. K. Baxter, "Cesarean skin closure preferences: a survey of obstetricians," Journal of Maternal-Fetal and Neonatal Medicine, vol. 26, no. 8, pp. 753–756, 2013.

[5] G. A. Hawker, S. Mian, T. Kendzerska, and M. French, "Measures of adult pain: Visual Analog Scale for Pain (VAS Pain), Numeric Rating Scale for Pain (NRS Pain), McGill Pain Questionnaire (MPQ), Short-Form McGill Pain Questionnaire (SF-MPQ), Chronic Pain Grade Scale (CPGS), Short Form-36 Bodily Pain Scale (SF-36 BPS), and Measure of Intermittent and Constant Osteoarthritis Pain (ICOAP)," Arthritis Care and Research, vol. 63, no. 11, pp. S240–S252, 2011.

[6] C. S. Rodriguez, "Pain measurement in the elderly: a review," Pain Management Nursing, vol. 2, no. 2, pp. 38–46, 2001.

[7] C. Sharma, A. Verma, A. Soni, M. Thusoo, V. K. Mahajan, and S. Verma, "A randomized controlled trial comparing cosmetic outcome after skin closure with 'staples' or 'subcuticular sutures' in emergency cesarean section," Archives of Gynecology and Obstetrics, vol. 290, no. 4, pp. 655–659, 2014.

[8] A. M. Coll, J. R. M. Ameen, and D. Mead, "Postoperative pain assessment tools in day surgery: literature review," Journal of Advanced Nursing, vol. 46, no. 2, pp. 124–133, 2004.

[9] A. D. Mackeen, V. Berghella, and M.-L. Larsen, "Techniques and materials for skin closure in caesarean section," Cochrane Database of Systematic Reviews, vol. 14, no. 11, Article ID CD003577, 2012.

[10] V. Berghella, J. K. Baxter, and S. P. Chauhan, "Evidence-based surgery for cesarean delivery," American Journal of Obstetrics and Gynecology, vol. 193, no. 5, pp. 1607–1617, 2005.

[11] F. Alderdice, D. McKenna, and J. Dornan, "Techniques and materials for skin closure in caesarean section," Cochrane Database of Systematic Reviews, vol. 2, Article ID CD003577, 2003.

[12] F. S. H. Clay, C. A. Walsh, and S. R. Walsh, "Staples vs subcuticular sutures for skin closure at cesarean delivery: a metaanalysis of randomized controlled trials," American Journal of Obstetrics and Gynecology, vol. 204, no. 5, pp. 378–383, 2011.

[13] A. D. Mackeen, M. Schuster, and V. Berghella, "Suture versus staples for skin closure after cesarean: a metaanalysis," American Journal of Obstetrics and Gynecology, vol. 212, no. 5, pp. 621.e1–621.e10, 2015.

[14] G. N. Frishman, T. Schwartz, and J. W. Hogan, "Closure of Pfannenstiel skin incisions. Staples vs. subcuticular suture," Journal of Reproductive Medicine for the Obstetrician and Gynecologist, vol. 42, no. 10, pp. 627–630, 1997.

[15] A. D. Mackeen, J. Fleisher, A. Khalifeh, C. M. Pettker, and V. Berghella, "Patient satisfaction and cosmetic outcome in a randomized study of cesarean skin closure," Obstetrics & Gynecology, vol. 123, pp. 4S–5S, 2014.

[16] I. Gaertner, T. Burkhardt, and E. Beinder, "Scar appearance of different skin and subcutaneous tissue closure techniques in caesarean section: a randomized study," European Journal of Obstetrics Gynecology and Reproductive Biology, vol. 138, no. 1, pp. 29–33, 2008.

[17] P. C. Tan, S. Mubarak, and S. Z. Omar, "Absorbable versus nonabsorbable sutures for subcuticular skin closure of a transverse suprapubic incision," International Journal of Gynecology and Obstetrics, vol. 103, no. 2, pp. 179–181, 2008.

Negative Pressure Incision Management System in the Prevention of Groin Wound Infection in Vascular Surgery Patients

Jan H. Koetje, Karsten D. Ottink, Iris Feenstra, and Wilbert M. Fritschy

Department of Vascular Surgery, Isala Zwolle, 8025 AB Zwolle, Netherlands

Correspondence should be addressed to Wilbert M. Fritschy; w.m.fritschy@isala.nl

Academic Editor: Axel Larena-Avellaneda

Objectives. Groin wounds following vascular surgery are highly susceptible to healing disturbances, with reported site infections reaching 30%. Negative pressure incision management systems (NPIMS) are believed to positively influence the prevention of surgical wound-healing disturbances (WHD) and surgical site infections (SSI). NPIMS placed directly after closure of the surgical wound is thought to result in fewer infections; we analysed its effect on postoperative wound infections in patients after vascular surgery via the groin. *Methods.* From May 2012 to March 2013 we included 90 surgical patients; 40 received a NPIMS. All patients with WHDs were labelled and subanalysed for surgical site infection in case of positive microbiological culture. These infections were graded according to Szilagyi. Number of WHDs and SSIs were compared across cohorts. *Results.* Patient and perioperative characteristics were equal, except for a significantly higher number of emergency procedures among non-NPIMS patients. We found no significant differences in number of WHDs, SSIs, or Szilagyi grades between the two cohorts. *Conclusion.* The equal number of SSIs across cohorts showed that NPIMS could not reduce the number of surgical site infections after vascular groin surgery.

1. Introduction

Negative pressure incision management systems (NPIMS), such as Prevena (KCI USA, Inc., San Antonio, TX), [1] are believed to have a positive effect in the prevention of surgical wound-healing disturbances and surgical site infection. Negative pressure treatment directly after closure of the surgical wound is thought to result in a better distribution of tensile forces on the wound edges, evacuation of subcutaneous seroma and haematoma, reduction of surgical site oedema, increased microvascular blood flow, prevention of influx and invasion of microorganisms, and protection and sealing of the wound [2].

It is known that groin wounds after vascular surgery are highly susceptible to wound-healing disturbances, with reported site infections varying up to 30% as reported in previous studies [3–6].

Several studies demonstrate the preventive effect of negative pressure wound management, for instance, after sternotomy, below knee amputations, and after surgery for blunt high energy trauma of the lower leg [7–10]. It is thought that vascular surgery in the groin region shows a high rate of wound problems due to disruption of lymphatics, proximity to the perineum, and the use of prosthetic material. Matatov et al. published recently a retrospective study on the use of NPIMS on groin wounds in vascular surgery patients [3]. They found a reduction from 30% site infections in the control group to 6% site infections in the NPIMS group ($P = .001$). Based on these promising data we started to apply NPIMS on groin wounds after vascular surgery. In this study, we will describe our first experience with this negative pressure wound management system.

2. Methods

Since early 2012, the Department of Vascular Surgery of our hospital has taken part in a Nationwide Hospital Quality Program for the registration of complications and surgical site infections by using a fixed protocol named "Prevention of Hospital bound Infections by Surveillance" (PREZIES) [11]. The registration of groin wound-healing disturbances (WHD) in vascular surgery patients was part of this program.

The NPIMS was introduced in May 2012. It was applied routinely to patients who underwent vascular surgery through a groin incision by two out of four vascular surgeons. No further randomisation was performed. After one year we analysed the data that were prospectively collected for PREZIES. We collected additional data from the hospital database and patient charts.

Ninety consecutive patients who underwent vascular surgery in the groin were included; 40 received the NPIMS on the surgical groin wound (NPIMS group). The remaining 50 patients did not receive NPIMS (non-NPIMS group). All patients underwent some kind of vascular operation on the common femoral artery, such as local endarterectomy or vascular bypass. They received preventive antibiotics 30 minutes prior to the start of operation, and the groin wounds were surgically closed by double-layer subcutaneous suturing and skin approximation with agraves. Patients suffering Rutherford 5 and 6 received routinely antibiotics perioperatively and at least one week after operation. In case of wound-healing disorders, a microbiological culture was taken and, if needed, antibiotic therapy was adjusted. Patients and nurses were instructed on the usage of the NPIMS. According to the instructions for use, the aim was to leave the NPIMS placed on the surgical wound for a minimum of four days. After discharge, follow-up took place during outpatient visits at the Department of Vascular Surgery.

All wounds with healing disorders (including erythema and swelling) and so clinical signs of infection were graded as "wound-healing disorder" (WHD). A WHD combined with positive microbiological culture was classified as a surgical site infection (SSI). These postoperative site infections were graded according to the Szilagyi classification system (Table 1) [12].

We have compared the number of WHDs and SSIs in the two patient cohorts (non-NPIMS group and NPIMS group). Based on the number of surgical site infections of the control group in the study of Matatov et al., we have calculated our required sample size, which seemed to be at least 40 subjects per group (95% confidence interval and power 0.8). Patient data were collected and analysed in SPSS.

For quality registration, we were obliged to collect data prospectively. We retrospectively analysed our results of the previously introduced NPIMS, without experimental base. Also, this study was performed by members of the treating medical team. For these reasons there was no need for gaining informed consent. The Institutional Review Board has approved our protocol, without further obligations.

3. Results

Of the 90 patients, 40 received the NPIMS on the groin (44%). Patient characteristics like age, BMI, smoking behaviour, diabetes mellitus, renal failure, end-stage renal disease, colonisation of microorganisms of preexisting wounds, preexisting colonisation with multiresistant microorganisms

TABLE 1: Szilagyi classification of surgical site infections.

Class	Description
Szilagyi I	Infection only involves the dermis
Szilagyi II	Infection extends into the subcutaneous tissue and does not invade the arterial implant
Szilagyi III	Arterial implant is involved in the infection

TABLE 2: Patient characteristics.

	Non-NPIMS	NPIMS	P value
Number of patients	50	40	
Gender			
Male[1]	34 (68.0%)	30 (75.0%)	.493[3]
Female[1]	16 (32.0%)	10 (25.0%)	.493[3]
Age[2]	71.5 ± 11.0	68.1 ± 8.6	.070[4]
BMI[2]	25.9 ± 5.8	27.4 ± 5.2	.130[4]
Smoking[1]	18 (36.0%)	23 (57.5%)	.056[3]
Diabetes mellitus[1]	15 (30.0%)	16 (40.0%)	.375[3]
Renal disorder[1]	22 (44%)	20 (50%)	.672[3]
End-stage renal disease[1]	2 (4.0%)	4 (10%)	.400[3]
Colonisation of preexisting wounds[1]	14 (28%)	10 (25%)	.814[3]
Preexisting multiresistant colonies[2]	3 (6.0%)	1 (2.5%)	.626[3]
ASA classification[1]			
I	0	0	.728[3]
II	19 (38.0%)	14 (35.0%)	"
III	31 (62.0%)	25 (62.5%)	"
IV	0	1 (2.5%)	"
Rutherford scale[1]			
I	11 (22.0%)	7 (17.5%)	.868[3]
II	2 (4.0%)	1 (2.5%)	"
III	7 (14.0%)	10 (25.0%)	"
IV	9 (18.0%)	7 (17.5%)	"
V	17 (34.0%)	12 (30.0%)	"
VI	4 (8.0%)	3 (7.5%)	

BMI: body mass index.
ASA classification: American Society of Anaesthesiologists' classification of physical health.
Data presented as either [1]number (percentage) or [2]mean ± standard deviation.
[3]P value using Fisher's Exact Test.
[4]P value using independent samples t-test.

(in this cohort only ESBL), ASA scores, and Rutherford classifications were compared. It was found that none of these parameters were significantly different between cohorts (Table 2). Perioperative characteristics were also compared, such as the use of prosthetic material (femoropopliteal bypass or aortobifemoral bypass), hybrid vascular surgery (endovascular procedure in combination with local endarterectomy of the common femoral artery), operating time, or whether the patient was operated in an emergency situation. Only the latter was found to be significantly different between cohorts;

TABLE 3: Perioperative characteristics.

	Non-NPIMS ($N = 50$)	NPIMS ($N = 40$)	P value
Procedure[1]			
Fem-pop Bypass	19 (38%)	14 (35%)	.455[3]
Hybrid endovascular surgery	9 (18%)	4 (10%)	"
Aortobifem-bifurcation	6 (12%)	3 (7.5%)	"
Endarterectomy	11 (22%)	10 (25%)	"
Other	5 (10%)	9 (22.5%)	"
Operating time (minutes)[2]	154.3 ± 51.3	162.6 ± 63.0	.154[4]
Emergency surgery[1]	17 (34%)	5 (12.5%)	.026[3]
Prosthetic material used[1]	13 (26%)	16 (40%)	.179[3]

Data presented as either [1]number (percentage) or [2]mean ± standard deviation.
[3]P value using Fisher's Exact Test.
[4]P value using independent samples t-test.

other perioperative factors were found to be comparable (Table 3).

A logistic regression was performed to analyse which patient or perioperative factors contributed to a WHD or a SSI. The analysis showed that there were no contributing patients or perioperative factors.

A WHD was found in 14.4% ($N = 13$) of analysed cases. Eight of them had positive microbiological cultures and were classified as surgical site infections (8.9%). The other WHDs were oedema, hematoma, or seroma, without bacterial infection. Of the patients with a WHD, 6 were found in the non-NPIMS group (12%) and 7 in the NPIMS group (17.5%, $P = .552$). SSIs with a positive microbiological culture were found in 3 patients in the non-NPIMS group (6%) and in 5 patients in the NPIMS group (12.5%, $P = .458$) (Table 4).

The site infections with positive microbiological cultures were scored according to the Szilagyi scale. Both cohorts displayed mainly superficial wound problems (Szilagyi grade 1). We found no significant differences in Szilagyi grades between cohorts ($P = 1.00$). Table 5 shows the different microbiological cultures from the groin infections in each cohort.

4. Discussion

Incisions in the inguinal region are known for an increased risk of surgical site infection. Wound problems after vascular groin operations especially lead to major morbidity (sepsis, limb amputation), prolonged hospital stay, increased costs, and even substantial mortality [5]. In 2007, Stewart et al. conducted a meta-analysis of 34 randomised controlled trials and concluded that, besides prophylactic antibiotics for vascular surgery, there are no surgical techniques for preventing groin wound-healing problems [13]. Because of our positive experience with the vacuum wound-closure system on open surgical wounds and some auspicious studies with this vacuum system on closed surgical wounds [3], we started using this system after the promising study of

TABLE 4: Incidence of postoperative infection and Szilagyi grades of infection.

	Non-NPIMS ($N = 50$)	NPIMS ($N = 40$)	P value
Wound-healing disorder[a,1]	6 (12.0%)	7 (17.5%)	.552[2]
Surgical site infection[b,1]	3 (6.0%)	5 (12.5%)	.458[2]
Szilagyi grade 1	2 (66.7%)	4 (80.0%)	1.000[2]
Szilagyi grade 2	0	0	"
Szilagyi grade 3	1 (33.3%)	1 (20.0%)	"

[a]Seroma/hematoma/dehiscence/erythema with or without microbiological culture.
[b]With positive microbiological culture.
Data presented as [1]number (percentage).
[2]P value using Fisher's Exact Test.

TABLE 5: Microbiological cultures of groin wound infections.

	Non-NPIMS ($N = 4$)	NPIMS ($N = 5$)
Staphylococcus aureus	4 (100%)	2[a] (40%)
Streptococcus hemolyticus	0	1[a] (20%)
Escherichia coli	0	1 (20%)
Pseudomonas aeruginosa	0	1 (20%)
Enterococcus faecalis	0	1[a] (20%)
Enterobacter cloacae	0	1[a] (20%)

[a]Found in multibacterial cultures (*Strept. hem.* and *Staph. aur.* and *Ent. face.* and *Ent. cloacae*).

Matatov et al. [3]. The NPIMS costs around 300 euros per single system, which would easily signify savings in the long run if SSIs could be prevented and hospital stay shortened.

Although some bias might be present by the selective use of the NPIMS by two out of four vascular surgeons, we have found that patient and perioperative characteristics were comparable, as shown by the analysis of the baseline characteristics of both patient cohorts. Known risk factors for wound-healing disturbances after vascular surgery, such as smoking, elevated body mass index, diabetes mellitus, and renal failure, were also found to be similar in both cohorts; even the distribution of Rutherford classification in patients operated for chronic limb ischemia was equally divided over the cohorts.

When comparing all parameters, only the number of emergency procedures differs significantly between the two groups, with higher numbers in the non-NPIMS group. This is also seen in the logistic regression that is performed. Elective surgery is a contributing factor in patients with NPIMS. This theoretically provides the NPIMS group an advantage, as emergency surgery is a risk factor for developing postoperative wound infection [5]. When subanalysing the elective operations only, we see equal results: more wound-healing disorders and surgical site infections in the NPIMS group.

In our daily practice, we have experienced failure of the NPIMS in different ways. The vacuum of the system was often failing, probably due to infolding in groin. Also movements of the leg did loosen the drape. Although there were several attempts to secure dry skin before applying the system, there were still several failures. If possible, we renewed the drape, in order to secure the vacuum. In an extra subanalysis, we found that failure of the NPIMS (which has led to application of less than four days and so did not meet the instructions for use) did not influence the number of SSIs.

Our study shows that, in any comparison of either surgical site infections or wound-healing problems, the NPIMS did not make a significant difference. Our hypothesis that wound-healing could be improved by the immediate evacuation of wound fluids through fast closure of the surgical wound under vacuum could not be demonstrated. The outcome of our study in combination with the sparse data in the literature does not support widespread application of the NPIMS on groin wounds after vascular surgery. Improvements of the system are advocated in order to avoid failure of the vacuum due to drape loosening, but, more importantly, prospective randomised clinical trials are needed to settle the value of vacuum wound management systems on closed (vascular) surgical wounds.

5. Conclusion

Our study on the prevention of wound-healing disturbances and surgical site infections after vascular surgery in the groin could not demonstrate any beneficial effect of the negative pressure incision management system. Improvements of the system are needed to achieve reliable and durable application of the vacuum, and prospective randomised trials are needed before widespread implementation of this costly wound dressing.

Conflict of Interests

The authors declare that there is no conflict of interests regarding the publication of this paper.

References

[1] KCI Licensing, *Incision Management System, Product Monograph*, Prevena, 2010.

[2] M. Pachowsky, J. Gusinde, A. Klein et al., "Negative pressure wound therapy to prevent seromas and treat surgical incisions after total hip arthroplasty," *International Orthopaedics*, vol. 36, no. 4, pp. 719–722, 2012.

[3] T. Matatov, K. N. Reddy, L. D. Doucet, C. X. Zhao, and W. W. Zhang, "Experience with a new negative pressure incision management system in prevention of groin wound infection in vascular surgery patients," *Journal of Vascular Surgery*, vol. 57, no. 3, pp. 791–795, 2013.

[4] A. L. J. Slappy, A. G. Hakaim, W. A. Oldenburg, R. Paz-Fumagalli, and J. M. McKinney, "Femoral incision morbidity following endovascular aortic aneurysm repair," *Vascular and Endovascular Surgery*, vol. 37, no. 2, pp. 105–109, 2003.

[5] D. F. Bandyk, "Vascular surgical site infection: risk factors and preventive measures," *Seminars in Vascular Surgery*, vol. 21, no. 3, pp. 119–123, 2008.

[6] A. J. Ploeg, J.-W. P. Lardenoye, M.-P. F. M. Vrancken Peeters, J. F. Hamming, and P. J. Breslau, "Wound complications at the groin after peripheral arterial surgery sparing the lymphatic tissue: a double-blind randomized clinical trial," *American Journal of Surgery*, vol. 197, no. 6, pp. 747–751, 2009.

[7] O. Grauhan, A. Navasardyan, M. Hofmann, P. Müller, J. Stein, and R. Hetzer, "Prevention of poststernotomy wound infections in obese patients by negative pressure wound therapy," *Journal of Thoracic and Cardiovascular Surgery*, vol. 145, no. 5, pp. 1387–1392, 2013.

[8] D. Masden, J. Goldstein, M. Endara, K. Xu, J. Steinberg, and C. Attinger, "Negative pressure wound therapy for at-risk surgical closures in patients with multiple comorbidities: a prospective randomized controlled study," *Annals of Surgery*, vol. 255, no. 6, pp. 1043–1047, 2012.

[9] J. P. Stannard, D. A. Volgas, R. Stewart, G. McGwin Jr., and J. E. Alonso, "Negative pressure wound therapy after severe open fractures: a prospective randomized study," *Journal of Orthopaedic Trauma*, vol. 23, no. 8, pp. 552–557, 2009.

[10] J. P. Stannard, D. A. Volgas, G. McGwin III et al., "Incisional negative pressure wound therapy after high-risk lower extremity fractures," *Journal of Orthopaedic Trauma*, vol. 26, no. 1, pp. 37–42, 2012.

[11] RIVM, "Strategisch beleidsplan PREZIES 2011–2015," 2013, http://www.rivm.nl/dsresource?objectid=rivmp:212486&type=org&disposition=inline&ns_nc=1.

[12] D. E. Szilagyi, R. F. Smith, J. P. Elliott, and M. P. Vrandecic, "Infection in arterial reconstruction with synthetic grafts," *Annals of Surgery*, vol. 176, no. 3, pp. 321–333, 1972.

[13] A. H. Stewart, P. S. Eyers, and J. J. Earnshaw, "Prevention of infection in peripheral arterial reconstruction: a systematic review and meta-analysis," *Journal of Vascular Surgery*, vol. 46, no. 1, pp. 148–155, 2007.

3

Evaluation of Early versus Delayed Laparoscopic Cholecystectomy in Acute Cholecystitis

Rati Agrawal, K. C. Sood, and Bhupender Agarwal

DNB (General Surgery), Department of General Surgery, Maharaja Agrasen Hospital (MAH), New Delhi 110026, India

Correspondence should be addressed to Rati Agrawal; drrati_agr@yahoo.com

Academic Editor: Akif Turna

Background. The role of early laparoscopic cholecystectomy for acute cholecystitis with cholelithiasis is not yet established. The aim of our prospective randomized study was to evaluate the safety and feasibility of early LC for acute cholecystitis and to compare the results with delayed LC. *Methods.* Between March 2007 to December 2008, 50 patients with diagnosis of acute cholecystitis were assigned randomly to early group, $n = 25$ (LC within 24 hrs of admission), and delayed group, $n = 25$ (initial conservative treatment followed by delayed LC, 6–8 weeks later). *Results.* We found in our study that the conversion rate in early LC and delayed LC was 16% and 8%, respectively, Operation time for early LC was 69.4 min versus 66.4 min for delayed LC, postoperative complications for early LC were 24% versus 8% for delayed LC, and blood loss was 159.6 mL early group versus 146.8 mL for delayed group. However early LC had significantly shorter hospital stay (4.1 days versus 8.6 days). *Conclusions.* Early LC for acute cholecystitis with cholelithiasis is safe and feasible, offering the additional benefit of shorter hospital stay. It should be offered to the patients with acute cholecystitis, provided that the surgery is performed within 96 hrs of acute symptoms by an experienced surgeon.

1. Introduction

For the management of acute cholecystitis with cholelithiasis the appropriate timing for laparoscopic cholecystectomy remains controversial [1]. Two approaches are available for the treatment of acute cholecystitis; the first approach is early (within 7 days of onset of symptoms) [2–5] laparoscopic cholecystectomy (LC) as definitive treatment after establishing diagnosis and surgical fitness of the patient in the same hospital admission. The second approach is conservative treatment which is successful in about 90% of the cases and then delayed cholecystectomy is performed in the second hospital admission after an interval of 6–12 weeks [6]. The choice of approach depends upon hospital infrastructure, surgical expertise, and patient's condition.

In the presence of acute inflammation, LC becomes more challenging and difficult because of edema, exudate, adhesions with adjoining structures, distension of gallbladder, friability of tissues, unclear and distorted ductal and vascular anatomy [7], hypervascularity, congestion, and dissemination of infection. These risk factors predispose for suboptimal outcome and high conversion rate to open cholecystectomy. As a result, the patient is deprived of potential benefits of LC which is now a "gold standard" for the management of symptomatic gallbladder stones [8].

Early open cholecystectomy had been established as the preferred treatment of acute cholecystitis to reduce morbidity, mortality, and total hospital stay [9]; however, with the advent of LC, the benefits of early surgery have been the subject of some contention [10]. Initial reports suggested that early LC for acute cholecystitis was associated with increased complication rates, prolonged operation time, and increased conversion rates (5%–35%) [1, 11–13]. As a consequence, initial conservative management with subsequent delayed or elective LC became accepted practice [9, 14, 15].

Delayed cholecystectomy potentially increases the chance of further gallstone-related complications [4] during the waiting interval and thus additional hospital admission. Recent evaluation has indicated early LC to be safe option in acute cholecystitis, although conversion to open cholecystectomy rates may be higher [11–13, 16].

2. Aims and Objectives

The aims and objectives of this study are as follows:

(1) to evaluate the results of early laparoscopic cholecystectomy in patients with acute cholecystitis with cholelithiasis in our setup with attention to clinical outcome,

(2) to compare the results of early with the delayed laparoscopic cholecystectomy for the treatment of acute cholecystitis with cholelithiasis.

3. Material and Methods

This prospective randomized study was undertaken in the Department of surgery at Maharaja Agrasen Hospital (MAH), New Delhi, between March 2007 and December 2008. Total of 50 patients were included in the study irrespective of their age and sex. Patients coming to the Emergency/Out Patient Department of MAH within 72 hrs of acute symptoms were diagnosed as a case of acute cholecystitis on the basis of clinical, laboratory (acute upper abdominal pain, right hypochondrial tenderness and/or guarding, fever >37.5°C and/or, white blood cell count greater than 10×10^9/L), and ultrasonographic criteria (thickened > 4 mm and edematous gallbladder (GB), distended gallbladder, positive sonographic Murphy's sign, pericholecystic fluid, and gallstones). According to *Tokyo guidelines 2013*, all our patients belong to *severity grade I (mild)*. Magnatic resonance cholangiopancreaticography (MRCP) was done in equivocal cases and findings correspond to the T2 single shot coronal image showing distended gallbladder, circumferential gallbladder wall thickening, and increased hyperintensity and T2 STIR axial image showing a distended gallbladder, cholelithiasis, and pericholecystic T2 hyperintense inflammation. Patients with acute symptoms present for >96 hrs prior to admission, previous upper abdominal surgery, patients unfit for general anaesthesia, coexisting common bile duct (CBD) stones as suggested by history of jaundice or fever with chills, icterus, raised alkaline phosphatase, or ultrasonographic evidence of CBD calculus, coexistent acute cholangitis, or pancreatitis were excluded from the study.

3.1. Workup of Patients. Eligible patients were talked to about the 2 options of treatment (early and delayed laparoscopic cholecystectomy) and informed consent was obtained. Patients were then randomized into two groups, "early" and "delayed" groups. Randomization was accomplished according to the patient's choice of treatment for some socioeconomic reasons. We used both the interview (for history and analgesic requirement) and the observation check list (for lab results, radiological and operative findings). In the early group, laparoscopic cholecystectomy was performed within 24 hours of randomization, that is, within 96 hours of acute symptoms, whereas in the delayed group conservative management with intravenous fluids and antibiotics was done. Patients who responded to the conservative management underwent an elective laparoscopic cholecystectomy 6–8 weeks after the acute episode.

3.2. Conduct of the Operation. The nature of the surgery, chance of conversion to open cholecystectomy, and the benefits likely to be achieved from LC were explained to the patients and the relatives in detail. After obtaining an informed written consent and randomization, patients were taken up for the surgery. Laparoscopic cholecystectomy, whether early or delayed, was performed by a consultant surgeon. The surgery was performed under general anaesthesia using endotracheal intubation in supine position.

Nasogastric tube was inserted to decompress the stomach. Pneumoperitoneum was created by blind puncture with Veress needle through a supraumblical incision. Confirmation of the intraperitoneal location of the needle tip is made by the saline drop test; once the needle is confirmed to be in the right position, the peritoneal cavity is insufflated, using carbon dioxide. To prevent problems of venous return, the pressure should never exceed 15 mm Hg. Four laparoscopic ports were made. The epigastric 10 mm port was for dissection or the suction and retrieval of specimen. Five mm port was made for telescope Three 5 mm ports were placed one in supraumblical region, one in right upper quadrant, and another in right flank at level of umbilicus were used for grasping forceps. If necessary, fifth port was added to improve exposure. Adhesions if present were cleared and gallbladder exposure was first undertaken; then the positions of gallbladder, the first part of the duodenum, common bile duct, Calots' triangle, and porta hepatis were ascertained. The gallbladder, if distended, was decompressed through suction needle to allow better grasping.

The gallbladder is held above the liver and the omentum and duodenum retracted caudally to define the neck of GB, Calot's triangle, and the common bile duct or lateral margin of the portal triad. Separation of the tissues to isolate structures in Calot's triangle by atraumatic manner is especially useful in AC.

The dissection is always started at the junction between the cystic duct and gallbladder at the inferior margin and carried out upwards close to the gallbladder neck on its posterior aspect with complimentary anterior dissection in Calot's triangle. Posterior window is created by separating the neck and part of body of the gallbladder all around. Next dissection is downward from the junction of gallbladder neck and the cystic duct, to define the cystic duct and the cystic artery. At the completion of this stage a critical view of safety is taken to ascertain that the two structures; that is, cystic duct and cystic artery are joining the gallbladder clearly. Dissection begins in the triangle of Calot taking small bands and strands of tissue. The cystic pedicle was dissected with curved dissector in order to isolate separately the cystic duct and artery. Both elements were then clipped and divided [7]. Gallbladder was dissected off its bed by to and fro retraction with a monopolar cautery hook. At the completion of the procedure, the gallbladder was placed into a retrieval bag if needed and extracted through the epigastric port, which was enlarged if necessary. Hemostasis was achieved in the gallbladder bed and after a thorough saline lavage, a suction drain was left in place if clinically indicated and the ports closed. When required, the conversion to open procedure was performed through a right subcostal incision.

3.3. Postoperative Assessment. Postoperatively, the patients were allowed oral intake 6–12 hrs after surgery if they had no nausea or vomiting. Pain relief was obtained by intramuscular diclofenac injection, which was changed to oral once patient was allowed orally. The severity of pain was documented by daily pain scoring using a visual analog scale (VAS 0: no pain; VAS 10: intolerable pain) for 3 days.

3.4. Study Parameters. Data was collected and entered in a predesigned proforma(Annexure-I) which included patient's demographics, timing of operation, operative findings, operative time, intra- or postoperative complications, and the length of hospital stay.

3.5. Statistical Analysis. Data was statistically analysed by using student t-test, Fisher's exact test, and Wilcoxon ranksum (Mann-whitney) test. A P value < 0.05 was considered significant.

4. Results

During the study period, a total of 50 patients with acute cholecystitis were included in the study. They were randomized in early and delayed groups with 25 patients in each group. The two groups were comparable in terms of age and sex, as well as clinical, laboratory parameters, and ultrasonographic findings (Table 1). No patient in delayed group required urgent surgery for failure of conservative treatment or recurrent symptoms during waiting period. Delayed laparoscopic cholecystectomy was performed at a mean interval of 47.32 days (6.76 weeks).

USG Finding on Initial Advice. See Table 1.

Modification of Technique. The various modifications in the techniques used in our studies are shown in Table 2.

Operation Time and Blood Loss. More modifications in the operative technique (Table 2) were required in early group than in the delayed group. The mean operating time was 60 min (range: 35–150 min) in early group and 60 min (range: 45–100 min) in delayed group, which is statistically not significant (P = 0.8004). The average blood loss in early LC was 159.6 mL (±58.1) and in delayed LC was 146.8 mL (±10.5). The difference in blood loss was statistically not significant (P = 0.418), and no patient required blood transfusion postoperatively.

Conversion to Open Cholecystectomy. In early group 21 cases were completed successfully by laparoscopy and 4 were converted to open cholecystectomy. Conversion rate was 16%. In delayed group 23 cases were successfully completed by laparoscopy and 2 were converted to open cholecystectomy. Conversion rate was 8%. The reasons for conversion in early group were as follows:

(1) unclear and distorted anatomy of ductal and vascular structures in Calot's triangle due to dense adhesions, edema, and exudates,

TABLE 1: USG findings in early and delayed group.

Group	Early (n = 25)	Delayed (n = 25)	P value
Thickened GB	13 (52%)	21 (84%)	0.032
Distended GB	23 (92%)	21 (84%)	0.667
Gall stones	25 (100%)	25 (100%)	0.463
Murphy's sign	14 (56%)	14 (56%)	0.999
Pericholecystic fluid	6 (24%)	5 (20%)	0.999

P value < 0.05 is statistically significant.
Used Fisher's exact test.

(2) tearing of GB at Hartmann's pouch because of friable tissue,

(3) bile leakage from cystic duct with suspicion of injury to common bile duct.

In our study, as shown in Table 3, conversion to open cholecystectomy was done in 4 patients due to dense adhesions; in two of them, on opening fundus, the first method was employed and anatomy was still unclear, so gallbladder was transected at the lower part of gallbladder neck, stones were removed, and the gallbladder wall was repaired. Patients recovered uneventfully. In the other two, structures could be defined clearly on opening and standard cholecystectomy was done.

In delayed group, only 2 patients were converted to open cholecystectomy. These patients had several previous episodes of acute cholecystitis and biliary pain and could be operated on earlier because of socioeconomic reasons. There were thickened dense adhesions and anatomy was unclear so conversion to open was done.

(i) One patient with bile leak had tear in the cystic duct and CBD was intact.

(ii) One patient with tearing of gallbladder neck was treated with standard open cholecystectomy.

Complications. There was no death in any of these two groups. The overall complication rate was 32% (8 of 25) in early group and 8% (2 of 25) in the delayed group. There was no major bile duct injury in any patient. In delayed group only one patient had chest infection and was managed with chest physiotherapy and intravenous antibiotics. There was high rate of wound infection in early group. Different complications are shown in Table 4.

Postoperative Analgesia. The average VAS score of postoperative analgesia was 2 in early group and 2 in delayed group, which was not statistically significant (P = 0.673).

Length of Hospital Stay (HS). The mean total HS was 4.16 (3–6 days) in the early and 8.6 (3–13 days). The difference in total HS between two groups was statistically significant (P = 0.0001), as shown in Table 5.

The overall comparison of the patients in the early and delayed groups is shown in Table 6.

In our study the parameters measured are depicted in Table 6. There is no statistically significant difference in both

TABLE 2: Various modifications of technique in early and delayed Group.

Technique	Early (n = 25)		Delayed (n = 25)		P value
	Frequency	Percentage	Frequency	Percentage	
GB decompression	16	64	3	12	0
Retrieval bag	4	16	1	4	0.349
Sub hepatic drain	7	28	2	8	0.138
Use of 5th port	1	4	0	0	0.999
Epigastric port enlargement	2	8	2	8	0.999

P value < 0.05 is statistically significant.
Used Fisher's exact test.

TABLE 3: Comparison of conversion to open cholecystectomy in early and delayed groups.

Procedure	Early (n = 25)	Delayed (n = 25)	P value
Successful LC	21	23	
Conversion to OC	4	2	
Conversion rate	16%	8%	0.667

P value < 0.05 is statistically significant.
Used Fisher's exact test.

groups except the total hospital stay which is less in early group being 4.16 ± 1.21 days in comparison to 8.6 ± 2.04 in delayed group.

5. Discussion

Laparoscopic cholecystectomy was started in 1987 and in few years became "gold standard" for the treatment of symptomatic cholelithiasis and was also used for acute cholecystitis as more experience was gained in the technique. However, the application of LC in the setting of acute cholecystitis is still controversial. In early years of laparoscopic surgery, acute cholecystitis was considered a relative contraindication to LC [4, 17]. However, some recent reports [1–6, 8, 18–26] have suggested that LC is feasible and safe procedure for acute cholecystitis also, although the complications and conversion rates are variable. However, more studies are required for conclusive results.

We, therefore, undertook a prospective randomized trial comparing early versus delayed LC for acute cholecystitis and also to evaluate feasibility and safety in our set up. The patients' population was well-matched in both groups and there was no significant difference in age, biochemical parameters, and radiological findings between 2 groups.

The mean operation time in our study was 69.4 min in early group and 66.4 min in delayed group. The difference was not statistically significant. This is in contrast to the reports from other trials which showed a significant difference in operative time between two groups.

There was no significant difference in blood loss between the two groups; the mean blood loss in early group was 159.6 mL and 146.8 mL in delayed group. Although there are not several studies which compared the difference in the blood loss, more blood loss in early group is due to highly vascular adhesions around inflammatory GB and oozing

from inflammatory GB bed; however, no patient in the study required blood transfusion.

More surgeons agree that in acute cholecystitis timing of cholecystectomy is an important factor in determining outcome. Ideally the surgery should be performed as soon after admission as possible. Although operation within golden 72 hrs from the onset of symptoms has been suggested, such an early surgery is not always possible in clinical practice because of logistic difficulties in operating such patients on an emergency basis. We perform the surgery for the patient in early group in the next available OT (elective list). >90% of our patients had surgery within 24 hrs of admission.

The technical difference of LC is related to operative findings during early surgery. A diseased GB containing infected bile is commonly seen in acute cholecystitis. We believe that several technical key points must be kept in mind while performing lap surgery for acute cholecystitis. For a good exposure of Calot's triangle, an additional port can be useful. Decompression of GB allows better grasping of GB by grasper. If available, ultrasonic dissector and coagulator should be used for adhesionolysis. In difficult cases with dense adhesions between the GB neck and porta hepatis, a partial cholecystectomy can be done leaving in place Hartmann's pouch and the cystic duct after confirming the absence of distal residual structures. The other technical rules are liberal use of subhepatic drain and a retrieval bag to remove spilled stones and perforated GB. In our study decompression of GB was required in 64% cases in early group and 12% cases in delayed group. Retrieval bag was used in 16% cases of early group and in 4% cases in delayed group. Subhepatic drain was placed in 28% pts of early group and 8% patients of delayed group.

Three questions have to be answered regarding LC in the setting of acute cholecystitis.

(1) Is Lap Chole for Acute Cholecystitis Safe? The overall complication rate in this study was 20%. It is comparable to that reported in other studies. Postoperative complication rate in early group was 24% and in delayed group was 8%. This difference was statistically not significant and was also reported the same by Johansson et al. [5] (18% versus 8%) and Kolla et al. [6] (20% versus 15%). Study by Lai et al. [17] showed no difference in the complication rate between the two groups (9% versus 8%).

However, another prospective controlled study by Lo et al. [4] (29%) and González-Rodríguez et al. [25] (17.7%)

TABLE 4: Comparison of operative complications in early and delayed groups.

Complications	Early (n = 25)		Delayed (n = 25)		P value
	Frequency	Percentage	Frequency	Percentage	
Intraoperative					0.353
Bile leak	1	4	0	0	
Perforation	1	4	0	0	
Postoperative					0.084
Chest infection	0	0	1	4	
Wound infection	6	24	1	4	
Total complications	8	32	2	8	

P value < 0.05 is statistically significant.
Used Fisher's exact test.

TABLE 5: Comparison of length of hospital stay in early and delayed group.

Hospital stay	Early (n = 25)		Delayed (n = 25)		P value
	Mean	SD	Mean	SD	
Postoperative HS	3	1	3.2	0.95	0.473
Total HS	4.16	1.21	8.6	2.04	0.0001

P value < 0.05 is statistically significant.
Used Wilcoxon rank-sum (Mann-Whitney) test.

TABLE 6: Overall comparison of early and delayed LC.

Groups	Early	Delayed	P value
Age	47.28 ± 14.57	50.96 ± 17.05	0.416
Sex	8 : 17	8 : 17	0.999
Duration of symptoms	35.44 ± 23.03	36.8 ± 21.30	0.209
TLC	10800 (6500–23200)	11200 (6600–18100)	0.341
Total bilirubin	0.76 (0.5–1.03)	1.8 (0.7–2.6)	0.05
SGOT	26 (15–94)	68 (14–99)	0.054
SGPT	28 (12–55)	97 (12–92)	0.095
Thickened GB	13 (52%)	21 (84%)	0.032
Distended GB	23 (92%)	21 (84%)	0.667
Murphy's sign	14 (56%)	14 (56%)	0.999
Pericholecystic fluid	6 (24%)	5 (20%)	0.999
Tense distended GB	18 (72%)	12 (48%)	0.085
Turbid bile/pus	4 (16%)	1 (4%)	0.349
Severe adhesions	3 (12%)	11 (44%)	0.059
GB decompression	16 (64%)	3 (12%)	0
Use of Retrieval bag	4 (16%)	1 (4%)	0.349
Subhepatic drain	7 (28%)	2 (8%)	0.138
Use of 5th port	1 (4%)	0	0.999
Epigastric port enlargement	2 (8%)	2 (8%)	0.999
Operation time	69.4 ± 29.59	66.4 ± 15.97	0.8004
Blood loss	159.6 ± 58.11	146.8 ± 52.69	0.418
Total hospital stay	4.16 ± 1.21	8.6 ± 2.04	0.0001
Conversion rate	16%	8%	0.667
Postoperative complications	24%	8%	0.084

had shown significantly higher complication in the delayed group than the early group.

The problem of biliary tract injury is the major concern in the routine use of the laparoscopic approach for acute cholecystitis. There was no mortality nor the major bile duct injuries in our study as were reported by Kum et al. [27] (5.5%) and Al-Hajjar et al. [28] (0.9%). Only the minor complications were more in early LC. These results suggest that the early LC is a safe procedure.

(2) Is LC for AC Feasible? In this study conversion rate in early group is more than the delayed group. It has been shown by many studies that LC for AC is feasible with conversion rate ranging from 6 to 35% [12, 13]. Although in our study conversion rate in early group is 16% which seems to be high, it reflects our safety concerns for the method and we feel that, with experience of these cases, the conversion rate will be lower in subsequent cases. The conversion rates in most of the studies lie in the acceptable range and are comparable to our study. So the procedure is feasible though the conversion rate in delayed cases is lower (8%) which has also been reported by various authors.

(3) Is Lap Chole for Acute Cholecystitis Beneficial to the Patients? The laparpscopic cholecystectomy for acute cholecystitis is definitely beneficial to the patient because of significantly shorter total hospital stay. The total hospital stay was significantly less for the early group (4.1 days) than the delayed group (8.6 days). Our study agrees with many other studies which also showed a significant difference in the hospital stay between both groups. There is socioeconomic advantage as well as prevention of recurrent attacks and complications during waiting period.

To conclude both early and delayed laparoscopic cholecystectomies are feasible and safe in acute cholecystitis; however, delayed lap chole is associated with lower conversion rate as compared to early LC; early cholecystectomy offers definitive treatment at the initial admission and avoids the problem of failed conservative management and recurrent symptoms which required emergency surgery. Furthermore, early LC is associated with a shorter total hospital stay as compared to delayed LC, which is a major economic benefit to the health care system especially in our country.

Conflict of Interests

The authors declare that there is no conflict of interests regarding the publication of this paper.

References

[1] T. Siddiqui, A. MacDonald, P. S. Chong, and J. T. Jenkins, "Early versus delayed laparoscopic cholecystectomy for acute cholecystitis: a meta-analysis of randomized clinical trials," *American Journal of Surgery*, vol. 195, no. 1, pp. 40–47, 2008.

[2] R. Sinha and N. Sharma, "Acute cholecystitis and laparoscopic cholecystectomy," *JSLS: Journal of the Society of Laparoendoscopic Surgeons/Society of Laparoendoscopic Surgeons*, vol. 6, no. 1, pp. 65–68, 2002.

[3] C.-M. Lo, C.-L. Liu, E. C. S. Lai, S.-T. Fan, and J. Wong, "Early versus delayed laparoscopic cholecystectomy for treatment of acute cholecystitis," *Annals of Surgery*, vol. 223, no. 1, pp. 37–42, 1996.

[4] C.-M. Lo, C.-L. Liu, S.-T. Fan, E. C. S. Lai, and J. Wong, "Prospective randomized study of early versus delayed laparoscopic cholecystectomy for acute cholecystitis," *Annals of Surgery*, vol. 227, no. 4, pp. 461–467, 1998.

[5] M. Johansson, A. Thune, A. Blomqvist, L. Nelvin, and L. Lundell, "Management of acute cholecystitis in the laparoscopic era: results of a prospective, randomized clinical trial," *Journal of Gastrointestinal Surgery*, vol. 7, no. 5, pp. 642–645, 2003.

[6] S. B. Kolla, S. Aggarwal, A. Kumar et al., "Early vs delayed laparoscopic cholecystectomy for acute cholecystitis: a prospective randomized trial," *Surgical Endoscopy*, vol. 18, no. 9, pp. 1323–1327, 2004.

[7] A. P. Nagle, N. J. Soper, and J. R. Hines, "Cholecystectomy (open and laproscopy)," in *Maingot's: Abdominal Operations*, M. J. Zinner and S. W. Asmhley, Eds., pp. 847–861, McGraw-Hill, New York, NY, USA, 11th edition, 2007.

[8] A. S. Serralta, J. L. Bueno, M. R. Planells, and D. R. Rodero, "Prospective evaluation of emergency versus delayed laparoscopic cholecystectomy for early cholecystitis," *Surgical Laparoscopy, Endoscopy and Percutaneous Techniques*, vol. 13, no. 2, pp. 71–75, 2003.

[9] W. Van Der Linden and G. Edlund, "Early versus delayed cholecystectomy: the effect of a change in management," *British Journal of Surgery*, vol. 68, no. 11, pp. 753–757, 1981.

[10] A. Cuschieri, F. Dubois, J. Mouiel et al., "The european experience with laparoscopic cholecystectomy," *The American Journal of Surgery*, vol. 161, no. 3, pp. 385–387, 1991.

[11] C. K. Kum, P. M. Y. Goh, J. R. Isaac, Y. Tekant, and S. S. Ngoi, "Laparoscopic cholecystectomy for acute cholecystitis," *British Journal of Surgery*, vol. 81, no. 11, pp. 1651–1654, 1994.

[12] R. G. Wilson, I. M. C. Macintyre, S. J. Nixon, J. H. Saunders, J. S. Varma, and P. M. King, "Laparoscopic cholecystectomy as a safe and effective treatment for severe acute cholecystitis," *British Medical Journal*, vol. 305, no. 6850, pp. 394–396, 1992.

[13] H. A. Graves Jr., J. F. Ballinger, and W. J. Anderson, "Appraisal of laparoscopic cholecystectomy," *Annals of Surgery*, vol. 213, no. 6, pp. 655–671, 1991.

[14] K. P. Koo and R. C. Thirlby, "Laparoscopic cholecystectomy in acute cholecystitis: what is the optimal timing for operation?" *Archives of Surgery*, vol. 131, no. 5, pp. 540–545, 1996.

[15] A. Cuschieri, "Approach to the treatment of acute cholecystitis: open surgical, laparoscopic or endoscopic?" *Endoscopy*, vol. 25, no. 6, pp. 397–398, 1993.

[16] T. Kiviluoto, J. Sirén, P. Luukkonen, and E. Kivilaakso, "Randomised trial of laparoscopic versus open cholecystectomy for acute and gangrenous cholecystitis," *The Lancet*, vol. 351, no. 9099, pp. 321–325, 1998.

[17] P. B. S. Lai, K. H. Kwong, K. L. Leung et al., "Randomized trial of early versus delayed laparoscopic cholecystectomy for acute cholecystitis," *British Journal of Surgery*, vol. 85, no. 6, pp. 764–767, 1998.

[18] A. K. Madan, S. Aliabadi-Wahle, D. Tesi, L. M. Flint, and S. M. Steinberg, "How early is early laparoscopic treatment of acute cholecystitis?" *The American Journal of Surgery*, vol. 183, no. 3, pp. 232–236, 2002.

[19] W. K. Peng, Z. Sheikh, S. J. Nixon, and S. Paterson-Brown, "Role of laparoscopic cholecystectomy in the early management of

acute gallbladder disease," *British Journal of Surgery*, vol. 92, no. 5, pp. 586–591, 2005.

[20] D. Bhattacharya and B. J. Ammori, "Contemporary minimally invasive approaches to the management of acute cholecystitis: a review and appraisal," *Surgical Laparoscopy, Endoscopy and Percutaneous Techniques*, vol. 15, no. 1, pp. 1–8, 2005.

[21] S. Shikata, Y. Noguchi, and T. Fukui, "Early versus delayed cholecystectomy for acute cholecystitis: a meta-analysis of randomized controlled trials," *Surgery Today*, vol. 35, no. 7, pp. 553–560, 2005.

[22] H. Lau, C. Y. Lo, N. G. Patil, and W. K. Yuen, "Early versus delayed-interval laparoscopic cholecystectomy for acute cholecystitis: a metaanalysis," *Surgical Endoscopy and Other Interventional Techniques*, vol. 20, no. 1, pp. 82–87, 2006.

[23] C. Papi, M. Catarci, L. D'Ambrosio et al., "Timing of cholecystectomy for acute calculous cholecystitis: a meta-analysis," *The American Journal of Gastroenterology*, vol. 99, no. 1, pp. 147–157, 2004.

[24] R. A. Casillas, S. Yegiyants, and J. C. Collins, "Early laparoscopic cholecystectomy is the preferred management of acute cholecystitis," *Archives of Surgery*, vol. 143, no. 6, pp. 533–537, 2008.

[25] F. J. González-Rodríguez, J. P. Paredes-Cotoré, C. Pontón et al., "Early or delayed laparoscopic cholecystectomy in acute cholecystitis? Conclusions of a controlled trial," *Hepato-Gastroenterology*, vol. 56, no. 89, pp. 11–16, 2009.

[26] T. C. Chang, M. T. Lin, M. H. Wu, M. Y. Wang, and P. H. Lee, "Evaluation of early vesus delayed laparoscopic cholecystectomy in the treatment of acute cholecystitis," *Hepatogastroenterology*, vol. 56, no. 89, pp. 26–28, 2009.

[27] C.-K. Kum, E. Eypasch, R. Lefering, A. Paul, E. Neugebauer, and H. Troidl, "Laparoscopic cholecystectomy for acute cholecystitis: is it really safe?" *World Journal of Surgery*, vol. 20, no. 1, pp. 43–49, 1996.

[28] N. Al-Hajjar, S. Duca, M. Géza, A. Vasilescu, and N. Nicolescu, "Incidents and postoperative complications of laparoscopic cholecystectomies for acute cholecystitis," *Romanian Journal of Gastroenterology*, vol. 11, no. 2, pp. 115–119, 2002.

4

Guidelines for Perioperative Management of the Diabetic Patient

Sivakumar Sudhakaran[1] and Salim R. Surani[2]

[1]*Texas A&M Health Science Center, 8447 State Highway 47, Bryan, TX 77807, USA*
[2]*Division of Pulmonary, Critical Care & Sleep Medicine, Texas A&M Health Science Center, Corpus Christi, 1177 West Wheeler Avenue, Suite 1, Aransas Pass, TX 78336, USA*

Correspondence should be addressed to Salim R. Surani; srsurani@hotmail.com

Academic Editor: Roland S. Croner

Management of glycemic levels in the perioperative setting is critical, especially in diabetic patients. The effects of surgical stress and anesthesia have unique effects on blood glucose levels, which should be taken into consideration to maintain optimum glycemic control. Each stage of surgery presents unique challenges in keeping glucose levels within target range. Additionally, there are special operative conditions that require distinctive glucose management protocols. Interestingly, the literature still does not report a consensus perioperative glucose management strategy for diabetic patients. We hope to outline the most important factors required in formulating a perioperative diabetic regimen, while still allowing for specific adjustments using prudent clinical judgment. Overall, through careful glycemic management in perioperative patients, we may reduce morbidity and mortality and improve surgical outcomes.

1. Introduction

Diabetes has classically been defined as a group of metabolic diseases characterized by hyperglycemia due to defects in insulin secretion, insulin action, or a combination of both [1]. The vast majority of diabetic cases can be classified as either type 1 or type 2 diabetes. Type 1 diabetes is generally due to β-cell destruction leading to absolute insulin deficiency. This form accounts for roughly 5–10% of diabetic cases, and individuals at increased risk can often be identified by evidence of autoimmune pathologic processes occurring at the pancreatic islets [1]. Type 2 diabetes is characterized by a progressive insulin secretory defect within a setting of insulin resistance [2]. Approximately 90–95% of diabetic cases are type 2 [1]. Management of glycemic levels in diabetic patients is critical, as persistent hyperglycemia may lend itself to a number of complications including cardiovascular disease, nephropathy, retinopathy, neuropathy, and various foot pathologies [2].

The prevalence and diagnostic criteria for diabetes are well defined. There are approximately 29.1 million people with diabetes in the United States (roughly 9.3% of the total population). Of these 29.1 million cases, around 27% or 8.1 million cases are undiagnosed [3]. Furthermore, a study funded by the World Health Organization (WHO) found that estimated 347 million people worldwide have diabetes [4]. Between 2010 and 2030, a 69% increase in the number of adults with diabetes in developing countries and a 20% increase in developed countries are predicted [5]. A diagnosis of diabetes may be confirmed through several different techniques. These diagnostic criteria include (1) hemoglobin A1c (A1c) ≥ 6.5%, (2) fasting plasma glucose ≥ 126 mg/dL (fasting is defined as no caloric intake for at least 8 hours), (3) 2-hour plasma glucose ≥ 200 mg/dL during an oral glucose tolerance test (OGTT), and (4) random plasma glucose ≥ 200 mg/dL in a patient with classic symptoms of hyperglycemia [2].

Proper glycemic control and attainment of other management goals (cholesterol, Body Mass Index (BMI), and blood pressure) are essential in prevention of long-term complications of diabetes as well as reduction of overall disease management costs [6]. In fact a recent study found that values of HbA1c that are either <6.5% or >9.0% may be associated with increased mortality within one year in clinical type 2 diabetes [7]. Tight glycemic control is becoming increasingly recognized as a perioperative goal in surgical patients [8–12]. However, there is still no overall consensus on the optimal perioperative management of the diabetic patient [13–21]. In this paper we hope to outline risk factors associated with hyperglycemia due to diabetes in the surgical patient, as well as review broad glucose management strategies during surgery as well as the pre- and postoperative stages.

2. Why Is Management of Diabetes Important in the Surgical Setting?

Surgical procedures may result in a number of metabolic perturbations that can alter normal glucose homeostasis. The resulting hyperglycemia due to abnormal glucose balance is a risk factor for postoperative sepsis [22], endothelial dysfunction [23], cerebral ischemia [24], and impaired wound healing [25, 26]. In addition, the stress response may also cause other diabetic pathologies including diabetic ketoacidosis [27] (DKA) or hyperglycemic hyperosmolar syndrome [28] (HHS) during surgery or postoperatively. However, recent evidence suggests that careful management of glucose levels in patients undergoing major surgeries, including cardiac [29] and orthopedic [30] procedures may minimize the aforementioned negative sequela and overall promote better outcomes. On average, diabetics require more hospitalizations, longer durations of stay, and cost more to manage than nondiabetics. The total estimated cost of managing diagnosed diabetes in 2012 was $245 billion, a 41% increase from the 2007 estimate, with the largest percentage (43% of the total medical cost) being spent on inpatient hospital care [31]. Hospitalized diabetics generally tend to be older, less active, and based on hemoglobin-AIC measurements and control their glycemic levels less aggressively [32]. Furthermore, diabetics undergo certain procedures and surgeries more commonly than nondiabetics and have increased morbidity and mortality rates when acutely compromised or ill [33–35].

Glycemic monitoring in the perioperative setting is done in a passive manner to combat any potential neuroglycopenic sequelae from underlying unrecognized hypoglycemia. Unmanaged hypoglycemia may result in a number of neurological complications including somnolence, unconsciousness, and seizures and depending on the duration, irreversible neurological insult, or death [35]. Recognition of the neurological manifestations of hypoglycemia while a patient is under general anesthesia or receiving sedatives/analgesics (with or without neuromuscular blocking agents) after completion of surgery is difficult, potentially leaving the hypoglycemic state unrecognized for a critical amount of time before proper management ensues [35]. Additionally, studies have suggested that hypoglycemia enhances morbidity/mortality in critically ill diabetic patients [36] and can prolong ICU/hospital stay [37]. In general, complications from surgical wounds are more prevalent in diabetics, and healing is impaired when glycemic levels are not well managed [38]. As diabetics tend to sustain increased perioperative morbidity and mortality, identification of diabetic patients is imperative in the surgical setting. Slightly more than a third of perioperative diabetics remain unrecognized or

untreated before surgery or admittance to the ICU [39, 40]; clinicians must remain alert to properly identify diabetes, glucose intolerance, insulin resistance, and associated diabetic pathologies. Overall, with the use of careful glucose management strategies, the primary outcome measures of surgery are similar between diabetic and nondiabetic patients [41].

3. A Brief Summary of the Metabolic Response to Surgery and Anesthesia

The trauma associated with surgery results in increased production of stress hormones, the magnitude of which depends on the severity of the surgery or any postoperative complications. In specific, the increases in cortisol and catecholamine levels related to surgery have been well documented [42, 43]. Increased cortisol and catecholamines reduce insulin sensitivity, while heightened sympathetic activity reduces insulin secretion while simultaneously increasing growth hormone and glucagon secretion [44, 45]. In the diabetic patient, insulin production is already marginalized; the metabolic changes outlined above that occur during surgery cause a marked catabolic state. Changes in normal metabolic patterns due to surgery trigger gluconeogenesis, glycogenolysis, proteolysis, lipolysis, and ketogenesis ultimately resulting in hyperglycemia and ketosis [46].

There are a number of anesthetic drugs, each of which has a variable effect on glycemic control. Most intravenous (IV) induction agents have a relatively negligible effect on blood glucose, although a notable exception is the induction agent etomidate. Etomidate is known to cause less hypotension during induction and generally fewer hangover-like effects upon recovery [47]. Review of the etomidate mechanism shows suppressed adrenocortical function mediated by blocking the activity of 11-beta-hydroxylase, ultimately causing decreased steroidogenesis [48]. In fact, the literature reports that acute adrenocortical insufficiency and crisis may occur after a standard induction dose of etomidate [49]. However, due to diminished cortisol secretion, etomidate triggers a subsequent decrease in the hyperglycemic response to surgery [47]. Additionally, if used in high doses during surgery, benzodiazepines decrease ACTH secretion. Benzodiazepines also stimulate release of growth hormone, while reducing sympathetic stimulation [50]. Opiates given in high doses such as during the postoperative recovery phase block the sympathetic nervous system as well as the hypothalamic-pituitary axis, essentially abolishing the hyperglycemic response to surgery [51]. In vitro studies revealed that volatile anesthetic agents such as halothane and isoflurane inhibit normal insulin production triggered by glucose in a dose dependent fashion, essentially resulting in a hyperglycemic response [52, 53]. Further studies must be completed in order to understand the full clinical effects of this response in diabetic patients undergoing surgery.

Whereas most anesthetic agents cause hyperglycemia, epidural anesthesia tends to have a nominal effect on glucose metabolism [54]. Epidural anesthesia inhibits catecholamine release (irrespective of spinal segmental level), as such noradrenaline and cortisol concentrations do not increase,

TABLE 1: Broad management goals across the perioperative timeline. Overall goals: (i) reduce patient morbidity and mortality, (ii) avoid clinically significant hyper- or hypoglycemia, (iii) maintain acid/base, electrolyte, and fluid balance, (iv) prevent ketoacidosis, and (v) establish blood glucose measurements less than 180 mg/dL in critical patients and less than 140 mg/dL in stable patients.

Preoperative management key points	Intraoperative management key points	Postoperative management key points
(i) Verify target blood glucose concentration with frequent glucose monitoring (ii) Use insulin therapy to maintain glycemic goals (iii) Discontinue biguanides, alpha glucosidase inhibitors, thiazolidinediones, sulfonylureas, and GLP-1 agonists (iv) Consider cancelling nonemergency procedures if patient presents with metabolic abnormalities (DKA, HHS, etc.) or glucose reading above 400–500 mg/dL	(i) Aim to maintain intraoperative glucose levels between 140 and 170 mg/dL (ii) Physicians must take length of surgery into account when determining an intraoperative glucose management strategy (iii) For minor surgery, preoperative glucose protocols may be continued (iv) IV insulin infusion is being promoted as a more efficient method of glycemic control for longer or more complex surgeries	(i) Target postoperative glycemic range between 140 and 180 mg/dL (ii) In the event a patient is hypoglycemic after surgery, begin a dextrose infusion at approximately 5–10 g/hour (iii) Ensure basal insulin levels are met, especially in type 1 diabetic patients (iv) Postprandial insulin requirements should be tailored according to the mode in which the patient is receiving nutrition (v) Supplemental insulin can be used to combat hyperglycemia and restore blood glucose values back to target range

Please note that the information presented in this table has been referenced in the text.

preventing elevation in blood glucose levels [55]. In addition, sympathetic efferent signal blockade with enhanced fibrinolytic activity blunts the surgical stress response normally responsible for hyperglycemia [56]. However, physicians must be cognizant of certain complications related to epidural and regional anesthetic use. For example, use of localized anesthesia in diabetic patients with autonomic neuropathy may result in deleterious consequences such as life-threatening hypotension. It is imperative that the anesthetic technique used allows for rapid recovery after surgery to prevent concealment of hyperglycemic or hypoglycemic coma [46].

In general, the response to neuromuscular blocking agents is normal in diabetic patients; however in patients with neuropathies or irregular transmission across the neuromuscular junction abnormalities may occur. Overall, the choice of neuromuscular blocking agent will be predicated on renal function, while anesthetic selection will be evaluated according to the degree of various systemic diseases such as diabetes, hypertension, and coronary artery disease. Finally, to insure proper postoperative management, clinicians should be aware that anesthetic agents tend to cause hyperglycemia [46].

4. Perioperative Assessment and Management Goals for the Diabetic Patient

Perioperative management of glucose levels revolves around several key objectives that are briefly elaborated on below:

(i) Reduction of overall patient morbidity and mortality [46, 57].

(ii) Avoidance of severe hyperglycemia or hypoglycemia [46, 57].

(iii) Maintenance of physiological electrolyte and fluid balance [46, 57].

(iv) Prevention of ketoacidosis [46, 57].

(v) Establishment of certain glycemic target levels [46, 57], less than 180 mg/dL in critical patients and less than 140 mg/dL in stable patients [58].

In surgical patients, careful blood glucose control has been associated with decreased mortality [59]. Additionally, ketoacidosis in diabetic patients undergoing surgery must be avoided. Treatment of patients with DKA uses significant healthcare resources accounting for 25% of healthcare dollars spent on direct medical care for adult patients with type 1 diabetes in the United States [60]. Lastly, optimizing glucose levels according to standard hospital protocols was associated with a 25.4% reduction in perioperative complications [61]. Specific strategies for glucose management differ during surgery as well as the preoperative and postoperative stages. All of the abovementioned goals as well as distinct strategies during each phase of surgery will be addressed below. Furthermore, a graphical diagram of the perioperative timeline can be seen in Table 1.

5. Preoperative Glycemic Management

In patients using insulin, frequent glucose monitoring should be utilized to ensure that glucose values are within normal ranges. Patients should monitor blood glucose levels vigilantly including before and after meals as well as before sleeping. Additionally, finger stick glucose monitoring should be completed every 4 to 6 hours in any patient who is nil per os (NPO), with supplemental insulin used to correct hyperglycemia back to normal values [57]. When using supplemental-scale coverage, short-acting insulin (humulin, novolin) has a shorter duration of action than human insulin and may be given subcutaneously every 4 to 6 hours; however to prevent insulin stacking regular human insulin should not be given more than every 6 hours to correct hyperglycemia [57]. Traditionally, long-acting insulin (glargine, ultralente) is discontinued two to three days prior to surgery; glucose levels are instead stabilized by a combination of intermediate insulin (NPH) with short-acting insulin twice daily or regular insulin before meals and intermediate-acting insulin at bedtime [62]. However, if glycemic control is well managed in a patient being treated with glargine, it is acceptable to continue the same insulin regimen until the day of surgery [63]. Finally, it is important to confirm the form of diabetes present, as patients with type 1 diabetes must continue a basal rate insulin replacement preoperatively (0.2 to 0.3 U/kg/day of a long-acting insulin) [57].

Along with careful insulin regulation, there are a number of oral glycemic control drugs that should be discontinued before surgery. Biguanides (metformin) sensitize specific tissues to insulin, mediating efficient uptake of glucose in muscle and fat while preventing hepatic glucose formation. Metformin usage is discontinued before surgery in the United States and Europe due to renal function complications that may arise intraoperatively (such as hemodynamic instability or decreased renal perfusion), increasing the risk of lactic acidosis [64, 65]. Alpha glucosidase inhibitors (acarbose, miglitol) weaken the effect of oligosaccharidases and disaccharidases in the intestinal brush border, effectively lowering the absorption of glucose after meals. However, in preoperative fasting states, this drug has no effect and thus should be discontinued until the patient resumes eating [66]. Thiazolidinediones (pioglitazone, rosiglitazone) mechanism of action is similar to that of metformin and however is not associated with lactic acidosis. Nevertheless, these drugs are generally discontinued as they are not insulin secretagogues and may also cause fluid retention in the postoperative phase [57, 67]. Sulfonylureas (glibenclamide, glimepiride, and glipizide) trigger insulin production and may induce hypoglycemia in a fasting preoperative patient. If a patient has mistakenly taken a sulfonylurea on the day of surgery, the operation may still be completed; however, careful glucose monitoring is imperative and IV dextrose may be required [65, 68]. Glucagon-like peptide-1 (GLP-1) agonists (exenatide, liraglutide) are held the day of surgery as they slow gastric motility and may delay restoration of proper gastrointestinal function during recovery. Finally, because dipeptidyl peptidase-4 (DPP-4) inhibitors (sitagliptin, linagliptin) work by a glucose dependent mechanism (reducing the risk of hypoglycemia even in fasting patients) they may be continued if necessary; however, these medications primarily reduce glycemic levels after meals and their effects will be greatly marginalized in preoperative NPO patients [57].

There currently exists no evidence-based guideline dictating when to cancel surgery due to hyperglycemia. As a rule, elective surgery should not be performed on patients in a compromised metabolic state (DKA, HHS, etc.). Although no strict standard for surgical cancellation has been determined, the Yale New-Haven Hospital recommends postponing surgery if glucose is greater than 400 mg/dL. Similarly, at Boston Medical Center, it is recommended to postpone nonurgent surgical procedures if glucose is >500 mg/dL. In the event surgical cancellation is required, physicians should first manage any metabolic pathologies if present. After resolution of any underlying metabolic abnormalities, clinicians may then aim to restore blood glucose back to target range using combination insulin therapy as described above [69].

6. Intraoperative Glycemic Management

As described above surgical stress as well as anesthesia promotes hyperglycemia in the diabetic patient. Although there currently exists no consensus target range, in general the literature suggests keeping glucose levels between 150 and 200 mg/dL (8 to 11 mmol/L) during surgery [13–21]. Moreover, a study discovered that intraoperative hyperglycemia (glucose greater than 200 mg/dL) as well as relative normoglycemia (glucose less than 140 mg/dL) was found to be associated with significant morbidity and mortality. In fact, the study found that glucose levels ranging from 140 to 170 mg/dL had the lowest risk of adverse outcomes [70]. During surgery, glycemic levels can be sufficiently monitored by utilizing blood glucose measurement systems designed for inpatient bedside use [17, 21]. Additionally, clinicians must take the approximate length of time required to complete a procedure into consideration when determining an intraoperative glycemic control strategy. For short, minor procedures, preoperative glucose maintenance protocols may still be employed [57]. For more complex procedures, variable rate IV insulin infusion has been highlighted as a more effective method for achieving glycemic control [16, 57, 71, 72].

Regular IV insulin remains physiologically active for approximately 1 hour but has a serum half-life of 7 minutes, as such it allows for tight glycemic control that can combat unexpected changes in blood glucose effectively [57]. In patients with type 1 diabetes the insulin infusion rate begins at roughly 0.5–1 U/hour (mix 100 U short-acting insulin in 100 mL normal saline; i.e., 1 U = 1 mL), whereas infusion rates are typically increased in type 2 diabetics to approximately 2-3 U/hour or higher [20]. There are a number of both static [73, 74] and adjustable [75] algorithms that can be used to adjust the rate of insulin infusion. It should be noted that there exists a continuous Glucose-Insulin-Potassium (GIK) infusion technique, which has been supported as an inotropic and metabolic therapy in several critical disease states [76]. The proposed mechanism of GIK therapy includes lowering circulating levels and subsequent myocardial uptake of free fatty acids (which are toxic to ischemic myocardium); increased myocardial energy production through exogenous glucose; and stabilization of intracellular potassium, which may be depleted during times of myocardial ischemia [77, 78]. However, this method does not allow for individual manipulation of glucose or insulin levels if required, as such this system may be better suited for blood glucose maintenance after achievement of a specific glycemic goal [20].

7. Postoperative Glycemic Management

Due to postoperative complications, anesthetic side effects, or a number of other reasons, glycemic control during the postoperative stage may be difficult. The foundation of good postoperative care is based on diligent blood glucose measurement. The Society of Thoracic Surgeons as well as the AACE/ADA consensus recommended a postoperative glycemic range between 140 and 180 mg/dL [79]. However, if patients are monitored in the acute care setting after surgery due to surgical complications or various underlying comorbidities, physicians should be cognizant of the stress hyperglycemic response (averaging roughly 180–220 mg/dL) and as such develop a more tolerant glucose management strategy [80]. If blood glucose levels remain low after surgery, a dextrose infusion rate of 5–10 g of glucose per hour should prevent hypoglycemia and concomitant ketosis [13]. Additionally, if a patient is unable to tolerate oral nourishment for a prolonged period of time, total parenteral nutrition (TPN) should be considered. However, enteral nutrition should be resumed as soon as possible, due to fewer infectious complications, decreased cost, earlier restoration of normal gut function, and reduced length of hospital stay when compared to TPN [81]. Physiologic replacement of insulin can be mediated by a long-acting basal insulin dose (regardless of alimentation status), short or rapid acting insulin dose following meals, and rapid acting supplemental insulin to combat hyperglycemia if needed. Finally, according to a randomized trial conducted in 2007, in noncritically ill hospitalized type 2 diabetics, use of basal/bolus insulin protocols (as outlined below) offers significantly better glycemic control than supplemental-scale insulin alone [82].

It is important to ensure that basal insulin levels remain stable after intraoperative IV insulin is discontinued. This is especially true in type 1 diabetes, as baseline insulin values must be met to prevent diabetic ketoacidosis. The basal insulin dosage can be calculated using the "Miami 4/12" rule or approximated to 50–80% of the intraoperative IV insulin total (assuming adequate glycemic control was achieved) [57]. For patients treated with intraoperative IV insulin, it may be easiest to continue IV insulin alongside a dextrose infusion until the patient can tolerate food without difficulty. After verifying the patient is able to consume food reliably, the intravenous drips can be terminated and glycemic control procedures employed before surgery may be reinstituted [83]. Again the literature does not report a clear consensus in management, as another source instead recommends transitioning from IV to subcutaneous insulin 12 to 24 hours prior to discontinuing the drip to insure a baseline insulin concentration in type 1 diabetics (significantly reducing the chances of diabetic ketoacidosis) and allowing for heightened glycemic control in type 2 diabetic patients [57].

Postprandial related insulin requirements must be tailored to the mode in which the patient is receiving nutrition. Moreover, patients should be given instructions on how to initiate subcutaneous insulin supplementation in the event of hyperglycemia. For clinicians, supplemental insulin compensation for hyperglycemic patients can be approximated by dividing the total daily insulin (TDI) dose by 30 for every 50 mg/dL (3 mmol/L) above the glycemic goal [83]. Take a patient with a TDI dose of 150 U with a blood glucose reading of 350 mg/dL. Subtracting the upper end of a normal glucose measurement (200 mg/dL) from the patients reading and diving by 50 mg/dL yields 3 [(350 − 200)/50 = 3]. Simply multiply this number by the TDI/30 (150/30 = 5) to determine the patient requires an additional 15 U of rapid acting insulin to restore blood glucose levels back into target range. Finally, glucose measurement during the perioperative period can generally be completed by either central-laboratory-device (CLD) or point-of-care (POC) devices [84]. Multiple studies recommend avoiding the POC device for glucose management during the perioperative period, instead favoring the use of CLD blood glucose measurements [84, 85]. A summary of key checkpoints regarding pre-, intra-, and postoperative glycemic control can be reviewed in Table 1.

8. Special Operative Conditions

There are a number of special operative conditions that should be taken into account when determining a glucose management plan. For minor outpatient surgeries, type 1 or type 2 diabetes can be managed by IV infusion or subcutaneous insulin strategies. Furthermore, type 2 diabetic patients who are taking oral glycemic control agents should follow similar management guidelines as described above [20]. For emergency surgery situations, blood glucose should be monitored frequently. Physicians should also note when the last dose of a sulphonylurea drug was taken, as progressive absorption may disturb glycemic control [46, 86]. Insulin requirements are generally much higher in cardiac procedures; recent studies suggest improved patient outcomes with tight glycemic control during and after cardiac surgery [87]. Finally, perioperative blood glucose levels must be carefully monitored in patients undergoing cesarean section. Hyperglycemia should be avoided during cesarean section to reduce the risk of neonatal hypoglycemia or wound infections in the mother. Before induction of labor, patients should follow their normal diabetic regimen; however if labor is prolonged and blood glucose levels fall below 100 mg/dL, a 5% dextrose infusion should be initiated [88].

9. Conclusion

A number of protocols defining perioperative glycemic control have been described in the literature. While clinical judgment must still be used to assess specific changes, we hope this paper has provided greater insight into the overall goals of glucose management during pre-, intra-, and postoperative periods. Healthcare providers should remember that glucose homeostasis during the perioperative period is extremely variable; blood glucose levels as well as electrolyte and acid-base status should be carefully monitored. Physicians should be mindful of a patient's normal diabetic regimen, and after making all necessary changes during the perioperative period, aid the patient's transition back to their normal glycemic management protocol. In closing, through careful perioperative glucose management, surgical complications as well as hyper- or hypoglycemic sequelae can be reduced, ultimately improving patient morbidity and mortality.

Conflict of Interests

The authors declare that they have no conflict of interests.

References

[1] American Diabetes Association, "Diagnosis and classification of diabetes mellitus," *Diabetes Care*, vol. 33, supplement 1, pp. S62–S69, 2010.

[2] American Diabetes Association, "Standards of medical care in diabetes—2014," *Diabetes Care*, vol. 37, supplement 1, pp. S14–S80, 2014.

[3] Centers for Disease Control and Prevention, *National Diabetes Statistics Report: Estimates of Diabetes and Its Burden in the United States*, US Department of Health and Human Services, Atlanta, Ga, USA, 2014.

[4] G. Danaei, M. M. Finucane, Y. Lu et al., "National, regional, and global trends in fasting plasma glucose and diabetes prevalence since 1980: systematic analysis of health examination surveys and epidemiological studies with 370 country-years and 2.7 million participants," *The Lancet*, vol. 378, no. 9785, pp. 31–40, 2011.

[5] J. E. Shaw, R. A. Sicree, and P. Z. Zimmet, "Global estimates of the prevalence of diabetes for 2010 and 2030," *Diabetes Research and Clinical Practice*, vol. 87, no. 1, pp. 4–14, 2010.

[6] M. W. Stolar, B. J. Hoogwerf, S. M. Gorshow, P. J. Boyle, and D. O. Wales, "Managing type 2 diabetes: going beyond glycemic control," *Journal of Managed Care Pharmacy*, vol. 14, no. 5, pp. s2–s19, 2008.

[7] J. Nicholas, J. Charlton, A. Dregan, and M. C. Gulliford, "Recent HbA1c values and mortality risk in type 2 diabetes. population-based case-control study," *PLoS ONE*, vol. 8, no. 7, Article ID e68008, 2013.

[8] G. van den Berghe, P. Wouters, F. Weekers et al., "Intensive insulin therapy in critically ill patients," *The New England Journal of Medicine*, vol. 345, no. 19, pp. 1359–1367, 2001.

[9] S. E. Capes, D. Hunt, K. Malmberg, and H. C. Gerstein, "Stress hyperglycaemia and increased risk of death after myocardial infarction in patients with and without diabetes: a systematic overview," *The Lancet*, vol. 355, no. 9206, pp. 773–778, 2000.

[10] C. T. Wass and W. L. Lanier, "Subspecialty clinics: anesthesiology: glucose modulation of ischemic brain injury: review and clinical recommendations," *Mayo Clinic Proceedings*, vol. 71, no. 8, pp. 801–812, 1996.

[11] D. Mesotten and G. van den Berghe, "Clinical potential of insulin therapy in critically ill patients," *Drugs*, vol. 63, no. 7, pp. 625–636, 2003.

[12] D. B. Coursin and M. J. Murray, "How sweet is euglycemia in critically ill patients?" *Mayo Clinic Proceedings*, vol. 78, no. 12, pp. 1460–1462, 2003.

[13] I. B. Hirsch and J. B. McGill, "Role of insulin in management of surgical patients with diabetes mellitus," *Diabetes Care*, vol. 13, no. 9, pp. 980–991, 1990.

[14] K. G. M. M. Alberti, G. V. Gill, and M. J. Elliott, "Insulin delivery during surgery in the diabetic patient," *Diabetes Care*, vol. 5, no. 1, pp. 65–77, 1982.

[15] C. Reynolds, "Management of the diabetic surgical patient. A systematic but flexible plan is the key," *Postgraduate Medicine*, vol. 77, no. 1, pp. 265–279, 1985.

[16] L. A. Gavin, "Perioperative management of the diabetic patient," *Endocrinology and Metabolism Clinics of North America*, vol. 21, no. 2, pp. 457–475, 1992.

[17] A. Peters and W. Kerner, "Perioperative management of the diabetic patient," *Experimental and Clinical Endocrinology & Diabetes*, vol. 103, no. 4, pp. 213–218, 1995.

[18] D. A. Fetchick and J. S. Fischer, "Perioperative management of the patient with diabetes mellitus undergoing outpatient or elective surgery," *Clinics in Podiatric Medicine and Surgery*, vol. 4, no. 2, pp. 439–443, 1987.

[19] P. J. Smail, "Children with diabetes who need surgery," *Archives of Disease in Childhood*, vol. 61, no. 4, pp. 413–414, 1986.

[20] J. B. Marks, "Perioperative management of diabetes," *American Family Physician*, vol. 67, no. 1, pp. 93–100, 2003.

[21] G. V. Gill and K. G. M. M. Alberti, "The care of the diabetic patient during surgery," in *International Textbook of Diabetes Mellitus*, John Wiley & Sons, New York, NY, USA, 2003.

[22] E. J. Rayfield, M. J. Ault, G. T. Keusch, M. J. Brothers, C. Nechemias, and H. Smith, "Infection and diabetes: the case for glucose control," *The American Journal of Medicine*, vol. 72, no. 3, pp. 439–450, 1982.

[23] A. Hempel, C. Maasch, U. Heintze et al., "High glucose concentrations increase endothelial cell permeability via activation of protein kinase Cα," *Circulation Research*, vol. 81, no. 3, pp. 363–371, 1997.

[24] W. A. Pulsinelli, D. E. Levy, B. Sigsbee, P. Scherer, and F. Plum, "Increased damage after ischemic stroke in patients with hyperglycemia with or without established diabetes mellitus," *The American Journal of Medicine*, vol. 74, no. 4, pp. 540–544, 1983.

[25] W. Marhoffer, M. Stein, E. Maeser, and K. Federlin, "Impairment of polymorphonuclear leukocyte function and metabolic control of diabetes," *Diabetes Care*, vol. 15, no. 2, pp. 256–260, 1992.

[26] J. F. McMurry Jr., "Wound healing with diabetes mellitus. Better glucose control for better wound healing in diabetes," *The Surgical Clinics of North America*, vol. 64, no. 4, pp. 769–778, 1984.

[27] M. Walker, S. M. Marshall, and K. G. M. M. Alberti, "Clinical aspects of diabetic ketoacidosis," *Diabetes/Metabolism Reviews*, vol. 5, no. 8, pp. 651–663, 1989.

[28] W. I. Brenner, Z. Lansky, R. M. Engelman, and W. M. Stahl, "Hyperosomolar coma in surgical patients: an iatrogenic disease of increasing incidence," *Annals of Surgery*, vol. 178, no. 5, pp. 651–654, 1973.

[29] G. A. Lee, S. Wyatt, D. Topliss, K. Z. Walker, and R. Stoney, "A study of a pre-operative intervention in patients with diabetes undergoing cardiac surgery," *Collegian*, vol. 21, no. 4, pp. 287–293, 2014.

[30] D. K. Wukich, "Diabetes and its negative impact on outcomes in orthopaedic surgery," *World Journal of Orthopedics*, vol. 6, no. 3, pp. 331–339, 2015.

[31] American Diabetes Association, "Economic costs of diabetes in the U.S. in 2012," *Diabetes Care*, vol. 36, no. 4, pp. 1033–1046, 2013.

[32] G. E. Umpierrez, S. D. Isaacs, N. Bazargan, X. You, L. M. Thaler, and A. E. Kitabchi, "Hyperglycemia: an independent marker of in-hospital mortality in patients with undiagnosed diabetes," *The Journal of Clinical Endocrinology & Metabolism*, vol. 87, no. 3, pp. 978–982, 2002.

[33] J. A. Galloway and C. R. Shuman, "Diabetes and surgery. A study of 667 cases," *The American Journal of Medicine*, vol. 34, no. 2, pp. 177–191, 1963.

[34] D. R. Goldmann, "Surgery in patients with endocrine dysfunction," *Medical Clinics of North America*, vol. 71, no. 3, pp. 499–509, 1987.

[35] G. Angelini, J. T. Ketzler, and D. B. Coursin, "Perioperative care of the diabetic patient," *ASA Refresher Courses in Anesthesiology*, vol. 29, no. 1, pp. 1–9, 2001.

[36] S. Finfer, R. Bellomi, D. Blair et al., "Intensive versus conventional glucose control in critically Ill patients," *The New England Journal of Medicine*, vol. 360, no. 13, pp. 1283–1297, 2009.

[37] A. Turchin, M. E. Matheny, M. Shubina, S. V. Scanlon, B. Greenwood, and M. L. Pendergrass, "Hypoglycemia and clinical outcomes in patients with diabetes hospitalized in the general ward," *Diabetes Care*, vol. 32, no. 7, pp. 1153–1157, 2009.

[38] A. Zacharias and R. H. Habib, "Factors predisposing to median sternotomy complications: deep vs superficial infection," *Chest*, vol. 110, no. 5, pp. 1173–1178, 1996.

[39] "Prevalence of diabetes and impaired fasting glucose in adults— United States, 1999-2000," *MMWR Morbidity and Mortality Weekly Report*, vol. 52, no. 35, pp. 833–837, 2003.

[40] K. M. V. Narayan, J. P. Boyle, T. J. Thompson, S. W. Sorensen, and D. F. Williamson, "Lifetime risk for diabetes mellitus in the United States," *Journal of the American Medical Association*, vol. 290, no. 14, pp. 1884–1890, 2003.

[41] A. Hjortrup, C. Sørensen, E. Dyremose, N. C. Hjortsø, and H. Kehlet, "Influence of diabetes mellitus on operative risk," *British Journal of Surgery*, vol. 72, no. 10, pp. 783–785, 1985.

[42] G. P. Zaloga, "Catecholamines in anesthetic and surgical stress," *International Anesthesiology Clinics*, vol. 26, no. 3, pp. 187–198, 1988.

[43] S. N. Madsen, A. Engquist, I. Badawi, and H. Kehlet, "Cyclic AMP, glucose and cortisol in plasma during surgery," *Hormone and Metabolic Research*, vol. 8, no. 6, pp. 483–485, 1976.

[44] M. R. Werb, B. Zinman, S. J. Teasdale, B. S. Goldman, H. E. Scully, and E. B. Marliss, "Hormonal and metabolic responses during coronary artery bypass surgery: role of infused glucose," *The Journal of Clinical Endocrinology & Metabolism*, vol. 69, no. 5, pp. 1010–1018, 1989.

[45] P. D. Wright and I. D. A. Johnston, "The effect of surgical operation on growth hormone levels in plasma," *Surgery*, vol. 77, no. 4, pp. 479–486, 1975.

[46] H. U. Rehman and K. Mohammed, "Perioperative management of diabetic patients," *Current Surgery*, vol. 60, no. 6, pp. 607–611, 2003.

[47] R. J. Fragen, C. A. Shanks, A. Molteni, and M. J. Avram, "Effects of etomidate on hormonal responses to surgical stress," *Anesthesiology*, vol. 61, no. 6, pp. 652–656, 1984.

[48] S. A. Forman, "Clinical and molecular pharmacology of etomidate," *Anesthesiology*, vol. 114, no. 3, pp. 695–707, 2011.

[49] J. B. Lundy, M. L. Slane, and J. D. Frizzi, "Acute adrenal insufficiency after a single dose of etomidate," *Journal of Intensive Care Medicine*, vol. 22, no. 2, pp. 111–117, 2007.

[50] J. P. Desborough, G. M. Hall, G. R. Hart, and J. M. Burrin, "Midazolam modifies pancreatic and anterior pituitary hormone secretion during upper abdominal surgery," *British Journal of Anaesthesia*, vol. 67, no. 4, pp. 390–396, 1991.

[51] G. M. Hall, S. Lacoumenta, G. R. Hart, and J. M. Burrin, "Site of action of fentanyl in inhibiting the pituitary-adrenal response to surgery in man," *British Journal of Anaesthesia*, vol. 65, no. 2, pp. 251–253, 1990.

[52] J. P. Desborough, P. M. Jones, S. J. Persaud, M. J. Landon, and S. L. Howell, "Isoflurane inhibits insulin secretion from isolated rat pancreatic islets of Langerhans," *British Journal of Anaesthesia*, vol. 71, no. 6, pp. 873–876, 1993.

[53] R. Lattermann, T. Schricker, U. Wachter, M. Georgieff, and A. Goertz, "Understanding the mechanisms by which isoflurane modifies the hyperglycemic response to surgery," *Anesthesia and Analgesia*, vol. 93, no. 1, pp. 121–127, 2001.

[54] A. R. Wolf, R. L. Eyres, P. C. Laussen et al., "Effect of extradural analgesia on stress responses to abdominal surgery in infants," *British Journal of Anaesthesia*, vol. 70, no. 6, pp. 654–660, 1993.

[55] A. E. Pflug and J. B. Halter, "Effect of spinal anesthesia on adrenergic tone and the neuroendocrine responses to surgical stress in humans," *Anesthesiology*, vol. 55, no. 2, pp. 120–126, 1981.

[56] R. J. Moraca, D. G. Sheldon, and R. C. Thirlby, "The role of epidural anesthesia and analgesia in surgical practice," *Annals of Surgery*, vol. 238, no. 5, pp. 663–673, 2003.

[57] L. F. Meneghini, "Perioperative management of diabetes: translating evidence into practice," *Cleveland Clinic Journal of Medicine*, vol. 76, no. 4, pp. S53–S59, 2009.

[58] E. S. Moghissi, M. T. Korytkowski, M. DiNardo et al., "American Association of Clinical Endocrinologists and American Diabetes Association consensus statement on inpatient glycemic control," *Diabetes Care*, vol. 32, no. 6, pp. 1119–1131, 2009.

[59] K. Giakoumidakis, R. Eltheni, E. Patelarou et al., "Effects of intensive glycemic control on outcomes of cardiac surgery," *Heart & Lung: The Journal of Acute and Critical Care*, vol. 42, no. 2, pp. 146–151, 2013.

[60] G. E. Umpierrez and A. E. Kitabchi, "Diabetic ketoacidosis: risk factors and management strategies," *Treatments in Endocrinology*, vol. 2, no. 2, pp. 95–108, 2003.

[61] M. McCavert, F. Mone, M. Dooher, R. Brown, and M. E. O'Donnell, "Peri-operative blood glucose management in general surgery—a potential element for improved diabetic patient outcomes—an observational cohort study," *International Journal of Surgery*, vol. 8, no. 6, pp. 494–498, 2010.

[62] M. Pietropaolo, "An 18-year-old patient with type 1 diabetes undergoing surgery," *PLoS Medicine*, vol. 2, no. 5, article e140, 2005.

[63] S. Clement, S. S. Braithwaite, M. F. Magee et al., "Management of diabetes and hyperglycemia in hospitals," *Diabetes Care*, vol. 27, no. 2, pp. 553–591, 2004.

[64] C. J. Bailey and R. C. Turner, "Metformin," *The New England Journal of Medicine*, vol. 334, no. 9, pp. 574–579, 1996.

[65] G. Williams, "Management of non-insulin-dependent diabetes mellitus," *The Lancet*, vol. 343, no. 8889, pp. 95–100, 1994.

[66] M. Toeller, "α-glucosidase inhibitors in diabetes: efficacy in NIDDM subjects," *European Journal of Clinical Investigation*, vol. 24, supplement 3, pp. 31–35, 1994.

[67] A. R. Saltiel and J. M. Olefsky, "Thiazolidinediones in the treatment of insulin resistance and type II diabetes," *Diabetes*, vol. 45, no. 12, pp. 1661–1669, 1996.

[68] L. C. Groop, "Sulfonylureas in NIDDM," *Diabetes Care*, vol. 15, no. 6, pp. 737–754, 1992.

[69] S. M. Alexanian, M. E. McDonnell, and S. Akhtar, "Creating a perioperative glycemic control program," *Anesthesiology Research and Practice*, vol. 2011, Article ID 465974, 9 pages, 2011.

[70] A. E. Duncan, A. Abd-Elsayed, A. Maheshwari, M. Xu, E. Soltesz, and C. G. Koch, "Role of intraoperative and postoperative blood glucose concentrations in predicting outcomes after cardiac surgery," *Anesthesiology*, vol. 112, no. 4, pp. 860–871, 2010.

[71] A. P. Furnary, K. J. Zerr, G. L. Grunkemeier, and A. Starr, "Continuous intravenous insulin infusion reduces the incidence of deep sternal wound infection in diabetic patients after cardiac surgical procedures," *The Annals of Thoracic Surgery*, vol. 67, no. 2, pp. 352–362, 1999.

[72] J.-Y. Li, S. Sun, and S.-J. Wu, "Continuous insulin infusion improves postoperative glucose control in patients with diabetes mellitus: undergoing coronary artery bypass surgery," *Texas Heart Institute Journal*, vol. 33, no. 4, pp. 445–451, 2006.

[73] L. Stockton, M. Baird, C. B. Cook et al., "Development and implementation of evidence-based guidelines for IV insulin: a statewide collaborative approach," *Insulin*, vol. 3, no. 2, pp. 67–77, 2008.

[74] L. J. Markovitz, R. J. Wiechmann, N. Harris et al., "Description and evaluation of a glycemic management protocol for patients with diabetes undergoing heart surgery," *Endocrine Practice*, vol. 8, no. 1, pp. 10–18, 2002.

[75] P. A. Goldberg, M. D. Siegel, R. S. Sherwin et al., "Implementation of a safe and effective insulin infusion protocol in a medical intensive care unit," *Diabetes Care*, vol. 27, no. 2, pp. 461–467, 2004.

[76] M. A. Puskarich, M. S. Runyon, S. Trzeciak, J. A. Kline, and A. E. Jones, "Effect of glucose-insulin-potassium infusion on mortality in critical care settings: a systematic review and meta-analysis," *Journal of Clinical Pharmacology*, vol. 49, no. 7, pp. 758–767, 2009.

[77] S. R. Mehta, S. Yusuf, R. Diaz et al., "Effect of glucose-insulin-potassium infusion on mortality in patients with acute ST-segment elevation myocardial infarction: the CREATE-ECLA randomized controlled trial," *The Journal of the American Medical Association*, vol. 293, no. 4, pp. 437–446, 2005.

[78] F. Fath-Ordoubadi and K. J. Beatt, "Glucose-insulin-potassium therapy for treatment of acute myocardial infarction: an overview of randomized placebo-controlled trials," *Circulation*, vol. 96, no. 4, pp. 1152–1156, 1997.

[79] T. Breithaupt, "Postoperative glycemic control in cardiac surgery patients," *Proceedings (Baylor University Medical Center)*, vol. 23, no. 1, pp. 79–82, 2010.

[80] P. E. Marik and R. Bellomo, "Stress hyperglycemia: an essential survival response!," *Critical Care*, vol. 17, no. 2, article 305, 2013.

[81] D. S. Seres, M. Valcarcel, and A. Guillaume, "Advantages of enteral nutrition over parenteral nutrition," *Therapeutic Advances in Gastroenterology*, vol. 6, no. 2, pp. 157–167, 2013.

[82] G. E. Umpierrez, D. Smiley, A. Zisman et al., "Randomized study of basal-bolus insulin therapy in the inpatient management of patients with type 2 diabetes (RABBIT 2 Trial)," *Diabetes Care*, vol. 30, no. 9, pp. 2181–2186, 2007.

[83] S. J. Jacober and J. R. Sowers, "An update on perioperative management of diabetes," *Archives of Internal Medicine*, vol. 159, no. 20, pp. 2405–2411, 1999.

[84] M. J. Rice, A. D. Pitkin, and D. B. Coursin, "Glucose measurement in the operating room: more complicated than it seems," *Anesthesia and Analgesia*, vol. 110, no. 4, pp. 1056–1065, 2010.

[85] B. Mraovic, E. S. Schwenk, and R. H. Epstein, "Intraoperative accuracy of a point-of-care glucose meter compared with simultaneous central laboratory measurements," *Journal of Diabetes Science and Technology*, vol. 6, no. 3, pp. 541–546, 2012.

[86] H. Kalimo and Y. Olsson, "Effects of severe hypoglycemia on the human brain. Neuropathological case reports," *Acta Neurologica Scandinavica*, vol. 62, no. 6, pp. 345–356, 1980.

[87] K. K. Haga, K. L. McClymont, S. Clarke et al., "The effect of tight glycaemic control, during and after cardiac surgery, on patient mortality and morbidity: a systematic review and meta-analysis," *Journal of Cardiothoracic Surgery*, vol. 6, no. 1, article 3, 2011.

[88] P. Kalra and M. Anakal, "Peripartum management of diabetes," *Indian Journal of Endocrinology and Metabolism*, vol. 17, supplement 1, pp. S72–S76, 2013.

5

Biomechanical Evaluation of a Mandibular Spanning Plate Technique Compared to Standard Plating Techniques to Treat Mandibular Symphyseal Fractures

Matthew Richardson,[1] **Jonathan Hayes,**[1] **J. Randall Jordan,**[1]
Aaron Puckett,[2] **and Matthew Fort**[1]

[1]University of Mississippi Medical Center, Department of Otolaryngology and Communicative Sciences,
 2500 N. State Street, Jackson, MS 39216, USA
[2]University of Mississippi Medical Center, Department of Biomedical Materials Science, 2500 N. State Street, Jackson,
 MS 39216, USA

Correspondence should be addressed to Matthew Richardson; mattrichardsonmd@gmail.com

Academic Editor: Antonio Boccaccio

Purpose. The purpose of this study is to compare the biomechanical behavior of the spanning reconstruction plate compared to standard plating techniques for mandibular symphyseal fractures. *Materials and Methods.* Twenty-five human mandible replicas were used. Five unaltered synthetic mandibles were used as controls. Four experimental groups of different reconstruction techniques with five in each group were tested. Each synthetic mandible was subjected to a splaying force applied to the mandibular angle by a mechanical testing unit until the construct failed. Peak load and stiffness were recorded. The peak load and stiffness were analyzed using ANOVA and the Tukey test at a confidence level of 95% ($P < 0.05$). *Results.* The two parallel plates' group showed statistically significant lower values for peak load and stiffness compared to all other groups. No statistically significant difference was found for peak load and stiffness between the control (C) group, lag screw (LS) group, and the spanning plate (SP1) group. *Conclusions.* The spanning reconstruction plate technique for fixation of mandibular symphyseal fractures showed similar mechanical behavior to the lag screw technique when subjected to splaying forces between the mandibular gonial angles and may be considered as an alternative technique when increased reconstructive strength is needed.

1. Introduction

The mandible is one of the most commonly fractured bones in the facial skeleton. Symphyseal and parasymphyseal fractures of the mandible have been reported to occur with a frequency of 9% to 57% [1, 2]. Treatment of mandible fractures is based on the restoration of form and function. This requires anatomic reduction of the mandible to its pretraumatic shape and proper fixation of the fracture to resist deformation. The anatomy of the mandible and vector of forces exerted by the suprahyoid, masseter, and temporalis muscles make symphysis fractures particularly problematic in this regard.

When the muscles of mastication contract to bite and clench, the mandible is bent in a sagittal plane. There is bilateral torsion of the mandibular bodies resulting in bending at the symphyseal region. This in turn leads to compression at the superior margin of the symphysis and tension at the inferior margin. Late in the power stroke of biting and clenching, lateral transverse bending occurs and the bending moment increases from back to front to reach its maximum magnitude near the symphysis. This lateral bending produces compressive stress at the buccal cortex and tensile stress at the lingual surface [3, 4]. In a patient with a symphyseal fracture, this results in the hemimandible being splayed outward. This is especially true in the setting of a mandibular symphysis fracture associated with a unilateral or bilateral mandibular subcondylar fracture. The symphyseal mandibular fracture with bilateral condylar or subcondylar fractures is a somewhat common fracture pattern and often a very difficult reconstructive problem [5]. In this setting, there is no longer posterior stability provided by the temporomandibular articulation and the mandibular gonial angles are flared [6] (Figure 1).

The various fixation techniques of mandibular fractures have evolved over time based on the patient's needs and the most recent scientific and surgical advances. For over thirty years, the treatment of choice has been open reduction with stable internal fixation. The lag screw technique, which was first described in 1970, was more recently shown by Madsen et al. to be mechanically superior to other commonly used techniques including the two-plate techniques [7].

A spanning reconstruction plate between the inferior borders of the mandibular body positions the long axis of the plate parallel with the splaying forces on the mandible. This offers a theoretical mechanical advantage, but the biomechanical behavior of the spanning reconstruction plate used in conjunction with two parallel plates' system has never been evaluated. Therefore, the purpose of this study is to evaluate the biomechanical behavior of the spanning reconstruction plate and compare it to the lag screw technique and the two parallel plates' technique. The parameters evaluated were peak load and stiffness. Peak load is the load at which permanent deformation of the system begins. Stiffness is a parameter used to describe the force needed to achieve a certain deformation of a structure (stiffness = the slope of the force divided by deformation).

2. Materials and Methods

A total of 25 human mandible replicas (Sawbones Foam Cortical Shell Mandibles, Pacific Research Laboratories, Vashon, Washington) were used in this study. These synthetic replicas were chosen to eliminate the variation in geometry and mechanical properties of human bone. They have been shown to be appropriate maxillofacial human bone substitutes for testing the stability of rigid fixation techniques [8].

Fixation materials consisted of 4-hole 0.6 mm thick straight titanium miniplates with spacer (Stryker Maxillofacial, 55-06704), 4-hole straight 1.5 mm thick titanium mandible miniplates with spacer (Stryker Maxillofacial, 55-10505), 12-hole 0.6 mm thick straight titanium plates (Stryker Maxillofacial, 55-06724), 30 mm 2.0 mm diameter titanium lag screws (Stryker Maxillofacial, 53-20430), 1.7 mm titanium monocortical bone screws each being 4 mm long (Stryker Maxillofacial, 50-17004), 2.0 mm titanium monocortical bone screws each being 10 mm long (Stryker Maxillofacial, 50-17004), and 2.0 mm 3D rectangular plates, 3 × 2 holes (Stryker Maxillofacial, 55-10532).

2.1. Sample Preparation. Five synthetic mandibles were unaltered and served as controls. Twenty synthetic mandibles were divided into four experimental groups with five mandibles in each group. Each experimental synthetic mandible was split evenly at the midline between the mandibular central incisors. The cuts were made with alloy steel blade coupled to a hand piece and a customized jig with saw guide was used to ensure uniformity of cuts. Each experimental group was fixed with a different technique (Table 1). Each reconstruction was performed using a customized jig made from epoxy resin to ensure consistent positioning of both mandibular segments.

The two parallel plates' (2PP) group was fixed with a 4-hole 0.6 mm thick miniplate secured to the superior border with four 1.7 mm outer diameter screws each being 4 mm long. The inferior border was fixed with the larger 4-hole 1.5 mm thick mandibular miniplate and secured with four 2.0 mm outer diameter screws each being 10 mm long (Figure 2). The 2PP plus spanning plate (SP1) group was fixed in a similar fashion as the two parallel plates' group with the addition of a straight 12-hole 1.5 mm thick plate spanning between the inferior borders of the mandibular body. This plate was secured using four 1.7 mm outer diameter screws each being 4 mm long (Figure 3). The second-spanning plate (SP2) group was fixed in a similar fashion to SP1 group with respect to the spanning plate, but with a 6-hole (3 holes × 2 holes) ladder plate rather than two parallel plates (Figure 4). The lag screw (LS) group was fixed with two 30 mm long 2.0 mm diameter self-tapping screws by the lag screw technique (Figure 5).

2.2. Load Testing. Biomechanical testing was performed on each synthetic mandible properly prepared with the respective fixation method. Each mandible was tested only once. Five uncut mandibles served as controls to define the limitations of the substrate (synthetic mandible replica). Each sample was placed in a custom fabricated jig consisting of two heavy-duty nylon straps. Each nylon strap was folded onto itself to create a loop. One nylon strap loop was placed over the condylar and coronoid heads and seated at the angle of the mandible on each side. The nylon strap loops were attached to the vertical arms of the mechanical testing unit. Each construct was preloaded with 0.5 lbs to provide enough tension between nylon strap loops such that the mandible would be suspended between them. Vertical loads were created and measured with a Sintech 2/G (MTS Corporation, Minneapolis, MN) servohydraulic materials testing unit (Figure 6). The vector force was therefore lateral to each mandibular angle simulating the physiologic splaying forces on the mandible from the suprahyoid, masseter, and temporalis muscles. The servohydraulic testing unit developed a linear displacement at a rate of 10 mm per minute, and 250 lbs load cell measured the resultant force. Loading was continued up to mechanical failure of each construct. Data were captured and analyzed with the TestWorks 4 (MTS Corporation, Minneapolis, MN) software. Means were calculated for peak load and stiffness of each test group (Table 2). The peak load and stiffness were analyzed using ANOVA and the Tukey test at a confidence level of 95% ($P < 0.05$). Results between groups were compared for statistical significance using the Mann-Whitney test allowing for nonparametric data analysis (Table 3). A two-tailed P less than 0.01 was considered significant.

TABLE 1: Groups.

Group	Fixation technique
Control	No simulated fractures or fixation
2 parallel plates (2PP)	Four-hole 0.6 mm miniplate secured with four 1.7 mm outer diameter screws 4 mm long to upper border of outer cortex + 4-hole 1.5 mm titanium plate secured with four 2.0 mm outer diameter screws 10 mm long to lower border of outer cortex
2PP + spanning plate (SP1)	Four-hole 0.6 mm miniplate secured with four 1.7 mm outer diameter screws 4 mm long to upper border of outer cortex + 4-hole 1.5 mm titanium plate secured with four 2.0 mm outer diameter screws 10 mm long to lower border of outer cortex + 12-hole 1.5 mm titanium plate spanning between the inferior borders of mandibular body secured with four 1.7 mm outer diameter screws 4 mm long
Ladder plate + spanning plate (SP2)	Six-hole 1.5 mm titanium ladder plate secured with four 2.0 mm outer diameter self-tapping screws 10 mm long to outer cortex + 12-hole 1.5 mm titanium plate spanning between the inferior borders of mandibular body secured with four 1.7 mm outer diameter self-tapping screws 4 mm long
Lag screw (LS)	Two 30 mm long 2.0 mm outer diameter self-tapping screws

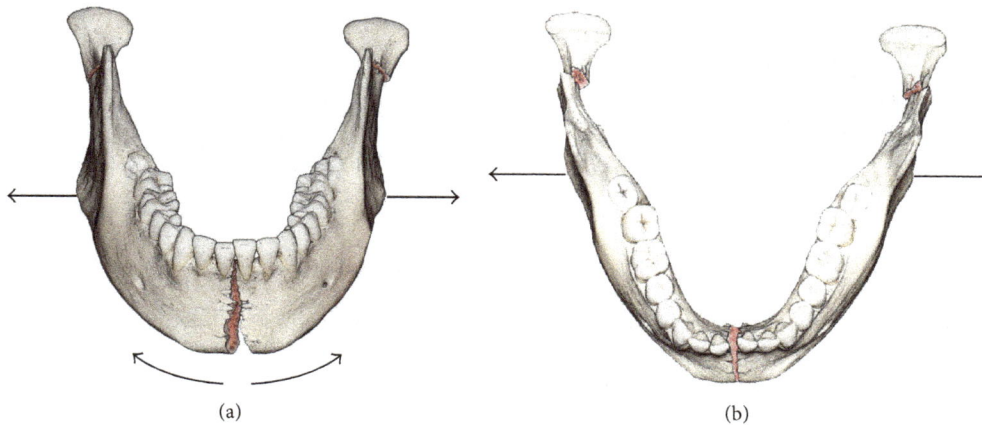

FIGURE 1: Illustration showing symphyseal fracture with bicondylar fractures and the resulting flaring (a) and widening (b) of the gonial angles.

TABLE 2: Summary of results (mean).

Group	Peak load (N)	Stiffness (force versus extension)
Control	55.8	187
2 parallel plates (2PP)	7.1	35.1
2PP + spanning plate (SP1)	32.1	102
Ladder plate + spanning plate (SP2)	40.6	126
Lag screw (LS)	34.5	97.8

TABLE 3: Statistical analysis summary.

Test	Between groups	Statistical significance	P value
Peak load	Control versus 2PP	Yes	0.004
Peak load	Control versus SP1	No	0.04
Peak load	Control versus LS	No	0.09
Peak load	2PP versus SP1	Yes	0.009
Peak load	2PP versus LS	Yes	0.009
Peak load	SP1 versus LS	No	0.92
Stiffness	Control versus 2PP	Yes	0.004
Stiffness	Control versus SP1	No	0.01
Stiffness	Control versus LS	No	0.01
Stiffness	2PP versus SP1	Yes	0.009
Stiffness	2PP versus LS	Yes	0.009
Stiffness	SP1 versus LS	No	0.92

$P < 0.01$ considered statistically significant.

3. Results

After statistical analysis of values for peak load, the results showed a statistically lower value for the two parallel plates' (2PP) group compared to the spanning plate (SP1) group, the lag screw (LS) group, and the control (C) group. No significant difference was found between the spanning plate (SP1) group, the lag screw (LS) group, and the control (C) group for peak load.

Similar results were found for stiffness values. Analysis revealed a statistically significant lower stiffness value for the two parallel plates' (2PP) group compared to the spanning

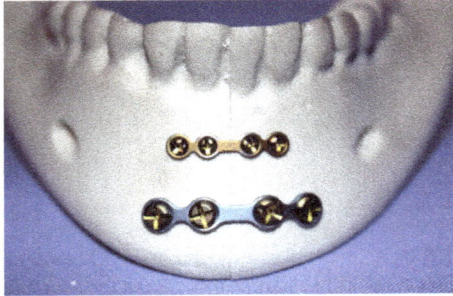

FIGURE 2: Two parallel plates (2PP).

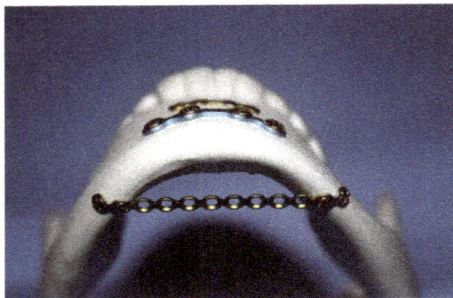

FIGURE 3: Two parallel plates plus spanning plate (SP1).

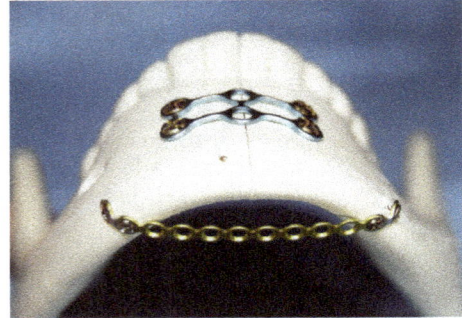

FIGURE 4: Ladder plate plus spanning plate (SP2).

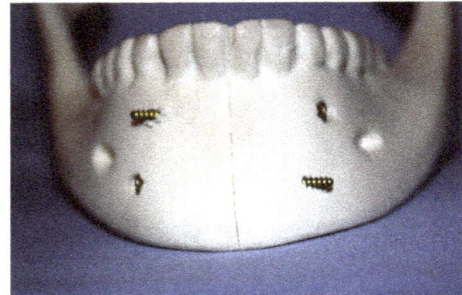

FIGURE 5: Lag screw (LS) group.

plate (SP1) group, the lag screw (LS) group, and the control (C) group. No significant difference was found between the spanning plate (SP1) group, the lag screw (LS) group, and the control (C) group for stiffness. SP2 group was added as an additional group in order to evaluate another potential plating combination with the spanning plate. This group was excluded from the Mann-Whitney statistical analysis comparison in order to avoid confusion over the role of the ladder plate versus the spanning plate in the overall construct strength. The rank order for peak load was (C) 55.8 N > (SP2) 40.6 N > (LS) 34.5 N > (SP1) 32.0 N > (2PP) 7.1 N. The rank order of stiffness was (C) 187 > (SP2) 126 > (SP1) 102 > (LS) 98 > (2PP) 35.

Observations were made regarding fracture pattern of each construct when system failure was reached. The unaltered synthetic mandibles in the control group all fractured in the symphyseal/parasymphyseal region when subjected to the splaying force during mechanical testing. The two parallel plates' (2PP) group showed the least resistance to deformity when tested. In each trial, failure occurred along the symphyseal fracture line with permanent deformation of the plating system or complete failure of the plating system due to fracture of the mandible in a separate location or screw pull-out. This is consistent with similar failure patterns of plate bending and screw pull-out (rather than plate fracture) that have been previously described [9]. In the lag screw (LS) group, failure occurred because of fracture of the synthetic mandible just lateral to where the lag screws penetrated the cortex in the parasymphyseal region. Similarly, failure in the spanning plate groups (SP1 and SP2 groups) occurred by fracture of the synthetic mandible at the fixation point of the spanning plate to the mandible.

4. Discussion

Mandible fractures that involve both the parasymphyseal-symphyseal region in combination with single or bilateral subcondylar fracture can lead to widening of the gonial angles if the mandibular arch is insufficiently reduced and stabilized [6]. As noted by Ellis III and Tharanon, particular attention should be given to the reduction and fixation of the buccal cortex in the symphyseal region. "Overreduction" of the fracture with a small gap at the buccal cortex can assure that the lingual cortex is adequately reduced. Overbending of the rigid fixation plate can also be effective. Several authors have investigated the relative strength of different techniques for stabilizing parasymphyseal fractures [7, 10]. The transverse lag screw technique has been found to offer increased stability and resistance to distortion when compared to plates or maxillomandibular fixation (MMF). The transverse lag screw technique can be technically difficult in some types of symphyseal fractures and is also dependent on the skill and experience of the surgeon as well as the availability of adequate length lag screws. We have sought a more universally applicable technique to provide improved stability against the deformational forces involved in this subset of mandible fractures. The use of additional "spanning" miniplate across the inferior border of the anterior mandibular arch in conjunction with traditional parallel upper and lower border plates was felt to be a potential candidate. The advantages of this approach are that it uses readily available plates and screws and is relatively simple to apply. The primary disadvantage is that it requires an external incision in the submental region, while other competing techniques may be performed through an intraoral approach.

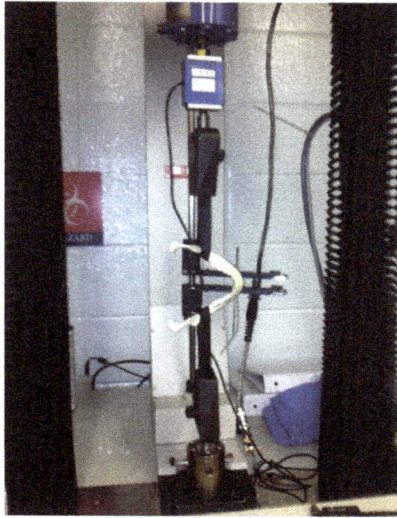

FIGURE 6: Sample positioned for mechanical testing in the Sintech 2/G servohydraulic materials testing unit.

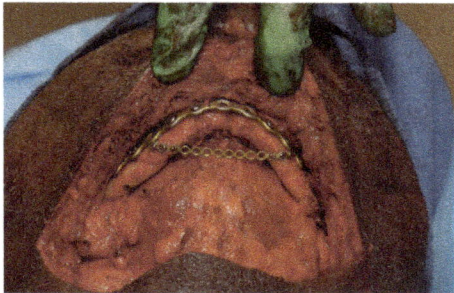

FIGURE 7: Spanning plate in a selected patient. Note that a different reconstructive plate was used on the anterior mandibular surface due to the multiple comminuted mandibular segments.

While this hardware is low profile, it remains potentially palpable, which is a risk with most facial reconstruction hardware. It also requires additional hardware compared to other techniques, which comes with increased financial cost.

The purpose of this study was to compare the biomechanical forces of the standard two parallel plates' (2PP) technique, lag screw (LS) technique, and the spanning plate techniques (SP1 and SP2 techniques). We attempted to mimic the splaying forces across the gonial angles with the use of a synthetic mandible model and servohydraulic mechanical testing unit. The synthetic mandible model has been investigated previously and found to be an adequate substitute for cadaveric mandibles for biomechanical testing purposes [8]. A variety of different constructs have been used for testing the various forces that are in play during mastication. A construct with perpendicular plates for symphyseal fractures has been previously tested [11]; however, this testing was focused on vertical bite forces rather than gonial angle splaying forces. The forces of mastication are varied and extremely complex [12, 13], but, for this particular application (the resistance to deforming forces causing widening of the gonial angles), we felt that direct application of force across the mandibular angles was the most accurate model. We do not represent that our testing construct accurately models all of the physiologic forces that are applied to the mandible during mastication, but it is limited to the splaying forces that we felt most representative of the issue at hand.

As noted in the Results, we found a statistically significant difference in the stiffness values between the lag screw (LS) group and two parallel plates' (2PP) group (97.8 versus 35.1, $P < 0.009$) as well as between the spanning plate (SP1) group and the two parallel plates' (2PP) group (102 versus 35.1, $P < 0.009$) with both the LS and SP1 groups exhibiting increased stiffness compared to the 2PP group. No significant difference was noted between the lag screw group and the spanning plate group (97.8 versus 102, $P < 0.92$). This finding indicates that the spanning plate technique is similar in strength to the lag screw technique. This could also support the use of either of these techniques in the treatment of mandible fractures involving both the symphyseal-parasymphyseal region and one or both subcondylar regions. Although excluded from the Mann-Whitney statistical analysis, the ladder plate and spanning plate (SP2) construct also resulted in higher peak load and stiffness values compared to the two parallel plates plus spanning plate (SP1) and lag screw (LS) groups, indicating another potentially strong construct utilizing a spanning plate.

The weaknesses of this study include the basic premise that this combination of fractures may lead to splaying of the gonial angles. While this may or may not be a common complication of this particular type of mandible fracture, its occurrence is documented in the report by Ellis III and Tharanon and is supported by the authors' experience [6]. In addition, while this study supports the use of lag screws and spanning plates in this fracture pattern, it may be that more conventional techniques such as properly applied parallel plates with or without MMF may be adequate for reduction and repair of these fractures. We do not advocate the use of the spanning plate techniques in all of these fractures, but when one desires increased stability of the repair, we offer that it may be considered as an alternative to the lag screw technique. Although not specifically described here, we have utilized the spanning plate technique clinically in select cases with positive outcomes (Figure 7).

In summary, the use of a spanning miniplate across the lower border of the anterior mandibular arch appears to offer increased stability to the deformational splaying forces at the gonial angles as compared to the traditional upper and lower parallel plate technique and is at least comparable to the transverse lag screw technique in this synthetic mandible model. Documentation of its use and efficacy in patients with this fracture pattern will require further study.

Conflict of Interests

The authors declare that there is no conflict of interests regarding the publication of this paper.

References

[1] P. Scolozzi and M. Richter, "Treatment of severe mandibular fractures using AO reconstruction plates," *Journal of Oral and Maxillofacial Surgery*, vol. 61, no. 4, pp. 458–461, 2003.

[2] A. S. Murthy and J. A. Lehman Jr., "Symptomatic plate removal in maxillofacial trauma: a review of 76 cases," *Annals of Plastic Surgery*, vol. 55, no. 6, pp. 603–607, 2005.

[3] R. T. Hart, V. V. Hennebel, N. Thongpreda, W. C. Van Buskirk, and R. C. Anderson, "Modeling the biomechanics of the mandible: a three-dimensional finite element study," *Journal of Biomechanics*, vol. 25, no. 3, pp. 261–286, 1992.

[4] J. Tams, J.-P. van Loon, F. R. Rozema, E. Otten, and R. R. M. Bos, "A three-dimensional study of loads across the fracture for different fracture sites of the mandible," *British Journal of Oral and Maxillofacial Surgery*, vol. 34, no. 5, pp. 400–405, 1996.

[5] G. Gerbino, P. Boffano, and G. F. Bosco, "Symphyseal mandibular fractures associated with bicondylar fractures: a retrospective analysis," *Journal of Oral and Maxillofacial Surgery*, vol. 67, no. 8, pp. 1656–1660, 2009.

[6] E. Ellis III and W. Tharanon, "Facial width problems associated with rigid fixation of mandibular fractures: case reports," *Journal of Oral and Maxillofacial Surgery*, vol. 50, no. 1, pp. 87–94, 1992.

[7] M. J. Madsen, C. A. McDaniel, and R. H. Haug, "A biomechanical evaluation of plating techniques used for reconstructing mandibular symphysis/parasymphysis fractures," *Journal of Oral and Maxillofacial Surgery*, vol. 66, no. 10, pp. 2012–2019, 2008.

[8] T. L. Bredbenner and R. H. Haug, "Substitutes for human cadaveric bone in maxillofacial rigid fixation research," *Oral Surgery, Oral Medicine, Oral Pathology, Oral Radiology, and Endodontics*, vol. 90, no. 5, pp. 574–580, 2000.

[9] T. A. Chiodo, V. B. Ziccardi, M. Janal, and C. Sabitini, "ailure strength of 2.0 locking versus 2.0 conventional Synthes mandibular plates: a laboratory model," *Journal of Oral and Maxillofacial Surgery*, vol. 64, no. 10, pp. 1475–1479, 2006.

[10] T. R. Vieira E Oliveira and L. A. Passeri, "Mechanical evaluation of different techniques for symphysis fracture fixation—an in vitro polyurethane mandible study," *Journal of Oral and Maxillofacial Surgery*, vol. 69, no. 6, pp. e141–e146, 2011.

[11] A. Kimura, T. Nagasao, T. Kaneko, J. Miyamoto, and T. Nakajima, "A comparative study of most suitable miniplate fixation for mandibular symphysis fracture using a finite element model," *Keio Journal of Medicine*, vol. 55, no. 1, pp. 1–8, 2006.

[12] T. M. G. J. Van Eijden, "Biomechanics of the mandible," *Critical Reviews in Oral Biology and Medicine*, vol. 11, no. 1, pp. 123–136, 2000.

[13] R. C. W. Wong, H. Tideman, L. Kin, and M. A. W. Merkx, "Biomechanics of mandibular reconstruction: a review," *International Journal of Oral and Maxillofacial Surgery*, vol. 39, no. 4, pp. 313–319, 2010.

6

Will Septal Correction Surgery for Deviated Nasal Septum Improve the Sense of Smell? A Prospective Study

Neelima Gupta, P. P. Singh, and Rahul Kumar Bagla

Department of Otorhinolaryngology, University College of Medical Sciences and GTB Hospital, Delhi 110095, India

Correspondence should be addressed to Neelima Gupta; write2drneelima@yahoo.com

Academic Editor: Jasvinder Singh

Background and Objectives. Nasal obstruction due to deviated nasal septum is a common problem bringing a patient to an otorhinolaryngologist. Occasionally, these patients may also complain of olfactory impairment. We proposed to study the effect of septal deviation on the lateralised olfactory function and the change in olfaction after surgery of the septum (septoplasty). *Methods.* Forty-one patients with deviated nasal septum were evaluated for nasal airflow, olfactory score, and nasal symptomatology. Septoplasty was done under local anesthesia. Pre- and postoperative olfactory scores, airflow and olfactory scores, and nasal symptomatology and olfactory scores were compared and correlated. *Results.* The range of preoperative composite olfactory score (COS) on the side of septal deviation was 4–14 (mean 7.90 ± 2.234) and on the nonobstructed side was 9–18 (mean 14.49 ± 2.378). Severity of deviated nasal septum and preoperative COS of diseased side were correlated and the correlation was found to be significant (rho $= -0.690$, $p = 0.000$ (<0.001)). The preoperative mean COS (7.90 ± 2.234) was compared with the postoperative mean COS (12.39 ± 3.687) and the improvement was found to be statistically significant ($p = 0.000$ (<0.001)). *Conclusion.* We found improvement in olfactory function in 70.6% patients after surgery, no change in 20.1%, and reduced function in 7.6%. With the limitation of a small sample size and a potential repeat testing bias, we would conclude that correction of nasal septal deviation may lead to improvement in sense of smell.

1. Introduction

Nasal obstruction is one of the most common problems bringing a patient to an otorhinolaryngologist's office, and septal deviation is a frequent structural etiology. Though nasal obstruction is the primary complaint in these patients, occasionally they may also complain of olfactory impairment. Higher olfactory thresholds as well as compromised olfactory identification have been documented on the deviated side of a septal deviation. Studies have shown that the structure of nasal cavity determines the pattern of airflow through the nose, thus affecting the number of odorant molecules transported to the olfactory epithelium. Leopold studied the relationship between nasal anatomy and human olfaction and found a relationship between changes in the structure of the upper nasal cavity and changes in olfactory ability [1]. Several other studies have focused on the relationship between the intranasal airflow and olfactory function [2, 3].

Damm et al. [2] assessed the intranasal volume and its relation to olfactory function in normosomic subjects using MRI scans. They found significant correlations between odor threshold measurements and volumes of the segment in the upper meatus directly below the cribriform plate and the anterior segment of inferior meatus.

Septoplasty most often improves the nasal respiratory airflow. Though studies have assessed the outcome of septal surgery in relation to nasal airflow, not many studies have focused on the change in olfaction following septal surgery. Also barring isolated studies [4], most studies have not directly correlated the uninasal airflow measurements and olfactory function before and after septal surgery. We proposed to study the effect of septal deviation on the lateralised olfactory function and correlate it with the visibility of the olfactory cleft and extent of posterior septal deviation. We also studied the change in olfaction after surgery of the septum. There are no reports from India about the effect of septal surgery on the olfactory function and in the presence of western reports about decrease in olfactory function following surgery due to direct trauma or vascular compromise to the olfactory epithelium [5]; it becomes imperative to investigate all septoplasty patients for this important aspect of nasal function.

2. Material and Methods

The study received approval by the institutional ethical committee. Forty-one patients presenting with nasal obstruction due to deviated nasal septum and impaired sense of smell were included in the study over one year. The age group was 15 to 45 years. Patients suffering from acute rhinitis, chronic rhinosinusitis, atrophic rhinitis, granulomatous diseases of nose, and nasal masses and patients having past history of nasal surgery were excluded from the study.

All patients were evaluated in detail with a history which included short form nasal questionnaire [6] for nasal symptomatology and visual analogue score (from 0 to 5) for subjective grading of their sense of smell, with grade of "5" being very poor and grade "0" being almost normal. Using short form nasal questionnaire (SFNQ), the symptoms graded were nasal obstruction (degree and duration), nasal stuffiness, excess mucus production, postnasal drip, snoring, and overall nasal symptoms on a scale of 0–4. For example, score 0 was given when there was no nasal obstruction and score 4 was given when the nasal obstruction was reported as very severe. The patients underwent test for olfaction, routine ENT examination with focus on anterior rhinoscopy, anterior rhinomanometry using nasal olives, and nasal endoscopy using a 0-degree nasal endoscope. The septal deviation was graded on anterior rhinoscopy as grade 1, mild septal deviation; grade 2, septum close to inferior turbinate; and grade 3, septum touching the inferior turbinate/lateral nasal wall.

Each side was graded separately and scores from each side were taken as "right nostril" and "left nostril" individual scores. The septal deviation and the visibility of olfactory cleft on endoscopy were recorded. According to the side of septal deviation, the nasal cavities were divided into diseased (obstructed) and nondiseased side.

Patients were worked up for septoplasty under local anaesthesia. Septal surgery was performed in which the deviated nasal septum was straightened with preservation of cartilaginous and bony parts of septum as much as possible. Nasal pack was removed after 48 hours and patients were kept under weekly follow-up.

Olfactory test, rhinomanometry, SFNQ, and VAS were repeated after four weeks of surgery.

2.1. Olfactory Test Methodology [7, 8]. The test comprised of two components: the olfactory threshold and identification.

2.1.1. Threshold Testing. The threshold test employed 1-butanol as the test odorant. The test kit contained nine glass bottles each containing ~20 mL of test solution (solutions one to nine) and another identical glass bottle filled with ~20 mL of sterile water. The 1-butanol solution was diluted by successive factors of three, the highest concentration being 4%, designated as solution one while the lowest concentration is 0.00061%, designated as solution nine. Participants received two bottles at a time, one with sterile water and one

with odorant. The test begins with the weakest solution in an ascending order of concentration to avoid desensitization. The lowest concentration of odorant that the patient correctly identifies on four successive occasions was defined as the threshold. Scores of one to nine were given depending on the lowest concentration of solution successfully identified. If the solution with the highest concentration was not identified, a score of zero was given. After determination of the threshold in one nostril, testing was done for the other nostril in the similar manner.

2.1.2. Odor Identification Testing. The odorant substances were kept in opaque plastic bottles and the patient's eyes were covered when the bottles were presented to them. To perform the test, the cap was removed by the examiner for approximately 3 seconds, and the tip of the bottle was placed approximately 2 cm in front of the nostril and patient was asked to sniff normally without any force. There was an interval of at least 30 seconds between successive presentations to prevent olfactory desensitization [9]. Patients were asked to choose from a list of four choices for each substance presented. Ten items were presented in random order for monorhinic smelling [10]. To restrict the stimulus to one nostril, the participant was asked to hold the other nostril closed. The total odor identification score was calculated by adding the number of substances correctly identified. The total score of the threshold test and the odor identification test was taken up as the combined olfactory score (COS) for the nostril being tested.

Substances for odor identification were asafoetida (heeng), naphthalene balls (moth balls), garlic (lahsun), Vicks VapoRub, rose water, cinnamon (dal chini), sandalwood oil, cardamom (elaichi), clove oil (laung), lemon, coffee, mint (pudina), camphor (kapur), and cumin seeds (jeera).

The combined olfactory score estimation using the threshold testing and odor identification testing has been previously validated in the Indian population [7]. The odors used for identification testing purposes have been selected after surveys and pilots and are according to Indian cultural preferences. The odors used in CCCRC are Johnson baby powder, chocolate, cinnamon, coffee, mothballs, peanut butter, Ivory bar soap, ammonia, Vicks VapoSteam, and wintergreen [10]. Since a few of these odors are not familiar to the Indian population, so we have used our previously validated "I-Smell" test.

For an objective assessment of nasal airflow we used anterior rhinomanometry. It is generally agreed that rhinomanometry with synchronous recording of flow rate and pressure drop across the nasal cavity during spontaneous breathing is the preferable and most reliable method for measuring nasal patency [11].

The HOMOTH-400 Rhinomanometer was used and Active Anterior Rhinomanometry (AAR) was done using nasal olives. The value of nasal airflow (NAF) at 150 pascals was taken for all assessments of nasal airflow.

2.2. Data Collection and Analysis. All relevant data were tabulated and systematically analysed using SPSS 17 statistical software. Wilcoxon's Sign Rank Test was used to compare the preoperative and postoperative olfactory score, short form nasal questionnaire score, and VAS score of olfaction. Spearman's/Pearson's correlation was used for correlation between olfactory score and rhinomanometry values both preoperative and postoperative and correlation between short form nasal questionnaire (SFNQ) and olfactory score. Paired t-test was used for comparing preoperative and postoperative flow rate values on rhinomanometry. p value <0.05 was considered significant.

3. Results

Over a period of 1 year, a total of 41 subjects with deviated nasal septum on presentation were prospectively recruited. The age of the subjects ranged from 15 to 45 years (mean 25.51 years). There were 27 males and 14 females with a male-to-female ratio of 1.9 : 1.

The mean preoperative SFNQ score was 16.20±3.494. The mean preoperative VAS score was 3.27 ± 0.633.

The olfactory cleft on diseased side was visible in 12 patients and on nondiseased side it was visible in 31 patients. On diseased side, posterior septal deviation was present in 10 patients, while it was absent in all patients on nondiseased side.

The range of COS on the diseased side was 4–14 (mean 7.90 ± 2.234); and on the nondiseased side it was 9–18 (mean 14.49 ± 2.378). Since we classified the side with the deviation of septum as the "diseased side," we further analyzed the parameters recorded on the obstructed/diseased side.

The severity of deviated nasal septum (DNS) on anterior rhinoscopy and preoperative COS of diseased side were correlated using Spearman's correlation and the correlation was found to be significant (rho = −0.690, p = 0.000 (<0.001)). The more severe the deviation was the less the COS was. The distribution of preoperative COS was compared with the olfactory cleft being visible or not visible using Mann-Whitney U test. The comparison was not significant (p = 0.134). Similarly the comparison between COS and posterior septal deviation being present or absent was insignificant (p = 0.042).

The preoperative mean score of SFNQ (16.20 ± 3.494) changed to postoperative mean score of SFNQ (7.78 ± 3.848), implying that there was decrease in the symptoms assessed on SFNQ after 4 weeks of follow-up and the improvement was found to be statistically significant (p = 0.000 (<0.001)).

The preoperative mean VAS (3.27 ± 0.633) was compared with postoperative mean VAS (1.56 ± 0.709) and the improvement was found to be statistically significant (p = 0.000 (<0.001)).

The preoperative mean COS (7.90 ± 2.234) on the diseased side was compared with the postoperative mean COS (12.39 ± 3.687), using the Wilcoxon Signed Rank Test and the improvement was found to be statistically significant (p = 0.000 (<0.001)). The improvement is shown in Figure 1.

All values of various parameters evaluated before and after surgery are shown in Table 1. The improvement in mean

TABLE 1: Mean ± standard deviation of variables studied (on the obstructed side).

Variable	Preoperative	Postoperative
COS	7.90 ± 2.234	12.39 ± 3.687
VAS	3.27 ± 0.633	1.56 ± 0.709
SFNQ	16.20 ± 3.494	7.78 ± 3.848
NAF (inspiration) (cm^3/sec)	219.24 ± 87.296	300.37 ± 143.652
NAF (expiration) (cm^3/sec)	252.40 ± 84.986	352.05 ± 164.484

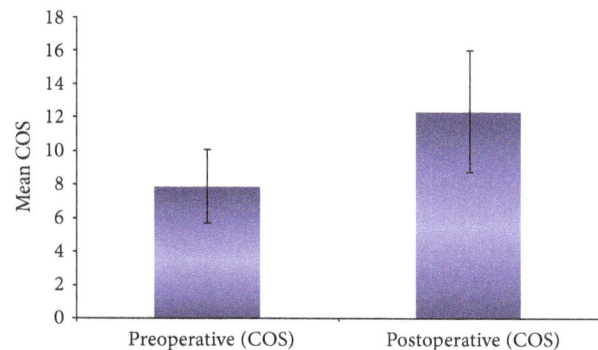

FIGURE 1: Preoperative and postoperative mean composite olfactory score (COS).

NAF after surgery was found to be statistically significant, both during inspiration and expiration (p < 0.001).

The preoperative VAS (3.27 ± 0.633) and preoperative COS (7.90 ± 2.234) of diseased side were correlated using Spearman's correlation and the correlation was found to be statistically significant (rho = −0.493, p = 0.001 (<0.001)), implying therefore that the objective olfaction test values correlated with the subjective sense of smell and there is a lateralised difference in olfactory score on the deviated side. The postoperative VAS and postoperative COS values of the diseased side showed a statistically significant inverse correlation (rho = −0.713, p = 0.000 (<0.001)). This indicates that after septal surgery, the subjective sense of smell improved (decreased mean VAS) and the composite olfactory score improved (increased mean COS) on the septal deviation side.

The preoperative COS (7.90 ± 2.234) correlated with the preoperative SFNQ (16.20 ± 3.494) scores significantly (rho = −0.436, p = 0.004 (<0.005)). More severe nasal symptoms were therefore found to be associated with decreased olfaction. And decrease in symptoms was associated with improved COS postoperatively (rho = −0.497, p = 0.001 (<0.001)).

The pre- and postoperative mean nasal air flow scores during inspiration and expiration were correlated with pre- and postoperative COS and the correlations were found to be significant. All correlations are shown in Table 2.

4. Discussion

The changes in olfactory ability following the correction of septal deviation is one way of evaluating how structural

TABLE 2: Correlation matrix between combined olfactory score on the obstructed side of the nose and rest of the variables, both pre- and postoperatively.

Variable	Preop COS (7.90 ± 2.234)	Postop COS (12.39 ± 3.687)
VAS	Rho = −0.493 ($p = 0.001$)	Rho = −0.713 ($p = 0.000$)
SFNQ	Rho = −0.436 ($p = 0.004$)	Rho = −0.497 ($p = 0.001$)
NAF (inspiration)	Rho = 0.440 ($p = 0.004$)	Rho = 0.739 ($p = 0.000$)
NAF (expiration)	Rho = 0.512 ($p = 0.001$)	Rho = 0.771 ($p = 0.000$)

changes in nasal anatomy relate to olfactory ability. Septal surgery produces a change in nasal airflow and also leads to improvement in the patient's olfactory abilities in majority of cases.

In our study, preoperatively, there was low composite olfactory score (COS) on the deviated nasal septum side. Objective assessments of preoperative nasal airflow correlated with the composite olfactory scores, showing that decreased airflow was associated with low COS. Previous study by Fyrmpas et al. also concluded that significant nasal septal deviation impairs the ability to identify a smell from the obstructed nostril [12].

In our set of patients, following septal surgery improvement of olfactory function was seen in 29 (70.6%); no change was seen in 5 (20.1%); and reduced olfactory function was observed in 3 (7.3%) patients. Four patients were lost to follow-up. In contrast Pade and Hummel [13] reported improvement in olfaction in 13%, no change in 81%, and decreased function in 7% of patients after septal surgery. They observed that patients exhibiting a postoperative decrease of olfactory function had significantly higher preoperative olfactory scores than patients who experienced improvement.

Different studies have reported variable outcomes of septal surgery on olfaction.

C. N. Stevens and M. H. Stevens [14] measured the olfactory thresholds before and after surgery in 100 patients. The primary surgical procedure of 63 patients was septoplasty, of 24 septorhinoplasty, of 3 turbinate reduction, and of 10 polypectomy. The authors concluded that all the surgical procedures improved the olfactory function; however, the data for each type of operation was not provided separately.

Pfaar et al. [15] in his landmark study produced three major findings: (1) before surgery odor thresholds were related to nasal obstruction, (2) during the postoperative period a significant decrease of odor discrimination was found, whereas there was no change in odor thresholds and odor identification, and (3) no significant change of olfactory function was reported after surgery. This type of inference was also drawn by Doty et al. [16] and Kimmelman [5], who reported a small proportion of patients (1.1%) showing anosmia 2–4 weeks after surgery.

These observations differ from what we observed in our study as we observed more cases with postoperative improvement. Also similar to our study, Damm et al. [17] in their study found improvement in odor identification and odor discrimination in 80% and improvement in odor threshold in 54% patients after septoplasty in combination with partial inferior turbinectomy. Our observations are limited on

the aspect of change in odor discrimination because we did not score odor discrimination.

Kimmelman [5] administered the UPSIT before and after septoplasty to 34 patients. The mean UPSIT scores of these largely normally functioning patients were essentially equivalent before and after the operation. However, in 15 rhinoplasty patients a small but statistically significant increase in performance was noted postoperatively. It was observed that since no control group was tested, a bias due to repeated testing may have accounted for the improvement after intervention. This is also a limitation of our study because we also did not have a control group.

Results of these various studies and our study suggest that septal surgery produces a variable outcome in terms of olfactory ability. Improvement in sense of smell can largely be attributed to an improvement in nasal airflow leading to a sense of improved ability to smell substances. A larger number of subjects with varying degrees of septal deviation, division of deviation into anatomical segments, and inclusion of a control group for lateralised difference in olfaction may bring out a better supported conclusion. Since we used composite olfactory score and not detection threshold and odor identification score separately we cannot comment on effect of septal deviation on suprathreshold olfactory function. However, we would like to conclude that even though the septal surgery is performed in an area remote from the olfactory epithelial area, changes in nasal airflow and intranasal volume can change the olfactory function of an individual.

Conflict of Interests

The authors declare that there is no conflict of interests regarding the publication of this paper.

References

[1] D. A. Leopold, "The relationship between nasal anatomy and human olfaction," *Laryngoscope*, vol. 98, no. 11, pp. 1232–1238, 1988.

[2] M. Damm, J. Vent, M. Schmidt et al., "Intranasal volume and olfactory function," *Chemical Senses*, vol. 27, no. 9, pp. 831–839, 2002.

[3] K. Zhao, P. W. Scherer, S. A. Hajiloo, and P. Dalton, "Effect of anatomy on human nasal air flow and odorant transport patterns: implications for olfaction," *Chemical Senses*, vol. 29, no. 5, pp. 365–379, 2004.

[4] D. E. Hornung and D. A. Leopold, "Relationship between uninasal anatomy and uninasal olfactory ability," *Archives of*

Will Septal Correction Surgery for Deviated Nasal Septum Improve the Sense of Smell? A Prospective Study

35

Otolaryngology—Head and Neck Surgery, vol. 125, no. 1, pp. 53–58, 1999.

[5] C. P. Kimmelman, "The risk of olfaction from nasal surgery," *Laryngoscope*, vol. 104, no. 8, pp. 981–988, 1994.

[6] N. Bhattacharyya and L. J. Kepnes, "Clinical effectiveness of coblation inferior turbinate reduction," *Otolaryngology: Head and Neck Surgery*, vol. 129, no. 4, pp. 365–371, 2003.

[7] N. Gupta, P. P. Singh, A. Goyal, and D. Bhatia, "Assessment of olfaction using the 'I-Smell' test in an indian population: a Pilot Study," *Indian Journal of Otolaryngology and Head and Neck Surgery*, vol. 65, no. 1, pp. 6–11, 2013.

[8] H. C. K. Lam, J. K. K. Sung, V. J. Abdullah, and C. A. V. Hasselt, "The combined olfactory test in a Chinese population," *Journal of Laryngology and Otology*, vol. 120, no. 2, pp. 113–116, 2006.

[9] M. Katotomichelakis, D. Balatsouras, G. Tripsianis, A. Tsaroucha, E. Homsioglou, and V. Danielides, "Normative values of olfactory function testing using the 'Sniffin Sticks'," *Laryngoscope*, vol. 117, no. 1, pp. 114–120, 2007.

[10] W. S. Cain, J. F. Gent, R. B. Goodspeed, and G. Leonard, "Evaluation of olfactory dysfunction in the Connecticut Chemosensory Clinical Research Center," *Laryngoscope*, vol. 98, no. 1, pp. 83–88, 1988.

[11] P. Panagou, S. Loukides, S. Tsipra, K. Syrigou, C. Anastasakis, and N. Kalogeropoulos, "Evaluation of nasal patency: comparison of patient and clinician assessments with rhinomanometry," *Acta Oto-Laryngologica*, vol. 118, no. 6, pp. 847–851, 1998.

[12] G. Fyrmpas, M. Tsalighopoulos, and J. Constantinidis, "Lateralised olfactory difference in patients with a nasal septal deviation before and after septoplasty," *Hippokratia*, vol. 16, no. 2, pp. 166–169, 2012.

[13] J. Pade and T. Hummel, "Olfactory function following nasal surgery," *Laryngoscope*, vol. 118, no. 7, pp. 1260–1264, 2008.

[14] C. N. Stevens and M. H. Stevens, "Quantitative effects of nasal surgery on olfaction," *American Journal of Otolaryngology*, vol. 6, no. 4, pp. 264–267, 1985.

[15] O. Pfaar, K. B. Hüttenbrink, and T. Hummel, "Assessment of olfactory function after septoplasty: a longitudinal study," *Rhinology*, vol. 42, no. 4, pp. 195–199, 2004.

[16] R. L. Doty, P. Shaman, and M. Dann, "Development of the University of Pennsylvania Smell Identification Test: a standardized microencapsulated test of olfactory function," *Physiology and Behavior*, vol. 32, no. 3, pp. 489–502, 1984.

[17] M. Damm, H. E. Eckel, M. Jungeholsing, and T. Hummel, "Olfactory changes at threshold and suprathreshold levels following septoplasty with partial inferior turbinectomy," *Annals of Otology, Rhinology and Laryngology*, vol. 112, no. 1, pp. 91–97, 2003.

7

Pharyngoesophageal Suturing Technique May Decrease the Incidence of Pharyngocutaneous Fistula following Total Laryngectomy

Mahmut Deniz, Zafer Ciftci, and Erdogan Gultekin

Department of Otorhinolaryngology, School of Medicine, Namik Kemal University, 59100 Tekirdag, Turkey

Correspondence should be addressed to Mahmut Deniz; mdeniz@nku.edu.tr

Academic Editor: Eelco de Bree

Objectives. A pharyngocutaneous fistula (PCF) following total laryngectomy is associated with increased morbidity and severe life threatening complications. We aimed to review our experience with the PCF following total laryngectomy and determine the impact of previously reported risk factors on the development of PCF in our patients. *Methods*. The medical records of 20 patients who had a total laryngectomy operation were retrospectively analyzed. The association between the proposed risk factors and the incidence of the PCF was investigated. *Results*. Comparison of the suture techniques used for the closure of the pharynx (either continuous Cushing type or interrupted) yielded that primary interrupted sutures had a significantly higher incidence of PCF formation ($p < 0.05$). Although it was not statistically significant, diabetes mellitus was also associated with increased PCF formation ($p > 0.05$). No significant difference was observed between the PCF and non-PCF groups in terms of other proposed risk factors ($p > 0.05$). *Conclusions*. The main risk factor associated with PCF was found to be the type of pharyngeal closure technique. A vertical closure with a Cushing type continuous suture may be more successful than interrupted sutures in preventing a PCF.

1. Introduction

In the recent years, the opportunity to preserve the functions of vocalization, swallowing, and natural airway respiration by organ preserving approaches led to a decrease in the number of total laryngectomy operations performed for laryngeal cancer [1]. However, for advanced stage tumors or recurrent disease, despite its significant morbidity and high complication rates, a total laryngectomy operation is usually employed [2]. Following total laryngectomy, a number of complications including, but not limited to, wound infection, swallowing difficulties, compromise of the airway, chyle leak, carotid rupture, and pharyngocutaneous fistula (PCF) may be seen in the early postoperative period [3]. Among these complications, the PCF merits special attention due to its significant negative impact on the recovery process of the patient and relatively high incidence rates ranging from 5 to 65 percent [4]. The PCF was found to be associated with increased hospitalization time, delayed adjuvant postoperative therapy, nutritional deterioration of the patient, and severe life threatening complications [5].

So far, in the literature, many factors were proposed to be significantly associated with the development of the PCF. Advanced primary tumor stage, preoperative radiotherapy, duration of surgery, transfusion requirement, patient comorbidities, prior tracheotomy, low perioperative albumin and hemoglobin, hypothyroidism, presence of tumor beyond resection margins, the type of the suture material, and the type of closure technique were implicated in the development of the PCF [2, 6, 7]. Despite the abundance of the series emphasizing the role of the various risk factors, the findings of these studies are usually inconsistent with the findings of the previous literature and a consensus regarding the identification of significant risk factors could still not be established.

TABLE 1: The main variables of the patients in both groups.

Risk factors	PCF group	Non-PCF group	Total
Interrupted suture	4	3	7
Continuous suture	0	13	13
DM* (+)	1	3	4
DM (−)	3	13	16
Hypoalbuminemia (+)	0	3	3
Hypoalbuminemia (−)	3	11	17
Preop. tracheotomy (+)	3	12	15
Preop. tracheotomy (−)	1	4	5
Neck dissection (+)	4	16	20
Neck dissection (−)	0	0	0
Preop. radiotherapy (+)	0	0	0
Preop. radiotherapy (−)	4	16	20
COPD** (+)	0	2	2
COPD (−)	4	14	18
Anemia (+)	0	3	3
Anemia (−)	4	13	17
CRF*** (+)	0	0	0
CRF (−)	4	16	20
Stage 4 cancer (+)	4	16	20
Stage 4 cancer (−)	0	0	0
Hypothyroidism (+)	0	0	0
Hypothyroidism (−)	4	16	20

*Diabetes mellitus: DM, **chronic obstructive pulmonary disease: COPD, and ***chronic renal failure: CRF.

The purpose of this retrospective analysis was to review our single-institute based experience with the PCF following total laryngectomy and determine the impact of previously reported risk factors on the development of PCF in our patients. The implications of our findings were also discussed within the scope of the existing literature.

2. Materials and Methods

The medical records of the patients, who underwent total laryngectomy for squamous cell carcinoma of the larynx in a tertiary referral center between 2010 and 2015, were retrospectively reviewed. Data regarding the age, gender, smoking habit, tumor stage, previous radiotherapy or chemotherapy, comorbid conditions including diabetes mellitus (DM), chronic obstructive pulmonary disease (COPD), chronic renal failure (CRF), perioperative hemoglobin, albumin, and thyroid hormone levels, prior tracheotomy, unilateral or bilateral neck dissection, the type of suture material used, and the type of closure technique were collected.

Patients who developed a PCF in the postoperative period (the PCF group) were considered as the study group and they were compared with the remaining patients (the non-PCF group). The main variables of the patients in both groups are listed in Table 1.

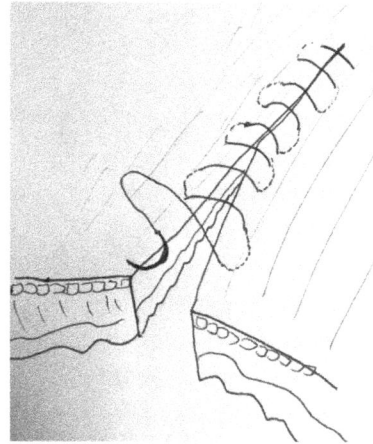

FIGURE 1: Cushing type continuous suture.

Total laryngectomy and pharyngeal closure were accomplished by the senior surgeons in all patients. Except for the type of suturing technique employed for creating the neopharynx, all patients underwent similar surgical interventions. All mucosal defects were closed by primary sutures and no patients required a flap procedure for the closure of the pharyngoesophageal segment. A 3/0 resorbable suture, "Surgicryl 910, HR-17 round bodied taper point needle 17 mm," manufactured from Polyglactine 910 was used as the suture material for all patients (SMI AG, Belgium). A vacuum drainage system was kept in place for 48 hours and a nasogastric tube was inserted. All patients received sulbactam/ampicillin 1 g/6 h i.v. after the procedure until 72 h later. For the creation of the neopharynx, either a vertical closure with a Cushing type continuous suture (Figures 1–3) or a T shaped closure with interrupted sutures was preferred.

For statistical analysis, SPSS for Windows, version 17, was used (SPSS Inc., Chicago, IL). The comparison of the qualitative data was conducted using Fisher's exact test. Results were considered as significant at the level where $p < 0.05$.

3. Results

The study population included 20 patients (1 female and 19 males) who underwent a total laryngectomy operation for stage 4 laryngeal cancer. The mean age of the patients was 58 years (range 51–68 years). The median follow-up time for all patients was 13.7 months (range 6.2–24.1 months). All patients had a history of smoking (at least 20 cigarettes per day for 20 years).

The PCF was observed in 4 of 20 patients (20%). Of these 4 patients, 1 patient was female and three were male. An additional surgical procedure was required to close the PCF in one patient and the remaining three patients had spontaneous closure of the PCF within one month.

13 patients had their pharyngeal closures with a Cushing type suture and none of them developed PCF in the postoperative period (0%). The pharyngeal closures of the remaining

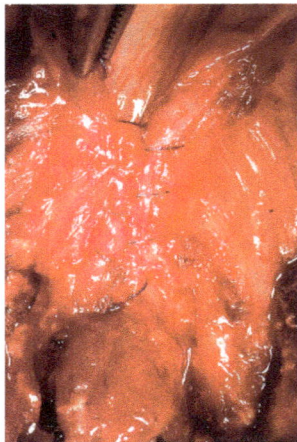

FIGURE 2: Closure of the pharyngoesophageal segment using a Cushing type continuous suture.

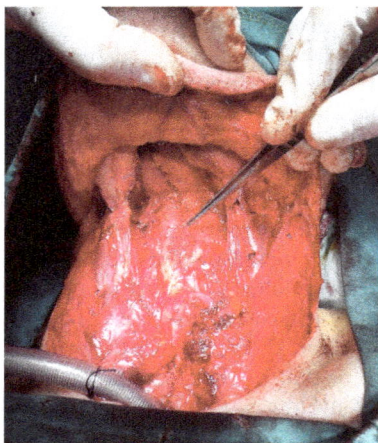

FIGURE 3: Reconstruction of the neopharynx was accomplished by a vertical closure using a Cushing type continuous suture.

7 patients were performed using interrupted sutures and, in this group of patients, 4 patients (57.14%) developed a PCF within the first postoperative week (Table 1). A statistically significant difference was observed between the two different suture groups in terms of PCF formation ($p = 0.007$, $p < 0.05$).

Four of 20 patients had a history of DM in the study group. Only one diabetic patient was in the PCF group (25%). In the non-PCF group, 3 patients were diabetic (18.75%). Although the incidence of PCF was slightly higher among the diabetic patients, the difference was not statistically significant ($p = 0.624$, $p > 0.05$).

Serum albumin levels were normal in 17 of 20 patients and 4 patients in this group had a PCF (23.52%). Hypoalbuminemia (serum albumin level <3.2 g/dL) was present in 3 of 20 patients (15%) and none of them had a PCF (0%) ($p = 0.596$, $p > 0.05$). Perioperative serum hemoglobin levels were found to be within normal range in 16 of 20 patients (80%) and 2 patients developed a PCF in this group (12.5%). Although the

remaining 4 patients had low hemoglobin levels, no patient in this group had a PCF in the postoperative period (0%). The association between low perioperative hemoglobin and development of a PCF was not statistically significant ($p = 0.491$, $p > 0.05$). Perioperative thyroid hormone levels were normal in all the patients.

15 of 20 patients were found to have a prior tracheotomy. Three of 15 patients (20%) with a prior tracheotomy and 1 of 5 patients (20%) without a prior tracheotomy were found to develop a PCF. The difference between the groups was statistically insignificant ($p = 0.751$, $p > 0.05$).

All patients in the study group had a bilateral neck dissection. None of the patients had a history of either chronic renal failure or preoperative chemotherapy or radiotherapy.

4. Discussion

In this research, we retrospectively investigated the impact of previously reported risk factors on the development of a PCF following total laryngectomy. Among these risk factors, although conflicting studies were reported in the literature, the type of suturing technique used for pharyngeal closure was suggested to be a significant risk factor [8, 9]. In this analysis, 57.14% of patients who had their pharyngeal closures with interrupted sutures were found to have a PCF. Strikingly, none of the patients who had a pharyngeal closure with a Cushing type continuous suture developed a PCF. This finding was also consistent with the previous reports emphasizing the high success rates and ease of application of a continuous type suturing technique following anastomosis or repair of the wall of the esophagus [10, 11]. In gastrointestinal system surgery, continuous suturing techniques (Connell and Cushing suture) are widely used for ileal, jejunal, and other colonic anastomoses either for cancer resection or traumatic perforations and successful results were presented in the literature [12, 13]. Pharyngoesophageal junction is the entry point for the gastrointestinal system; therefore, it is reasonable to assume that using Cushing type suture to join the pharyngeal and esophageal segments should be more successful than interrupted sutures in the prevention of a PCF following total laryngectomy.

The presence of a comorbid medical condition including DM, COPD, and CRF was proposed to be a significant risk factor for the development of the PCF [14]. However, such an association could not be demonstrated by others [15]. The PCF incidence in patients with a history of DM, although statistically insignificant, was higher in our study. On the contrary, none of the patients who developed a PCF had a history of either COPD or CRF. Larger series should be conducted to establish such an association.

The impact of low perioperative hemoglobin and albumin levels on the PCF incidence was also extensively reviewed in the literature [16]. However, in our study, perioperative anemia and hypoalbuminemia were not significantly associated with the PCF formation ($p > 0.05$).

Addition of neck dissection to total laryngectomy is another suggested contributing factor for the development of a PCF [17, 18]. In one study, the incidence of the PCF was reported to be increased from 11.3% to 17.5% when neck dissection is combined with total laryngectomy [19]. In our study, all patients in the PCF and non-PCF groups had a bilateral neck dissection and the impact of neck dissection on the incidence of the PCF could not be investigated.

Another factor that was proposed to increase the incidence of a PCF was having a prior chemotherapy or radiotherapy. It was suggested that preoperative chemotherapy or radiotherapy was also associated with longer hospital stays and the necessity for a second surgical operation for the closure of PCF was higher in preoperatively irradiated patients [20–22]. Other authors, however, could not find such an association [23, 24]. In our study, the impact of preoperative chemo- or radiotherapy on the PCF incidence could not be evaluated because none of the patients in our study group had a preoperative treatment.

A preoperative tracheotomy was found to be responsible for the increased rates of PCF following laryngectomy [25, 26]. In the present study, we could not reveal such an association because no statistically significant difference was present between the two different groups of patients in terms of PCF formation ($p > 0.05$). We are of the opinion that larger series should be conducted to further analyze such an association.

5. Conclusion

Pharyngocutaneous fistula is one of the most common postoperative complications among the patients who underwent total laryngectomy. The development of the PCF significantly increases the length of the hospital stay and the incidence of severe life threatening complications in this group of patients. In our research, the main factor associated with the occurrence of this complication was found to be the type of suturing technique used for pharyngeal closure. A vertical closure with a Cushing type continuous suture may be more successful than a T shaped closure with interrupted sutures in decreasing the incidence of a PCF following total laryngectomy.

Ethical Approval

All procedures performed in studies involving human participants were in accordance with the 1964 Declaration of Helsinki and the 2013 National Code on Clinical Researches.

Disclosure

This research received no specific grant from any funding agency, commercial or not-for-profit sectors.

Conflict of Interests

The authors declare that there is no conflict of interests regarding the publication of this paper.

Acknowledgment

The authors would like to acknowledge Birol Topcu, Assistant Professor, from the Department of Biostatistics in Namik Kemal University, School of Medicine, for his contributions in the statistical analysis of the data.

References

[1] M. Nakayama, O. Laccourreye, F. C. Holsinger, M. Okamoto, and K. Hayakawa, "Functional organ preservation for laryngeal cancer: past, present and future," *Japanese Journal of Clinical Oncology*, vol. 42, no. 3, pp. 155–160, 2012.

[2] E. M. Benson, R. M. Hirata, C. B. Thompson et al., "Pharyngocutaneous fistula after total laryngectomy: a single-institution experience, 2001–2012," *The American Journal of Otolaryngology—Head and Neck Medicine and Surgery*, vol. 36, no. 1, pp. 24–31, 2015.

[3] I. Ganly, S. Patel, J. Matsuo et al., "Postoperative complications of salvage total laryngectomy," *Cancer*, vol. 103, no. 10, pp. 2073–2081, 2005.

[4] H. N. White, B. Golden, L. Sweeny, W. R. Carroll, J. S. Magnuson, and E. L. Rosenthal, "Assessment and incidence of salivary leak following laryngectomy," *Laryngoscope*, vol. 122, no. 8, pp. 1796–1799, 2012.

[5] M. A. Erdag, S. Arslanoglu, K. Onal, M. Songu, and A. O. Tuylu, "Pharyngocutaneous fistula following total laryngectomy: Multivariate analysis of risk factors," *European Archives of Oto-Rhino-Laryngology*, vol. 270, no. 1, pp. 173–179, 2013.

[6] R. P. Morton, H. Mehanna, F. T. Hall, and N. P. McIvor, "Prediction of pharyngocutaneous fistulas after laryngectomy," *Otolaryngology—Head and Neck Surgery*, vol. 136, no. 4, supplement, pp. S46–S49, 2007.

[7] J. A. Virtaniemi, E. J. Kumpulainen, P. P. Hirvikoski, R. T. Johansson, and V.-M. Kosma, "Backside first in head and neck surgery?: preventing pressure ulcers in extended length surgeries," *Head & Neck*, vol. 23, no. 1, pp. 25–28, 2001.

[8] D. Akduman, B. Naiboğlu, C. Uslu et al., "Pharyngocutaneous fistula after total laryngectomy: incidence, predisposing factors, and treatment," *Kulak Burun Boğaz Ihtisas Dergisi*, vol. 18, no. 6, pp. 349–354, 2008.

[9] L. Soylu, M. Kiroglu, B. Aydogan et al., "Pharyngocutaneous fistula following laryngectomy," *Head & Neck*, vol. 20, no. 1, pp. 22–25, 1998.

[10] R. Bardini, L. Bonavina, M. Asolati, A. Ruol, C. Castoro, and E. Tiso, "Single-layered cervical esophageal anastomoses: a prospective study of two suturing techniques," *The Annals of Thoracic Surgery*, vol. 58, no. 4, pp. 1087–1089, 1994.

[11] S. Law, D. T. K. Suen, K.-H. Wong, K.-F. Kwok, and J. Wong, "A single-layer, continuous, hand-sewn method for esophageal anastomosis: prospective evaluation in 218 patients," *Archives of Surgery*, vol. 140, no. 1, pp. 33–39, 2005.

[12] Y. Chen, N. Ke, C. Tan et al., "Continuous versus interrupted suture techniques of pancreaticojejunostomy after pancreaticoduodenectomy," *Journal of Surgical Research*, vol. 193, no. 2, pp. 590–597, 2015.

[13] H. Singh, D. Krishnamurthy, R. Tayal, M. Singh, and K. Singh, "Colonic anastomosis in calves: an experimental study," *Acta Veterinaria Hungarica*, vol. 37, no. 1-2, pp. 167–177, 1989.

[14] P. Boscolo-Rizzo, G. De Cillis, C. Marchiori, S. Carpenè, and M. C. Da Mosto, "Multivariate analysis of risk factors for

pharyngocutaneous fistula after total laryngectomy," *European Archives of Oto-Rhino-Laryngology*, vol. 265, no. 8, pp. 929–936, 2008.

[15] A. A. Mäkitie, R. Niemensivu, M. Hero et al., "Pharyngocutaneous fistula following total laryngectomy: a single institution's 10-year experience," *European Archives of Oto-Rhino-Laryngology*, vol. 263, no. 12, pp. 1127–1130, 2006.

[16] J. W. Liang, Z. D. Li, S. C. Li, F. Q. Fang, Y. J. Zhao, and Y. G. Li, "Pharyngocutaneous fistula after total laryngectomy: a systematic review and meta-analysis of risk factors," *Auris Nasus Larynx*, vol. 42, no. 5, pp. 353–359, 2015.

[17] N. Violaris and M. Bridger, "Prophylactic antibiotics and post laryngectomy pharyngocutaneous fistulae," *Journal of Laryngology and Otology*, vol. 104, no. 3, pp. 225–228, 1990.

[18] J. A. Paydarfar and N. J. Birkmeyer, "Complications in head and neck surgery: a meta-analysis of postlaryngectomy pharyngocutaneous fistula," *Archives of Otolaryngology—Head and Neck Surgery*, vol. 132, no. 1, pp. 67–72, 2006.

[19] E. C. Horgan and H. H. Dedo, "Prevention of major and minor fistulae after laryngectomy," *Laryngoscope*, vol. 89, no. 2, pp. 250–260, 1979.

[20] M. Sayles, S. L. Koonce, L. Harrison, N. Beasley, A. R. McRae, and D. G. Grant, "Pharyngo-cutaneous fistula complicating laryngectomy in the chemo-radiotherapy organ-preservation epoch," *European Archives of Oto-Rhino-Laryngology*, vol. 271, no. 6, pp. 1765–1769, 2014.

[21] C. Righini, T. Lequeux, O. Cuisnier, N. Morel, and E. Reyt, "The pectoralis myofascial flap in pharyngolaryngeal surgery after radiotherapy," *European Archives of Oto-Rhino-Laryngology*, vol. 262, no. 5, pp. 357–361, 2005.

[22] N. Süslü, R. T. Senirli, R. Ö. Günaydın, S. Özer, J. Karakaya, and A. Ş. HoŞal, "Pharyngocutaneous fistula after salvage laryngectomy," *Acta Oto-Laryngologica*, vol. 135, no. 6, pp. 615–621, 2015.

[23] K. D. Markou, K. C. Vlachtsis, A. C. Nikolaou, D. G. Petridis, A. I. Kouloulas, and I. C. Daniilidis, "Incidence and predisposing factors of pharyngocutaneous fistula formation after total laryngectomy. Is there a relationship with tumor recurrence?" *European Archives of Oto-Rhino-Laryngology*, vol. 261, no. 2, pp. 61–67, 2004.

[24] L. O. R. de Zinis, L. Ferrari, D. Tomenzoli, G. Premoli, G. Parrinello, and P. Nicolai, "Postlaryngectomy pharyngocutaneous fistula: incidence, predisposing factors, and therapy," *Head & Neck*, vol. 21, no. 2, pp. 131–138, 1999.

[25] U. A. Patel, B. A. Moore, M. Wax et al., "Impact of pharyngeal closure technique on fistula after salvage laryngectomy," *The JAMA Otolaryngology—Head and Neck Surgery*, vol. 139, no. 11, pp. 1156–1162, 2013.

[26] R. A. Dedivitis, F. T. Aires, C. R. Cernea, and L. G. Brandão, "Pharyngocutaneous fistula after total laryngectomy: a systematic review of risk factors," *Head & Neck*, 2014.

8

Surgical Audit of Patients with Ileal Perforations Requiring Ileostomy in a Tertiary Care Hospital in India

Hemkant Verma, Siddharth Pandey, Kapil Dev Sheoran, and Sanjay Marwah

Department of Surgery, Pt. B.D. Sharma, PGIMS, Rohtak 124001, India

Correspondence should be addressed to Siddharth Pandey; sid1420@gmail.com

Academic Editor: Pramateftakis Manousos-Georgios

Introduction. Ileal perforation peritonitis is a frequently encountered surgical emergency in the developing countries. The choice of a procedure for source control depends on the patient condition as well as the surgeon preference. *Material and Methods*. This was a prospective observational study including 41 patients presenting with perforation peritonitis due to ileal perforation and managed with ileostomy. Demographic profile and operative findings in terms of number of perforations, site, and size of perforation along with histopathological findings of all the cases were recorded. *Results*. The majority of patients were male. Pain abdomen and fever were the most common presenting complaints. Body mass index of the patients was in the range of 15.4–25.3 while comorbidities were present in 43% cases. Mean duration of preoperative resuscitation was 14.73 + 13.77 hours. Operative findings showed that 78% patients had a single perforation; most perforations were 0.6–1 cm in size and within 15 cm proximal to ileocecal junction. Mesenteric lymphadenopathy was seen in 29.2% patients. On histopathological examination, nonspecific perforations followed by typhoid and tubercular perforations respectively were the most common. *Conclusion*. Patients with ileal perforations are routinely seen in surgical emergencies and their demography, clinical profile, and intraoperative findings may guide the choice of procedure to be performed.

1. Introduction

Ileal perforation peritonitis is a frequently encountered surgical emergency in the developing countries [1]. Typhoid is the most common cause for this dreaded complication while tuberculosis, trauma, and nonspecific enteritis follow close suit [2]. The incidence of perforation in typhoid fever has been reported to be 0.8% to 18% [3]. Tuberculosis accounts for 5–9% of all small intestinal perforations in India and it is the second commonest cause after typhoid fever [4]. These cases of perforation peritonitis often require ileostomy as a lifesaving measure. However, in the Western countries, indications for ileostomy are altogether different and include inflammatory bowel disease, familial adenomatous polyposis, colorectal cancer, pelvic sepsis, trauma, diverticulitis, fistula, ischemic bowel disease, radiation enteritis, fecal incontinence, and paraplegia [5].

The standard source control measure for secondary peritonitis due to hollow viscus perforation is resuscitation followed by laparotomy. The methods of source control for ileal perforations include primary closure, resection, and anastomosis of small gut or diverting stoma, depending on the site and number of perforations, severity of peritonitis, and general condition of the patient. Thereafter, the patient is managed with antibiotics and continued postoperative care. Ileostomy serves the purpose of diversion, decompression, and exteriorization. Primary ileostomy has been found to be superior to other surgical procedures as far as the morbidity and mortality are concerned and especially so in moribund patients presenting late in course of their illness, where it proves to be a lifesaving procedure [6]. These are the types of patients that usually come to our surgical emergencies in India.

Though ileostomy is a lifesaving procedure in such cases, it may result in significant number of complications as well. A small intestinal diverting stoma carries significant morbidity, mostly due to fluid/electrolyte imbalance and nutritional depletion. Peristomal skin irritation is perhaps

TABLE 1: Criteria for deciding the type of operative procedure.

Operative procedure	Criteria
Primary closure	Patient presenting within 24 hrs of perforation, being hemodynamically stable, having minimal or no resuscitation required preoperatively, localized peritonitis, mild enteritis, single perforation, and no other areas of impending perforation
Resection and anastomosis	Patient presenting within 24 hrs of perforation, being hemodynamically stable, having minimal or no resuscitation required preoperatively, localized peritonitis, mild to moderate enteritis, multiple perforations, and areas of impending perforation
Ileostomy	Patient presenting > 24 hrs after perforation, being hemodynamically unstable, having resuscitation required preoperatively, generalized peritonitis, severe enteritis, multiple perforations, and areas of impending perforation

TABLE 2: Demographic and clinical profiles of patients.

Mean age (years)	38.31 ± 18.99
Sex (male/female)	34/7
Pain n (%)	41 (100)
Vomiting n (%)	37 (92)
Constipation n (%)	30 (73)
Shock n (%)	41 (100)
Fever n (%)	35 (85.3)
Dehydration n (%)	32 (78.1)
Distension n (%)	29 (70.7)
Abdominal tenderness n (%)	41 (100)
Abdominal guarding n (%)	38 (95.1)
Average time of resuscitation (hours)	14.7
Body mass index n (BMI)	19.6 ± 1.66

the commonest complication of ileostomy leading to skin excoriation [7]. Other complications after ileostomy are bleeding, ischemia, obstruction, prolapse, retraction, stenosis, para-stomal herniation, fistula formation, residual abscess, wound infection, and incisional hernia. In addition, ileostomy is known to adversely affect the quality of life due to physical restrictions and psychological problems [8].

The present study is aimed to analyze the epidemiology and presentation of such cases undergoing ileostomy for perforation peritonitis.

2. Material and Methods

The present study was a prospective observational study conducted in the Department of Surgery, Postgraduate Institute of Medical Sciences, Rohtak, a tertiary care center in North India. The study was conducted over a period of two and a half years (August 2011 to December 2013) after getting approval from the institutional ethical committee. Forty-one patients admitted with perforation peritonitis due to ileal perforation and undergoing emergency laparotomy with ileostomy were included in the study. Those cases of ileal perforation managed by primary closure or small gut resection and anastomosis were excluded from the study. The criteria used for deciding the type of operative procedure are given in Table 1.

All patients were thoroughly evaluated with detailed history, clinical examination, and blood investigations including complete blood counts, blood urea, X-ray chest in erect position, Widal test, and blood culture. The procedure was explained to the patients and written consent was taken regarding the stoma formation. All the cases were managed with intravenous fluids for resuscitation, nasogastric tube for gut decompression, urethral catheterization for monitoring urine output, third generation cephalosporins, and analgesics. After initial resuscitation in emergency department, patients underwent emergency laparotomy through midline incision. The intraoperative findings, namely, site, number, and size of perforations, extent of peritonitis, condition of gut, status of lymph nodes, and mesentery, were recorded and thorough peritoneal lavage was done. End or loop ileostomy was created as per the standard methods. Patients were monitored postoperatively and their histopathology reports were compiled.

3. Results

A total of 41 patients suffering from generalized peritonitis due to ileal perforation and managed with ileostomy were included in the study and their demographic and clinical profile was analyzed (Table 2). The majority of these cases belonged to the age group of 21–30 years with 34 (82.9%) being males. Moreover, 80% of the patients were from rural background. At the time of presentation, the patients had pain abdomen (100%), vomiting (92.7%), fever (85.3%), and obstipation (73%). On examination, there was abdominal tenderness (100%), guarding (95.1%), absent bowel sounds (85.4%), and abdominal distension (70.7%).

Mean body mass index (BMI) was 19.6 ± 1.66 with a range of 15.4–25.3. Only one patient (2.4%) was moderately obese, whereas 22% cases were underweight. Comorbidities were recorded in all the cases with chest infection being the commonest (22%) followed by heart diseases (9.7%), diabetes (4.8%), and hypertension (2.4%). Most of the patients were chronic smokers. Among other comorbidities, one patient had hypothyroidism, carcinoma base of tongue (after chemoradiation), and hepatitis B.

Blood investigations showed that 51.2% patients had total leucocyte counts more than $11,000/mm^3$ whereas only one patient had counts less than $4000/mm^3$. Preoperative blood urea was raised in majority of the patients. Widal test was positive in 36.6% patients while only one patient had a positive blood culture, with the isolate being *Citrobacter*.

On chest X-ray (erect film), thirty-seven patients (90.2%) had air under diaphragm suggestive of gut perforation. Four patients had associated pleural effusion and two had changes suggestive of pneumonitis. Four patients had normal skiagram. In view of clinical suspicion of perforation peritonitis in these four cases, contrast enhanced computerized tomography (CECT) scan of the abdomen was done that confirmed the diagnosis. All the patients were hemodynamically unstable and required resuscitation before surgery with intravenous fluids and inotropes. Resuscitation period ranged from 4 to 72 hours with a mean duration of 14.7 hours. The majority of the patients required preoperative resuscitation for 7–12 hours.

On exploration, all the patients had generalized peritonitis and diffuse enteritis with multiple perforations in the distal ileum (100%). Mesenteric edema and thickening were seen in more than half the patients (65.9%) whereas almost a quarter of patients had mesenteric lymphadenopathy (27.8%). Histopathological examination of resected gut specimen revealed nonspecific inflammation (56%), typhoid perforation (24.4%), and tubercular inflammation (19.5%) (Table 2).

In postoperative period, various complications seen were stomal discoloration (14.6%), peristomal skin excoriation (41.4%), wound sepsis (24.3%), intra-abdominal abscess (17%), and burst abdomen (4.8%). Three patients had postoperative septicemia and expired (7.3%).

4. Discussion

Peritonitis due to hollow viscus perforation is commonly encountered in surgical practice. It is caused by the introduction of infection into the otherwise sterile peritoneal environment through perforation of bowel. The spectrum of aetiology of perforation in tropical countries continues to be different from its Western counterpart. In contrast to Western countries where lower gastrointestinal tract perforations predominate, upper gastrointestinal tract perforations constitute the majority of cases in India [1]. Spontaneous ileal perforation remains a formidable surgical condition in developing countries. Typhoid fever is the predominant cause of nontraumatic ileal perforation while other causes include tuberculosis, nonspecific inflammation, obstruction, radiation enteritis, and Crohn's disease.

Though surgery is accepted as the definite treatment, the choice of exact surgical procedure remains controversial. Most series report simple closure of the perforation or resection and anastomosis as choice of procedure. These procedures though appealing are not free of complications especially in an emergency setup. Of all the postoperative complications reported, faecal fistula remains the most life-threatening; the rate of its occurrence has been reported to be around 12% with a very high mortality rate [14]. In view of this alarming situation, a shift in favour of a defunctioning protective ileostomy has been observed in recent years. Ileostomy is a lifesaving procedure, particularly in those cases where there are fulminant enteritis and generalized peritonitis of long duration. Various criteria used for deciding the type of operative procedure can be based on preoperative conditions and intraoperative findings in such cases (Table 1).

In most of the studies from Asia, mean age of the patients presenting with ileal perforation is around 35 to 40 years and the findings in the present study were the same [1, 15–17]. According to Mock et al., morbidity and mortality increase as age advances possibly due to comorbidities and poor immunity [18]. Park et al. [19] also had similar observations but only for early complications; late complications did not correlate with age.

The incidence of perforation peritonitis due to ileal perforation is significantly more in male population as seen in the present and the previous similar studies. In most of the studies, male patients contributed more than 75% of total cases [1, 15–17]. This is possibly because males indulge in outdoor activities and are more prone to GI infections and its attendant complications including perforation peritonitis. However, Park et al. found that there was no relation between sex and complications in these cases [19]. The majority of the patients in the present study and previous similar studies presented with pain abdomen, vomiting, constipation, and fever. Fever is a common symptom in cases of typhoid perforation peritonitis and ileal perforation is usually seen in the third week of illness. Shock and dehydration were seen more in our patients compared to other studies, indicating that patients in the present study were sicker and underwent ileostomy as a lifesaving measure. The clinically stable cases underwent primary closure/resection anastomosis of small gut and were excluded from the present study.

Associated comorbid illnesses seen in Western population included cardiac diseases and diabetes mellitus whereas, in our study, most of the patients had poor chest condition as most the common comorbidity, probably because of smoking habits and associated chronic obstructive pulmonary disease (COPD). Patients of COPD are more prone to postoperative complications like pneumonitis, poor healing, and wound dehiscence.

Compared to our study, the patients in previous studies had a normal BMI or were obese. Chun et al. [12] encountered more than 65% patients with BMI >25. They found that obesity was a significant risk factor for overall ileostomy complications, outpatient complications, and severe peristomal skin problems that required additional care. Moreover, in their study, patients with a BMI >30 had the highest number of ileostomy related complications. Leong et al. [20] suggested that, in obese patients, an end ileostomy may be the only option that provides sufficient length for the stoma to extend through the abdominal wall without tension because of the short thickened fatty mesentery. Park et al. [19] found that there is no significant relation in BMI and early or late complications. Faunø et al. [13] found a weak association between high BMI and parastomal hernia. Most of the patients in our study were poorly nourished and had BMI ranging from 15.4 to 25.3, with a mean of 19.6 ± 1.66. In our study, complications like parastomal skin excoriation, wound sepsis, stomal retraction, and prolapse had no significant correlation with BMI (Table 3).

Most patients with ileal perforation peritonitis have one or two perforations. Sometimes, there may be multiple perforations especially in immune-compromised patients [21]. Mock et al. [18] in their series of 221 patients found that the increased number of perforations was associated with a significantly higher mortality rate. In the present study, all the patients had multiple perforations with severe enteritis and postoperative mortality occurred in three cases (7.3%).

TABLE 3: Mean BMI of patients in various studies.

Study (number of patients)	Mean BMI
Arumugam et al., 2003 [9] ($n = 97$)*	24.5 ± 4.66
El-Hussuna et al., 2012 [10] ($n = 159$)*	27 ± 5.12
Sharma et al., 2013 [11] ($n = 5401$)	25.5
Chun et al., 2012 [12] ($n = 123$)*	29.6
Faunø et al., 2012 [13] ($n = 700$)*	28 ± 5.32
Our study ($n = 41$)	19.6 ± 1.66

(*Ileostomy done electively for colorectal cancer, polyposis coli, and inflammatory bowel disease.)

5. Conclusion

Temporary defunctioning protective ileostomy in moribund cases of peritonitis due to ileal perforation is a lifesaving procedure. Apart from reducing mortality, it plays a vital role in decreasing the incidence of complications like faecal fistula. While some advocate primary repair or anastomosis as methods of source control in these cases, ileostomy may be a more prudent alternative in an Indian setting where most of the patients have low BMI and usually present late with severe sepsis and generalized peritonitis. It is essential that an emergency surgeon be well versed in all the techniques of source control in such cases and choose the appropriate source control measure.

Conflict of Interests

The authors declare that there is no conflict of interests regarding the publication of this paper.

References

[1] R. S. Jhobta, A. K. Attri, R. Kaushik, R. Sharma, and A. Jhobta, "Spectrum of perforation peritonitis in India—review of 504 consecutive cases," World Journal of Emergency Surgery, vol. 1, article 26, 2006.

[2] T. Hussain, S. N. Alam, and M. Salim, "Outcome of ileostomy in cases of small bowel perforation," Pakistan Journal of Surgery, vol. 21, pp. 65–71, 2005.

[3] S. T. Edino, A. A. Yakubu, A. Z. Mohammed, and I. S. Abubakar, "Prognostic factors in typhoid ileal perforation: a prospective study of 53 cases," Journal of the National Medical Association, vol. 99, no. 9, pp. 1042–1045, 2007.

[4] V. K. Kapoor, "Abdominal tuberculosis: the Indian contribution," Indian Journal of Gastroenterology, vol. 17, no. 4, pp. 141–147, 1998.

[5] I. Ashraf, G. Muammad, R. S. Noon, M. Ashraf, H. Haider, and K. J. Abid, "To compare the outcome of ileostomy versus primary repair in enteric perforation," Pakistan Journal of Medical and Health Sciences, vol. 4, no. 4, pp. 523–525, 2010.

[6] M. Bashir, T. Nadeem, J. Iqbal, and A. Rashid, "Ileostomy in typhoid perforation," Annals of King Edward Medical College, vol. 9, pp. 221–225, 2003.

[7] O. G. Ajao, "Typhoid perforation: factors affecting mortality & morbidity," International Surgery, vol. 67, no. 4, pp. 317–319, 1982.

[8] A. M. Malik, A. A. Laghari, Q. Mallah et al., "Different surgical options and ileostomy in typhoid perforation," World Journal of Medical Sciences, vol. 1, pp. 112–116, 2006.

[9] P. J. Arumugam, L. Bevan, L. Macdonald et al., "A prospective audit of stomas-analysis of risk factors and complications and their management," Colorectal Disease, vol. 5, no. 1, pp. 49–52, 2003.

[10] A. El-Hussuna, M. Lauritsen, and S. Bülow, "Relatively high incidence of complications after loop ileostomy reversal," Danish Medical Journal, vol. 59, no. 10, pp. 4517–4522, 2012.

[11] A. Sharma, A.-P. Deeb, A. S. Rickles, J. C. Iannuzzi, J. R. T. Monson, and F. J. Fleming, "Closure of defunctioning loop ileostomy is associated with considerable morbidity," Colorectal Disease, vol. 15, no. 4, pp. 458–462, 2013.

[12] L. J. Chun, P. I. Haigh, M. S. Tam, and M. A. Abbas, "Defunctioning loop ileostomy for pelvic anastomoses: predictors of morbidity and nonclosure," Diseases of the Colon and Rectum, vol. 55, no. 2, pp. 167–174, 2012.

[13] L. Faunø, C. Rasmussen, K. K. Sloth, A. M. Sloth, and A. Tøttrup, "Low complication rate after stoma closure. Consultants attended 90% of the operations," Colorectal Disease, vol. 14, no. 8, pp. e499–e505, 2012.

[14] A. A. Khan, I. R. Kha, U. Najeeb, and A. J. Shaikh, "Comparison between primary repair and exteriorization in cases of typhoid perforation," Annals of King Edward Medical College, vol. 11, no. 3, pp. 226–227, 2005.

[15] V. Patil, A. Vijayakumar, M. B. Ajitha, and S. L. Kumar, "Comparison between tube ileostomy and loop ileostomy as a diversion procedure," ISRN Surgery, vol. 2012, Article ID 547523, 5 pages, 2012.

[16] M. Z. Ali, K. Munir, A. Zaffar, and M. I. Anwar, "Surgical audit of emergency ileostomies," Journal of Rawalpindi Medical College, vol. 16, no. 1, pp. 45–47, 2012.

[17] P. Batra, D. Gupta, S. Rao, R. Narang, and R. Batra, "Spectrum of gastrointestinal perforation peritonitis in rural central India," Journal of Mahatma Gandhi Institute of Medical Sciences, vol. 18, no. 1, pp. 44–48, 2013.

[18] C. N. Mock, J. Amaral, and L. E. Visser, "Improvement in survival from Typhoid ileal perforation," Annals of Surgery, vol. 215, no. 3, pp. 244–249, 1992.

[19] J. J. Park, A. Del Pino, C. P. Orsay et al., "Stoma complications: the cook county hospital experience," Diseases of the Colon and Rectum, vol. 42, no. 12, pp. 1575–1580, 1999.

[20] A. P. K. Leong, E. E. L. Schimmer, and R. K. S. Phillips, "Life-table analysis of stomal complications following ileostomy," British Journal of Surgery, vol. 81, no. 5, pp. 727–729, 1994.

[21] F. G. Siddiqui, J. M. Shaikh, A. G. Soomro, K. Bux, A. S. Memon, and S. A. Ali, "Outcome of ileostomy in the management of ileal perforation," Journal of the Liaquat University of Medical and Health Sciences, vol. 7, no. 3, pp. 168–172, 2008.

9

Superior Mesenteric Artery Syndrome: Clinical and Radiological Considerations

M. Ezzedien Rabie,[1] **Olajide Ogunbiyi,**[2] **Abdullah Saad Al Qahtani,**[1] **Sherif B. M. Taha,**[1] **Ahmad El Hadad,**[2] **and Ismail El Hakeem**[1]

[1]*Department of Surgery, Armed Forces Hospital, Southern Region, Khamis Mushait, Saudi Arabia*
[2]*Department of Radiology, Armed Forces Hospital, Southern Region, Khamis Mushait, Saudi Arabia*

Correspondence should be addressed to M. Ezzedien Rabie; ezzedien@hotmail.com

Academic Editor: Michael Hünerbein

Background. Superior mesenteric artery (SMA) syndrome is a rare condition of duodenal obstruction, caused by the overlying SMA. *Aim.* To report on our experience with the management of SMA syndrome, drawing the attention to its existence. *Material and Methods.* We reviewed our records to identify cases diagnosed with SMA syndrome, in the period from October 1995 to January 2012. *Results.* Seven patients were identified, one male and six females. Their mean age was 17.1 years. Vomiting and abdominal pain were the presenting complaints in all patients and history of weight loss was present in six of them. In no patient was the diagnosis suspected initially on clinical grounds. Only after radiological investigations was the diagnosis declared. Radiology took the form of gastrografin/barium meal only in four patients and both gastrografin/barium meal and computerized tomography scan in the remaining three. Four patients responded to medical treatment and surgery was performed in the remaining three, with open duodenojejunostomy in two patients and laparoscopic dissection of the ligament of Treitz in the third. Long lasting improvement was sustained in all patients except one in the surgery group who, despite initial improvement, still has infrequent attacks of abdominal pain. *Conclusion.* Although the clinical manifestations of SMA syndrome are shared with many other disease entities, it has unique radiological as well as endoscopic features, which enables a confident diagnosis to be made. Once diagnosed, conservative treatment with nutritional support and positioning should be tried first. In case of unresponsiveness, surgery may give a lasting cure.

1. Introduction

Superior mesenteric artery (SMA) syndrome was first described by Professor Rokitansky in 1842 [1, 2]. Only relatively recently has it established itself as a disease entity. The clinical picture is caused by compression of the 3rd part of the duodenum between the SMA and aorta, which exert a clam-like or striding action on it. Virtually, any condition associated with weight reduction may be followed by the syndrome. Tuberculosis [3], brucellosis [2], diabetes mellitus [4], anorexia nervosa [5], blunt abdominal trauma [6], and burns [7] are only few to mention. It has also been reported after spinal surgery [8], application of body casts [9], and bed confinement in the supine position [10]. Moreover, it may complicate weight reduction following bariatric surgery [11], a pertinent fact to consider after the current surge of this type of surgery.

2. Material and Methods

We reviewed our records to identify cases of SMA syndrome, diagnosed in our hospital, a 609-bed tertiary referral hospital, serving a population of 1 million individuals, in the period from October 1995 to January 2012. Patients' files were retrieved and data were collected which included patients' demographics, their clinical presentation, how the diagnosis was substantiated, the treatment offered, and the response to treatment.

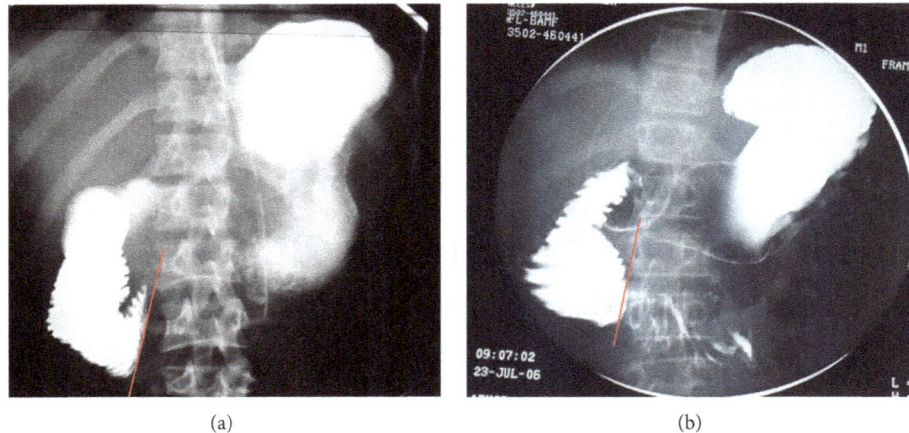

FIGURE 1: (a) and (b) Dilation of the duodenum with abrupt cut-off at its third part, coinciding with the line of the SMA (red line).

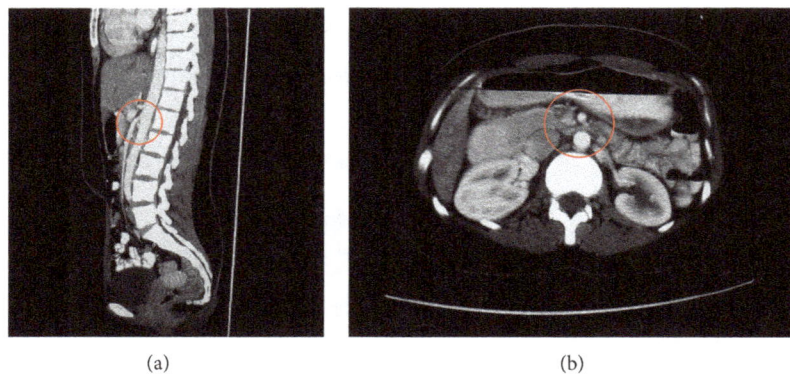

FIGURE 2: Narrow aortomesenteric angle (10°) and aortomesenteric distance (6 mm) (red circles in (a) and (b), resp.), compressing the duodenum in between.

3. Results

In this period, we were able to retrieve the files of seven patients, one male and six females, with a mean age of 17.1 years (range 9–25, SD 5.3).

All patients had vomiting and all of them had abdominal pain which was acute in three cases and chronic in the other four. Weight loss was spontaneous in five patients and it followed a weight reduction program in one, while in the seventh patient no history of weight loss was obtained. Associated comorbidities were present in two patients, one with tuberculous interstitial nephritis and another with traumatic paraplegia, while the rest had no comorbidities.

Out of the 7 patients, only three underwent upper endoscopy and in none of them was it diagnostic.

The diagnosis was not suspected on clinical grounds. Rather, it was revealed after radiological investigations performed to explore the patients' complaints. This took the form of gastrografin/barium meal only in four patients (Figure 1), while both gastrografin/barium meal and computerized tomography (CT) scan were used in the remaining three (Figure 2).

Four patients responded to medical treatment, the essential elements of which were initial gastroduodenal decompression through a nasogastric tube, followed by nutritional support with total parenteral nutrition (TPN) or, if tolerated, small frequent oral meals, aided by positioning of the patient in the right recumbent or prone positions to relieve the compressed duodenum. In the remaining three, surgery was performed. In two patients, it was the primary treatment in the form of side to side duodenojejunostomy, while in the third patient, it followed unresponsiveness to medical treatment and took the form of laparoscopic dissection of the ligament of Treitz.

All patients improved with no further admissions with the same complaints except one patient who received primary duodenojejunostomy, in whom vomiting recurred and was admitted several times with left iliac fossa pain with no obvious reason despite repeated investigations, including a psychiatric evaluation. The clinical and radiological features of the patients as well as the treatment given are shown in Tables 1 and 2.

4. Discussions

Wilkie described the clinical and pathophysiological characteristics of the syndrome as well as its management

TABLE 1: Clinical, radiological, and endoscopic features of individual patients in the series.

Patient	Age (years)/ sex	Clinical presentation	Diagnosis on gastrografin/ barium meal*	Diagnosis on CT scan**	Upper endoscopy
1st	17/♀	Chronic abdominal pain, vomiting, and weight loss	Yes	Not done	Done, not diagnostic
2nd	16/♀	Chronic abdominal pain, nausea, repeated vomiting, persistent hunger, and weight loss	Yes	Yes	Done, not diagnostic
3rd	18/♀	Acute abdominal pain, vomiting, and weight loss	Yes	Not done	Not done
4th	25/♂	Acute abdominal pain, vomiting, sense of distension, and weight loss	Yes	Yes	Done, not diagnostic+
5th	13/♀	Chronic abdominal pain after meals, vomiting, and weight loss	Yes	Not done	Not done
6th	9/♀	Acute abdominal pain, nausea, and repeated vomiting	Yes	Not done	Not done
7th	22/♀	Chronic abdominal pain, vomiting, and weight loss	Yes	Yes	Not done

*Dilation of the duodenum with abrupt cut-off at its third part, coinciding with the line of the SMA.
**Narrow aortomesenteric angle and aortomesenteric distance.

TABLE 2: Treatment and its result.

Patient	Treatment	Result
1st	Duodenojejunostomy	Recurrence of vomiting
2nd	Medical treatment	Improved
3rd	Duodenojejunostomy	Improved
4th	Medical treatment	Improved
5th	Laparoscopic dissection of the ligament of Treitz	Improved
6th	Medical treatment	Improved
7th	Medical treatment	Improved

approach, in a series of 64 patients [12, 13], giving the syndrome its eponym "Wilkie's syndrome." Many other eponyms, including chronic duodenal ileus, megaduodenum, aortomesenteric artery compression, arteriomesenteric duodenal obstruction, cast syndrome, and chronic duodenal pseudoobstruction, have also been used [10, 14]. The diagnosis requires a high index of suspicion in the proper clinical context and entails a detailed radiologic evaluation.

Clinically, the patient with a predisposing illness presents with features of gastric outlet obstruction. Sense of fullness, postprandial epigastric pain, belching, and vomiting are characteristic features. Radiologically, barium meal and CT scan show dilatation of the stomach and proximal duodenum with an abrupt cut-off across its third part, together with a decreased aortomesenteric distance as well as aortomesenteric angle. These findings, in the proper clinical sitting, virtually establish the diagnosis. Ultrasound (US) has also been used to aid in the diagnosis. The findings include to and fro movements across the duodenum in the supine, left recumbent, and sitting positions, with facilitation of the flow through the jejunum and elongation of the aortomesenteric

distance when the patient assumes the right recumbent position [15]. These findings confirm the diagnosis and establish the role of positioning in providing a symptomatic relief in such cases. Despite its confirmatory role, US was not used in any of our patients to substantiate the diagnosis, probably due to its inability to provide clear anatomic details, compared to barium meal or CT scan.

The syndrome has specific anatomic basis. The SMA takes off from the abdominal aorta at the level of the first lumbar vertebra with an average angle of 42.4° (range 18° to 70°) and a distance of 10–28 mm. Suspended by the ligament of Treitz, which is attached to its 4th part or to its junction with the jejunum, the duodenum crosses the abdomen at the level of the third lumbar vertebra [10]. Minor anatomic alterations predispose to the clinical manifestations of the syndrome. A narrow aortomesenteric angle of 15.2° (range 1°–40°) and a narrow aortomesenteric distance of 2 to 8 mm have been observed in individuals with SMA syndrome [10]. As seen in Figures 2 and 3, CT in a formatted sagittal view could easily document these measures in individuals with clinical evidence of the syndrome, thus establishing the diagnosis.

Thinning out of the fat pad between SMA and aorta, consequently upon weight loss, narrows the aortomesenteric angle and distance, thereby compressing the duodenum and thus producing the clinical manifestations of the syndrome. Other contributory factors include an abnormally low origin of SMA, excessive lumbar lordosis, and hypertrophied or shortened ligament of Treitz or its multiple attachments to the duodenum [10]. High fixation of the duodenum by the ligament of Treitz or an anomalous SMA crossing directly over the aorta as the latter transects the duodenum [16] has also been incriminated.

When performed, endoscopy may reveal narrowing of the 3rd part of the duodenum due to external compression [2]. This was not noticed in our series where upper endoscopy

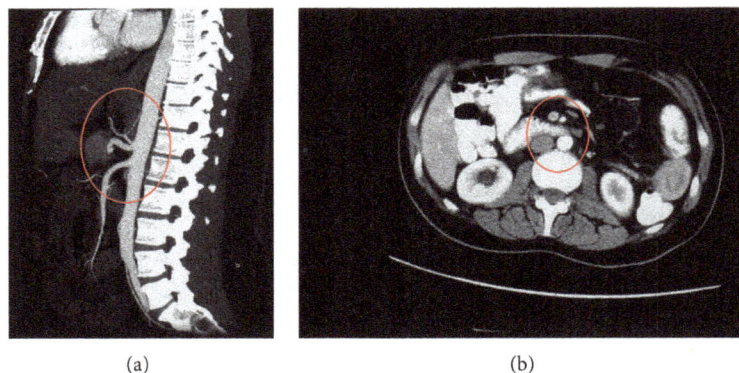

(a)   (b)

FIGURE 3: (a) and (b) Wide aortomesenteric angle and distance in a normal individual with no duodenal compression (red circles).

was performed in only three cases, probably due to the unfamiliarity of the endoscopist with the condition or the inability to reach the 3rd part of the duodenum.

As noticed in our series, upper gastrointestinal series utilizing barium or gastrografin will show dilatation of the stomach and duodenum down to the 3rd part, with a sudden cut-off distally, conforming to the anatomical position of the superior mesenteric artery. In addition, CT scan will show the anatomical configuration of the region with the clam-like action of the SMA and aorta across the third part of the duodenum, resulting in the abrupt cut-off. On sagittal reconstruction of the CT images, a narrowed aortomesenteric distance and angle can be easily depicted, substantiating the diagnosis.

Unrelieved, duodenal perforation may ensue [17]. For established cases of SMA syndrome, medical and surgical options do exist. It is intuitive to start with the medical lines first which include decompression of the stomach and duodenum with a nasogastric tube, correction of nutritional and electrolytes deficiencies, through TPN [2], or preferably, if possible, enteral feeding with a nasojejunal tube past the point of compression, which facilitates the nutritional management while avoiding TPN complications. When tolerated, oral feeding may be resumed. This helps build up the fat cushion between the SMA and aorta and, hence, reversing the situation. Additionally, as it lies in the root of the mesentery, SMA may be dragged by the small bowel, to drop off the duodenum when the patient assumes the prone or right recumbent position, as proved by ultrasound studies [15]. This might bring about symptomatic relief till the fat pad builds up.

Failing appropriate medical treatment, surgical intervention may be considered. The essence is to bypass the site of obstruction by anastomosing the bowel below the bowel above it, thus resuming the functional integrity of the bowel. This may take the form of gastrojejunostomy or duodeno-jejunostomy, by the open [18] or laparoscopic means [19]. Dissection of the ligament of Treitz, with mobilization of the 3rd and 4th parts of the duodenum, releasing the compression, has also been reported [20, 21]. More recently, robotic duodenojejunostomy has been utilized with success [22].

In our series, four patients successfully responded to conservative treatment, one patient failed to respond and received laparoscopic dissection of the ligament of Treitz, and the remaining two received duodenojejunostomy without a proper trial of medical treatment. Although both improved postoperatively, one of them has had repeated emergency room visits for left iliac fossa pain with no obvious reason. In this regard, surgery should not be offered before a proper trial of conservative management.

Other pathological conditions with similar clinical presentation, including diabetic gastroparesis, scleroderma with duodenal involvement [23], hereditary megaduodenum [24], megaduodenum due to aganglionosis [25], have been rarely reported. The distinction between these entities and SMA syndrome is of utmost importance when embarking on treatment, especially the surgical option.

The apparent rarity of SMA syndrome may reflect its true rare nature or, alternatively, unawareness of its existence. Published articles are mainly case reports and, rarely, small case series. This limits our understanding of the disease. Keeping a high index of suspension, followed by the utilization of appropriate radiology, may bring more cases to light.

5. Conclusion

SMA syndrome is a rarely diagnosed condition. Keeping a high index of suspicion followed by the utilization of appropriate radiology is essential for its diagnosis. Although the clinical manifestations of SMA syndrome are shared with many other disease entities, it has unique radiological as well as endoscopic features, which enable a confident diagnosis to be made. Once diagnosed, conservative treatment with nutritional support and positioning should be tried first. In case of unresponsiveness, surgery may give a lasting cure.

Ethical Approval

This research has been conducted in accordance with national and international standards of ethics, and the approval of the medical research ethics committee has been granted before conducting the study.

Conflict of Interests

The authors of this paper have no conflict of interests to declare and did not receive funding for this research project.

References

[1] C. Rokitansky, *Handbook der Pathologischen Anatomie*, vol. 3, Braunmuller and Seidel, Wien, Austria, 1st edition, 1842.

[2] S. Prasad, R. Lingadakai, K. Chethan, and Z. Abdul, "Superior mesenteric artery syndrome secondary to brucellosis—a case report," *Indian Journal of Surgery*, vol. 72, no. 3, pp. 265–267, 2010.

[3] C. S. Limaye, S. P. Karande, S. P. Aher, and K. A. Pati, "Superior mesenteric artery syndrome secondary to tuberculosis induced cachexia," *The Journal of the Association of Physicians of India*, vol. 59, pp. 670–671, 2011.

[4] M.-C. Wu, I.-C. Wu, J.-Y. Wu, D.-C. Wu, and W.-M. Wang, "Superior mesenteric artery syndrome in a diabetic patient with acute weight loss," *World Journal of Gastroenterology*, vol. 15, no. 47, pp. 6004–6006, 2009.

[5] C. W. Lee, M. I. Park, S. J. Park et al., "A case of superior mesenteric artery syndrome caused by anorexia nervosa," *The Korean Journal of Gastroenterology*, vol. 58, no. 5, pp. 280–283, 2011.

[6] J. L. Falcone and K. O. Garrett, "Superior mesenteric artery syndrome after blunt abdominal trauma: a case report," *Vascular and Endovascular Surgery*, vol. 44, no. 5, pp. 410–412, 2010.

[7] T. J. Lescher, K. R. Sirinek, and B. A. Pruitt Jr., "Superior mesenteric artery syndrome in thermally injured patients," *Journal of Trauma*, vol. 19, no. 8, pp. 567–571, 1979.

[8] A. I. Tsirikos, R. E. Anakwe, and A. D. L. Baker, "Late presentation of superior mesenteric artery syndrome following scoliosis surgery: a case report," *Journal of Medical Case Reports*, vol. 2, article 9, 2008.

[9] D. T. Hutchinson and G. S. Bassett, "Superior mesenteric artery syndrome in pediatric orthopedic patients," *Clinical Orthopaedics and Related Research*, no. 250, pp. 250–257, 1990.

[10] C. M. Townsend and J. J. Naoum, "Vascular compression of the duodenum," in *Mastery of Surgery*, J. E. Fischer, Ed., pp. 955–961, Lippincott Williams & Wilkins, 5th edition, 2007.

[11] D. Goitein, D. J. Gagné, P. K. Papasavas et al., "Superior mesenteric artery syndrome after laparoscopic Roux-en-Y gastric bypass for morbid obesity," *Obesity Surgery*, vol. 14, no. 7, pp. 1008–1011, 2004.

[12] D. P. Wilkie, "Chronic duodenal ileus," *British Journal of Surgery*, vol. 9, no. 34, pp. 204–214, 1921.

[13] A. Roy, J. J. Gisel, V. Roy, and E. P. Bouras, "Superior mesenteric artery (Wilkie's) syndrome as a result of cardiac cachexia," *Journal of General Internal Medicine*, vol. 20, no. 10, pp. C3–C4, 2005.

[14] M. Sturtevant, "Megaduodenum and duodenal obstruction. Criteria for diagnosis," *Radiology*, vol. 33, no. 2, pp. 185–188, 1939.

[15] M. Kodama, H. Yamada, Y. Matsumoto et al., "Usefulness of ultrasonography for diagnosis and treatment in case of superior mesenteric artery (SMA) syndrome," *Journal of Japanese Society of Gastroenterology*, vol. 107, no. 8, pp. 1283–1289, 2010.

[16] L. B. Cohen, S. P. Field, and D. B. Sachar, "The superior mesenteric artery syndrome. The disease that isn't, or is it?" *Journal of Clinical Gastroenterology*, vol. 7, no. 2, pp. 113–116, 1985.

[17] E. Kandil, H. Alabbas, A. C. Harbin, and H. R. Neitzschman, "Superior mesenteric artery syndrome," *Journal of the Louisiana State Medical Society*, vol. 161, no. 5, pp. 285–286, 2009.

[18] U. Baltazar, J. Dunn, C. Floresguerra, L. Schmidt, and W. Browder, "Superior mesenteric artery syndrome: an uncommon cause of intestinal obstruction," *Southern Medical Journal*, vol. 93, no. 6, pp. 606–608, 2000.

[19] G. Munene, M. Knab, and B. Parag, "Laparoscopic duodenojejunostomy for superior mesenteric artery syndrome," *The American Surgeon*, vol. 76, no. 3, pp. 321–324, 2010.

[20] R. Mosalli, B. El-Bizre, M. Farooqui, and B. Paes, "Superior mesenteric artery syndrome: a rare cause of complete intestinal obstruction in neonates," *Journal of Pediatric Surgery*, vol. 46, no. 12, pp. E29–E31, 2011.

[21] W. Z. Massoud, "Laparoscopic management of superior mesenteric artery syndrome," *International Surgery*, vol. 80, no. 4, pp. 322–327, 1995.

[22] S. M. Ayloo, M. A. Masrur, F. M. Bianco, and P. C. Giulianotti, "Robotic roux-en-Y duodenojejunostomy for superior mesenteric artery syndrome: operative technique," *Journal of Laparoendoscopic and Advanced Surgical Techniques*, vol. 21, no. 9, pp. 841–844, 2011.

[23] F. H. Anderson, "Megaduodenum: a case report and literature review," *American Journal of Gastroenterology*, vol. 62, no. 6, pp. 509–515, 1974.

[24] G. Basilisco, "Hereditary megaduodenum," *The American Journal of Gastroenterology*, vol. 92, no. 1, pp. 150–153, 1997.

[25] W. T. Newton, "Radical enterectomy for hereditary megaduodenum," *Archives of Surgery*, vol. 96, no. 4, pp. 549–553, 1968.

10

Perioperative Evaluation of Patient Outcomes after Severe Acid Corrosive Injury

Ming-Ho Wu and Han-Yun Wu

Department of Surgery, Tainan Municipal Hospital, 670 Chung-Te Road, Tainan 701, Taiwan

Correspondence should be addressed to Ming-Ho Wu; m2201@mail.ncku.edu.tw

Academic Editor: Baran Tokar

We reviewed 64 patients with perforation or full-thickness injury of the alimentary tract after acid ingestion. Based on our classification of laparotomy findings, there were class I ($n = 15$); class II ($n = 13$); class III ($n = 16$); and class IV ($n = 20$). Study parameters were preoperative laboratory data, gastric perforation, associated visceral injury, and extension of the injury. End points of the study were the patients' mortality and length of hospital stay. All these patients underwent esophagogastrectomy with ($n = 16$) or without ($n = 24$) concomitant resection, esophagogastroduodenojejunectomy with ($n = 4$) or without ($n = 13$) concomitant resection, and laparotomy only ($n = 7$). Concomitant resections were performed on the spleen ($n = 10$), colon ($n = 2$), pancreas ($n = 1$), gall bladder ($n = 1$), skipped areas of jejunum ($n = 4$), and the first portion of the duodenum ($n = 4$). The study demonstrates five preoperative risk factors, female gender, shock status, shock index, pH value, and base deficit, and four intraoperative risk factors, gastric perforation, associated visceral injury, injury beyond the pylorus, and continuous involvement of the jejunum over a length of 50 cm. The overall mortality rate was 45.3%, which increased significantly with advancing class of corrosive injury.

1. Introduction

Corrosive injury could be accidental or suicide attempt. Ingested agents include acid or alkali [1]. Acid ingestion is one of the most frequent means of attempted suicide in Taiwan. Ingestion of strong acids often results in a corrosive injury to the upper alimentary tract [2, 3]. Isolated gastric outlet obstruction will be detected several weeks later in some moderately injured patients [4]. In some severely injured patients, associated injuries of intra-abdominal organs, such as the pancreas, gall bladder, spleen, colon, diaphragm, and skipped areas of jejunum, occur frequently. Aggressive surgery may save the life of extensively injured patients during the acute stage [5–13]. However, the mortality rate varies in surgically treated patients, ranging from 40% to 77.7% [7, 10, 11, 14]. It is clinically important to identify intraoperative risk factors and to form subgroups according to risk of death so that injuries can be categorized. In the study, the preoperative clinical data, intraoperative risk factors, surgical procedures, outcomes, and follow-up data of patients with extensive corrosive injuries were reviewed retrospectively from medical charts.

The obtained data were analyzed to categorize laparotomy findings to evaluate the patient outcomes.

2. Materials and Methods

2.1. Management of Acute Corrosive Injury. During the acute stage of extensive corrosive injury, treatment includes fasting, nasogastric tube decompression, intravenous fluid replacement, and correction of any acid-base imbalance and antibiotics and H_2-blockers. Complete blood cell counts, leukocyte differential counts, blood biochemistry analysis, and chest and plain abdominal film studies are routinely conducted. Arterial blood gases are regularly monitored. Endoscopy is performed only on patients who do not require immediate surgery. Comatose or hypoxic patients are intubated immediately for airway security. Ventilatory support is provided for patients with respiratory failure.

2.2. Selection of Patients for Laparotomy. An early exploratory laparotomy is mandatory in the presence of generalized

TABLE 1: Classification of severe acid corrosive injury.

Class I	Isolated gastric full-thickness injury
Class II	(1) Gastric perforation or (2) Full-thickness injury extending from the stomach to the duodenum
Class III	(1) Injury extending from the stomach to the duodenum with perforation or (2) Full-thickness injury extending from the stomach up to 50 cm of the jejunum
Class IV	(1) Injury extending from the stomach beyond the duodenum with perforation or (2) Injury extending from the stomach beyond 50 cm of the jejunum

peritoneal signs, continuous gastrointestinal bleeding, endoscopic findings of severe burns of the esophagus and stomach, pleural effusion, hydropneumothorax, or pneumoperitoneum determined by radiographic examination, or pH < 7.0 [5] or a base deficit > 16 mmol/L on initial arterial blood gases (ABG) analysis.

2.3. Definition of Severe Corrosive Injury.
In this study, severe corrosive injury is defined as perforation or full-thickness injury of the alimentary tract.

2.4. Classification of Severe Acid Corrosive Injury Based on Laparotomy Findings (Table 1).
The associated visceral injury represents the tissue damage of the pancreas, gall bladder, spleen, colon, diaphragm, liver, or skipped areas of jejunum. In cases of previous subtotal gastrectomy associated with gastrojejunostomy, the jejunum connected to the stomach was considered as a continuous involvement when it was injured. An estimate of the injury in patients who had had a previous gastrectomy appeared to have been defined a little differently. In gastrectomy patients, continuous involvement of the jejunum longer than 30 cm was comparable to injury beyond the pylorus in normal individuals, that longer than 50 cm was comparable to injury beyond the duodenum, and that longer than 100 cm was comparable to beyond 50 cm of the jejunum in the normal individual.

2.5. Methods.
Medical records were reviewed retrospectively on preoperative (Table 2) and intraoperative (Table 3) risk factors. The parameters were age (<45 versus ≥45 years), gender, shock (BP < 90 mmHg), shock index (<1 versus ≥1), white blood cell count (<15000 versus ≥15000/μL), hemoglobin (<13.5 versus ≥13.5 g/dL), pH (<7.23 versus ≥7.23), base deficit (<14 versus ≥14 mmol/L), amylase (<130 versus ≥130 IU/L), gastric perforation, associated visceral injury, injury beyond the pylorus, and continuous involvement of the jejunum over a length of 50 cm. The selection of the cut-off values for white blood cell count, hemoglobin, pH, base deficit, amylase, and length of the jejunum was based on a median of the respective data. Analysis was performed mainly to identify the above four intraoperative risk factors. The patients in the series were categorized by using the laparotomy findings according to

TABLE 2: Analysis of preoperative risk factors in 64 severely injured patients.

	Survivor	Death	p value
Age (years)			NS
<45	21	12	
≥45	14	17	
Gender			0.016
Male	20	8	
Female	15	21	
Shock (BP < 90 mmHg)			0.01
Yes	0	6	
No	35	23	
Shock index			0.005
≥1	3	11	
<1	32	18	
White blood cell count (/μL)			NS
<15000	14	15	
≥15000	19	13	
Platelet (k/L)*			NS
<150	16	15	
≥150	15	12	
pH*			0.027
<7.23	11	16	
≥7.23	21	12	
Base deficit (mmol/L)*			0.009
<14	21	10	
≥14	9	18	
Amylase (IU/L)*			NS
<130	11	11	
≥130	12	11	

*Some data not available.
NS: not significant.

TABLE 3: Analysis of intraoperative risk factors in 64 severely injured patients.

	Survivor	Death	p value
Injury beyond pylorus			0.000
Yes	14	29	
No	21	0	
Continuous involvement of jejunum			0.000
<50 cm	6	3	
≥50 cm	1	15	
Associated visceral injury			0.000
Yes	11	22	
No	24	7	
Gastric perforation			0.001
Yes	19	27	
No	16	2	

the rule described above. End points of the study were the patients' mortality and their length of hospital stay.

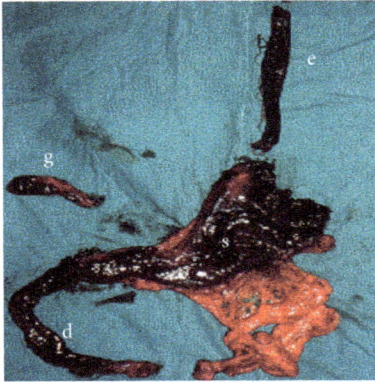

FIGURE 1: These organs were resected from a 32-year-old woman with severe acid corrosive injury; e: esophagus, s: perforated stomach, g: gall bladder, and d: duodenum.

2.6. Statistical Analysis. Continuous variables are expressed as the mean ± the standard error. The Chi-square test was used to determine the significance of the difference between categorical variables, including the preoperative and intraoperative variables, surgical procedures, outcomes, and length of hospital stay. A value of $p < 0.05$ was considered as statistically significant. These analyses were performed using the SPSS 12.0 software package for Windows (SPSS, Inc., Chicago, IL).

3. Results

3.1. Patients Who Underwent Emergency Surgery for Extensive Corrosive Injury. A total of 426 patients with acid corrosive injuries were treated in a period of 14 years. Of those, 84 (19.7%) underwent surgery in the acute stage according to the selection criteria described above. Twenty (4.6%) patients who underwent gastrostomy and jejunostomy only, not recognized as a severe injury, were excluded from the study. The remaining 64 (15%) patients (28 men and 36 women) ranged from 16 to 78 years old (mean + SEM, 46.3 ± 1.9 years old). All these patients had ingested acid in a liquid form, mostly hydrochloric acid. The volume of acid ingested varied from 50 to 450 mL in 10~30% concentrations. Sixty-one (95.3%) of the patients ingested the caustics in suicidal attempts. The interval between the injury and laparotomy was 14.6 ± 2.6 hours.

3.2. Operative Procedure. The surgical procedures consisted of esophagogastrectomy with or without concomitant resection, esophagogastroduodenojejunectomy with or without concomitant resection (Figure 1), and exploratory laparotomy only. Concomitant resection of the associated viscera was performed as indications stipulated. Cervical esophagostomy and feeding jejunostomy were also performed in cases of resection. All resections were performed via midline laparotomy and oblique neck incision. The esophagectomy was initially performed via the transhiatal route in all patients. Because thrombosis of the periesophageal vessels always

occurred and there was no obvious esophageal perforation following acid ingestion in this series, only one patient needed a thoracotomy as a result of massive intrathoracic bleeding.

3.3. Postoperative Care and Follow-Up. All patients received postoperative care in an intensive care unit either until they were weaned from ventilators and their vital signs were stable or until death. Once patients had had a bowel movement or a flatus passage, feeding via jejunostomy was started. Total parenteral nutrition was reserved for patients who had a paralytic ileus or intestinal complications. We continued regular outpatient follow-up after discharge and subsequently performed esophageal reconstruction for survivors.

The study demonstrated five preoperative risk factors, namely, female gender, shock status, shock index ≥ 1, pH value < 7.23, and base deficit > 14 mmol/L, and four intraoperative risk factors, namely, gastric perforation, associated visceral injury, injury beyond the pylorus, and continuous involvement of the jejunum over a length of 50 cm. Among these 64 patients, 15 (23.4%) were class I, 13 (20.3%) were class II, 16 (25.0%) were class III, and 20 (31.3%) were class IV (Table 4). They all underwent esophagogastrectomy with ($n = 16$, 25.0%) or without ($n = 24$, 37.5%) concomitant resection, esophagogastroduodenojejunectomy with ($n = 4$, 6.3%) or without ($n = 13$, 20.3%) concomitant resection, and laparotomy only ($n = 7$, 10.9%). Concomitant resections were performed on the spleen ($n = 10$), colon ($n = 2$), pancreas ($n = 1$), gall bladder ($n = 1$), skipped areas of jejunum ($n = 4$), and the first portion of the duodenum ($n = 4$). The intraoperative risk factors, including the gastric perforation, associated visceral injury, injury beyond the pylorus, and continuous involvement of the jejunum over a length of 50 cm, and operative procedure correlate significantly with death in each class of injury ($p = 0.044$, 0.000, 0.000, 0.000, and 0.000, resp.). The overall mortality rate was 45.3% (29/64), which increased significantly with advancing class of corrosive injury (class I, 0.0%; class II, 23.1%; class III, 56.3%; and class IV, 85.0%, $p = 0.000$). These 29 patients died between days 1 and 64 (average 14.4 days), including 12 (41.3%) who died within 24 hours after surgery. Four deaths received cardiopulmonary resuscitation during surgery. The major causes of death were multiple organ failure ($n = 20$) and sepsis ($n = 9$). The average hospital stay of 35 (54.7%) survivors was 44.8 ± 7.1 days, with a significant increase with advancing class of injury ($p = 0.000$). The range of follow-up for survivors was from 6 months to 9 years, with a median of 3.9 years. Twenty-nine (45.3%) patients subsequently underwent reconstruction of the esophagus, from 2.5 months to 8 months (average of 3.5 months) after an esophagogastrectomy ($n = 25$) or an esophagogastroduodenojejunectomy ($n = 4$).

4. Discussion

All of the series of patients had extensive corrosive injuries after ingesting strong acids. Their presentations, management, and injury patterns were different from those of patients with alkali injury, which commonly occurs in western countries. Previous reports [14, 15] revealed that most deaths from

TABLE 4: Intraoperative risk factors, operative procedures, and patient outcome in different classes of severe corrosive injury.

	Class I (n = 15)	Class II (n = 13)	Class III (n = 16)	Class IV (n = 20)	Total (n = 64)	p value
Gastric perforation	7	9	12	18	46	0.044
Associated injury	0	7	10	16	33	0.000
Injury beyond pylorus	0	6	15	20	43	0.000
Continuous involvement of jejunum						0.000
>50 cm	0	0	0	16	16	
<50 cm	0	0	5	4	11	
Operative procedure						0.000
Esophagogastrectomy	14	6	4	0	24	
Esophagogastrectomy + concomitant resection	1	7	7	1	16	
Esophagogastroduodenojejunectomy	0	0	5	8	13	
Esophagogastroduodenojejunectomy + concomitant resection	0	0	0	4	4	
Laparotomy only	0	0	0	7	7	
Mortality rate	0	3	9	17	29	0.000
Hospital stay of survivors (day)	26.1 ± 3.7	33.9 ± 6.0	56.4 ± 15.8	144.0 ± 27.2	44.8 ± 7.1	0.000
Esophageal reconstruction subsequently	13	9	6	1	29	0.000

alkali injury are due to associated intrathoracic organ injuries, such as tracheobronchial necrosis or esophagoaortic fistula. In our series, females had a higher risk of death. Probably, females ingested larger amounts of the corrosive agent (255.6 ± 18.6 mL versus 229.7 ± 16.5 mL, $p = 0.356$). A shock index ≥ 1 and coma in the emergency room were two ominous signs [7, 10, 15] for a poor prognosis because they were an indication of associated intra-abdominal organ injuries. A shock index ≥ 1 indicated severe fluid loss from the third space of the abdominal cavity. Most of these patients were in poor general condition as a result of extensive associated organ injuries. Patients with irreversible coma usually die quite soon. Patients presenting with a shock index ≥ 1 in the emergency room should undergo aggressive perioperative fluid resuscitation and acid-base correction, followed by adequate resection of injured organs as soon as possible, although the mortality rate is extremely high.

In acid-injured patients, a blood pH value < 7.0 usually indicates the necessity for esophagogastrectomy [7]. In this study, a blood pH value < 7.23 was significantly related to deaths compared to a pH value ≥ 7.23. A base deficit in vivo or within the extracellular fluid has long been used as the index of a nonrespiratory acid-base imbalance [16]. In our animal experiment [17], obvious gastric perforation, which caused intra-abdominal organ injuries, occurred in animals that had a base deficit of more than 16 mmol/L. In the present study, a base deficit of more than 14 mmol/L is a significant predictor of death ($p = 0.009$). We highly recommend that patients with a base deficit of more than 14 mmol/L on initial ABG also undergo early surgery. Endoscopy has been used for routine evaluation of corrosive injury [18]. In our institute, the endoscopy is performed only on patients who do not require immediate surgery.

The present study showed that four intraoperative findings were well correlated to the deaths in each class of acid corrosive injury. These findings were (1) gastric perforation which reflects severe injury of the gastric wall; (2) associated visceral injury which reflects extra-alimentary extension of injury; (3) injury beyond the pylorus, and (4) continuous involvement of the jejunum over a length of 50 cm, the last two findings reflecting intra-alimentary extension of the injury. Any combination of the above findings always made the treatment more complicated and the patient outcome worse. According to the analysis of the intraoperative risk factors and the surgeon's experience, categorization of severe acid corrosive injury should be mandatory.

In the series, 56.5% (26 of 46) of gastric perforations had associated visceral injuries, compared to 38.8% (7/18) of nongastric perforations which had associated visceral injuries (odds ratio for associated injury = 2.043, $p = 0.204$). Obviously, the associated injuries were caused either by outflow or by direct infiltration of caustic agents.

In our experience, upper and lower abdominal pain were the most common presentation, while peritoneal signs or muscle guarding was detected less often. To improve the survival rate, we emphasize that patients with an obvious abdominal presentation should undergo early exploratory laparotomy. Left pleural effusion indicates gastric fundus perforation and also helps in the decision for surgery. In some patients, severe acid injury could have been blocked by prepyloric spasm [19] causing early perforation of the stomach, especially on the posterior wall of the fundus and body. The associated injury of the pancreas and retroperitoneal tissues precluded adequate resection. These patients often had persistent metabolic acidosis or early acute renal failure postoperatively and subsequently died from multiple organ failure.

Some developed repeated internal bleeding from necrosis of the retroperitoneal tissues. Diffuse oozing in the abdominal cavity made surgical homeostasis unsuccessful. One should preserve the omentum as far as possible to cover these injured tissues to attenuate this complication. Although associated visceral injury was a major risk factor for death, some patients could be saved if the injured organs could be resected completely [20].

The esophagectomy was initially performed via the transhiatal route in all patients to lessen the morbidity and mortality [21–23]. Thoracotomy for esophagectomy was reserved for those patients who had esophageal perforation or had complications such as esophageal disruption or massive bleeding during transhiatal esophageal stripping. In the case of previous subtotal gastrectomy associated with gastrojejunostomy when the jejunum was injured, which is recognized as continuous involvement, the injury should not be ignored. In the series, three patients, with a history of subtotal gastrectomy associated with gastrojejunostomy, had continued jejunum involvement of 20 cm, 29 cm, and 120 cm, respectively. Combined diaphragm injury seemed to delay the morbidity of the survivors and some of them required repeat surgery for subphrenic, pleural, and gastro- or colobronchial fistula complications. Wide and adequate resection of injured organs is still the only way to block the process of acid injury and to improve the survival rate [8, 12, 20].

Injuries that required duodenectomy actually had a significantly poor prognosis compared to those without duodenectomy ($p = 0.000$). Most deaths were due to respiratory or intra-abdominal complications that resulted from a technically difficult surgery and complicated postoperative course [8, 9, 12]. Adequate debridement of an injured pancreas head after duodenectomy with multiple intra-abdominal and intraluminal drainage (pancreatic duct and jejunum) was performed in this series. Although pancreaticojejunostomy leakage was still found in more than one-third of the patients, 41.1% (7/17) of our patients who underwent esophagogastroduodenojejunectomy survived. However, the patients who required continuous resection of the alimentary tract beyond 50 cm of the jejunum usually had a much higher mortality, namely, 93.8% (15/16), compared to those with less than 50 cm of the jejunum involved, namely, 33.3% (3/9), $p = 0.001$.

In the early deaths, the patients had multiple visceral damage, thrombosis of the visceral vessels resulting from spreading out of the ingested agent, or extensive alimentary tract injury. Surgical procedures were halted owing to persistent unstable vital signs or disseminated bleeding. For most of those patients devitalization of all abdominal viscera made radical resection impossible [6, 7, 22]. These patients manifested diffuse abdominal pain, either with early peritoneal signs or without rebounding as seen in ischemic bowel disease, and usually died shortly after surgery.

A poor patient outcome is significantly increased in the advanced class of corrosive injury, which reflects that the risk of death is increased in severely injured patients. In the study, 29 (45.3%) patients died between days 1 and 64 (average 14.4 days), including 12 (41.3%) who died within 24 hours after surgery. Hence, only 35 (54.7%) survivors were enrolled to analyze the hospital stay, which increased significantly with advancing class of injury ($p = 0.000$).

5. Conclusions

Surgery remains the only way to save the life of patients with extensive corrosive injuries. Gastric perforation, associated visceral injury, and extension of the alimentary injury are well correlated with the mortality rate among each class of injury. The severity classification of acid corrosive injuries based on laparotomy findings firstly designed by us is useful to predict the probability of survival when a laparotomy is performed.

Conflict of Interests

The authors declare that there is no conflict of interests regarding the publication of this paper.

References

[1] M. T. Rajabi, G. Maddah, R. Bagheri, M. Mehrabi, H. Shabahang, and F. Lorestani, "Corrosive injury of the upper gastrointestinal tract: review of surgical management and outcome in 14 adult cases," *Iranian Journal of Otorhinolaryngology*, vol. 27, pp. 15–21, 2015.

[2] G. C. Chong, O. H. Beahrs, and W. S. Payne, "Management of corrosive gastritis due to ingested acid," *Mayo Clinic Proceedings*, vol. 49, no. 11, pp. 861–865, 1974.

[3] J. B. Dilawari, S. Singh, P. N. Rao, and B. S. Anand, "Corrosive acid ingestion in man: a clinical and endoscopic study," *Gut*, vol. 25, no. 2, pp. 183–187, 1984.

[4] R. Lebeau, A. Coulibaly, S. Kountélé Gona et al., "Isolated gastric outlet obstruction due to corrosive ingestion," *Journal of Visceral Surgery*, vol. 148, no. 1, pp. 59–63, 2011.

[5] O. Gago, F. N. Ritter, W. Martel et al., "Aggressive surgical treatment for caustic injury of the esophagus and stomach," *Annals of Thoracic Surgery*, vol. 13, no. 3, pp. 243–250, 1972.

[6] A. Estrera, W. Taylor, L. J. Mills, and M. R. Platt, "Corrosive burns of the esophagus and stomach: a recommendation for an aggressive surgical approach," *Annals of Thoracic Surgery*, vol. 41, no. 3, pp. 276–283, 1986.

[7] Ö. P. Horváth, T. Oláh, and G. Zentai, "Emergency esophagogastrectomy for treatment of hydrochloric acid injury," *The Annals of Thoracic Surgery*, vol. 52, no. 1, pp. 98–101, 1991.

[8] M.-H. Wu and W.-W. Lai, "Surgical management of extensive corrosive injuries of the alimentary tract," *Surgery Gynecology & Obstetrics*, vol. 177, no. 1, pp. 12–16, 1993.

[9] L.-B. B. Jeng, H.-Y. Chen, S.-C. Chen et al., "Upper gastrointestinal tract ablation for patients with extensive injury after ingestion of strong acid," *Archives of Surgery*, vol. 129, no. 10, pp. 1086–1090, 1994.

[10] J. M. Su, H. K. Hsu, H. C. Chang, and W. H. Hsu, "Management for acute corrosive injury of upper gastrointestinal tract," *Chinese Medical Journal*, vol. 54, no. 1, pp. 20–25, 1994.

[11] K. H. Lai, B. S. Huang, M. H. Huang et al., "Emergency surgical intervention for severe corrosive injuries of the upper digestive tract," *Chinese Medical Journal*, vol. 56, no. 1, pp. 40–46, 1995.

[12] M.-H. Wu, W.-W. Lai, T.-L. Hwang, S.-C. Lee, H.-K. Hsu, and T.-S. Lin, "Surgical results of corrosive injuries involving

esophagus to jejunum," *Hepato-Gastroenterology*, vol. 43, no. 10, pp. 846–850, 1996.

[13] B. Berthet, P. Castellani, M. I. Brioche, R. Assadourian, and A. Gauthier, "Early operation for severe corrosive injury of the gastrointestinal tract," *European Journal of Surgery*, vol. 162, pp. 951–955, 1996.

[14] M. M. Kirsh, A. Peterson, J. W. Brown, M. B. Orringer, F. Ritter, and H. Sloan, "Treatment of caustic injuries of the esophagus: a ten year experience," *Annals of Surgery*, vol. 188, no. 5, pp. 675–678, 1978.

[15] E. Sarfati, D. Gossot, P. Assens, and M. Celerier, "Management of caustic ingestion in adults," *British Journal of Surgery*, vol. 74, no. 2, pp. 146–148, 1987.

[16] J. W. Severinghaus and P. B. Astrup, "History of blood gas analysis. II. pH and acid-base balance measurements," *Journal of Clinical Monitoring*, vol. 1, no. 4, pp. 259–277, 1985.

[17] M.-H. Wu, S. C. Chan, N.-S. Chou, M.-Y. Lin, and W.-W. Lai, "Blood pH change and base deficit as severity indices of acid corrosive injury: observation in an experimental study," *Journal of Surgical Association Republic of China*, vol. 28, no. 2, pp. 89–94, 1995.

[18] L. S. Lu, W. C. Tai, M. L. Hu, K. L. Wu, and Y. C. Chiu, "Predicting the progress of caustic injury to complicated gastric outlet obstruction and esophageal stricture, using modified endoscopic mucosal injury grading scale," *BioMed Research International*, vol. 2014, Article ID 919870, 6 pages, 2014.

[19] C. A. R. Schulenburg, "Corrosive stricture of stomach: without involvement of the esophagus," *The Lancet*, vol. 238, no. 6161, pp. 367–368, 1941.

[20] P. Cattan, N. Munoz-Bongrand, T. Berney, B. Halimi, E. Sarfati, and M. Celerier, "Extensive abdominal surgery after caustic ingestion," *Annals of Surgery*, vol. 231, no. 4, pp. 519–523, 2000.

[21] J. G. Brun, M. Celerier, F. Koskas, and C. Dubost, "Blunt thorax oesophageal stripping: an emergency procedure for caustic ingestion," *British Journal of Surgery*, vol. 71, no. 9, pp. 698–700, 1984.

[22] T. L. Hwang, S. M. Shen-Chen, and M.-F. Chen, "Nonthoracotomy esophagectomy for corrosive esophagitis with gastric perforation," *Surgery Gynecology & Obstetrics*, vol. 164, no. 6, pp. 537–540, 1987.

[23] M. B. Orringer, B. Marshall, and M. C. Stirling, "Transhiatal esophagectomy for benign and malignant disease," *The Journal of Thoracic and Cardiovascular Surgery*, vol. 105, no. 2, pp. 265–277, 1993.

11

Local Anaesthetic Infiltration and Indwelling Postoperative Wound Catheters for Patients with Hip Fracture Reduce Death Rates and Length of Stay

William D. Harrison, Deborah Lees, Jamie A'Court, Thomas Ankers, Ian Harper, Dominic Inman, and Mike R. Reed

Orthopaedic Department, Wansbeck General Hospital, Northumbria Healthcare Trust, Woodhorn Lane, Ashington, Northumberland NE63 9JJ, UK

Correspondence should be addressed to William D. Harrison; will.d.harrison@gmail.com

Academic Editor: Ahmed H. Al-Salem

Background. An analgesic enhanced recovery (ER) protocol for patients with a hip fracture was introduced. It was hypothesised that the ER would reduce pain, length of stay and improve clinical outcomes. The protocol used intraoperative infiltration of levobupivacaine followed by ongoing wound infusions. *Methods.* Consecutive patients admitted to two hospitals were eligible for the ER protocol. Numerical Reporting Scale pain scores (0–10) were recorded alongside opiate requirements. 434 patients in the ER group (316 full ER, 90 partial ER, and 28 no ER) were compared to a control group (CG) of 100 consecutive patients managed with traditional opiate analgesia. *Results.* Mean opiate requirement was 49.2 mg (CG) versus 32.5 mg (ER). Pain scores were significantly reduced in the full ER group, $p < 0.0001$. Direct discharge home and mean acute inpatient stay were significantly reduced ($p = 0.0031$ and $p < 0.0001$, resp.). 30-day mortality was 15% (CG) versus 5.5% (ER), $p = 0.0024$. *Conclusions.* This analgesic ER protocol for patients with a hip fracture was safe and effective and was associated with reduced inpatient stay and mortality.

1. Introduction

Enhanced recovery initiatives for orthopaedic surgery have been shown to improve patient outcomes and effectively reduce service demand and costs [1–3]. Hip fracture is the most common trauma admission in the United Kingdom and is expected to become more common with an ageing population [4]. The general approach to hip fracture management has changed over the last decade with a drive to improve the associated morbidity and mortality. Recognising the multisystem needs of this at-risk patient group is crucial and is the focus of quality improvement programmes within the United Kingdom National Health Service.

Local infiltration of anaesthetic (LIA) intraoperatively and subsequent indwelling catheter infusion (CATH) for postoperative arthroplasty pain management are gaining popularity in the enhanced recovery setting. The combination of LIA and CATH is more accepted in total knee arthroplasty

than in elective hip arthroplasty [5]. Results from studies looking specifically at LIA in hip arthroplasty have shown no clinical benefit compared to multimodal oral analgesia [6–9]. Early evidence from LIA and CATH for knee arthroplasty surgery demonstrates lower opiate requirements and overall pain scores when compared to intrathecal morphine [10]. LIA and CATH in conjunction with other pharmacological, procedural, and behavioral adaptations for an enhanced recovery protocol for knee arthroplasty demonstrated an increased patient satisfaction, reduced blood transfusions, reduced length of stay, and decreased mortality [3].

Level 1 evidence has demonstrated lower requirement for breakthrough opiates following LIA in hip arthroplasty [11, 12]. Busch et al. demonstrated a reduction of patient controlled opiate analgesia and reduced pain on activity, in their level 1 study of 64 patients [13]. However, there is conflicting evidence from other randomized studies that have demonstrated that LIA and particularly CATH have no short-term benefit in elective primary total hip replacement [5–7, 9]. The differences between the pain experienced after elective total hip replacement and the pain experienced after hip fracture fixation or hemiarthroplasty are speculative. Pain originating from the local damage to soft tissues and the fracture itself from trauma are more acute than the chronic pain experienced prior to elective arthroplasty surgery. Whether the nociceptive stimuli of trauma and arthritis respond differently to local anaesthetic infusions is not known.

Patients with hip fracture often have cognitive impairment and often receive an inequality of pain relief [14]. One aim of this analgesic enhanced recovery programme was to reduce this inequality and provide standard multimodal analgesia for all patients.

Other benefits of LIA and CATH are to reduce the volume of opiates and subsequently reduce the adverse side effects [12, 15, 16]. Opiates are renally excreted and the elderly are at risk of significant opiate sensitivity leading to respiratory depression, hypoxia, lower respiratory tract infection, delirium, and constipation. There are however potential risks of using high doses of local anaesthetic in this frail elderly group with possible systemic local anesthetic toxicity with central nervous or cardiorespiratory compromise [2, 17, 18].

The aim of this study is to establish if local infiltration of anaesthetic (LIA) and indwelling anaesthetic catheter infusions (CATH) are superior to standard analgesia used in a control group (CG) for management of patients with a hip fracture.

2. Method

This is a study of consecutive patients presenting to two separate acute hospitals between April 2010 and May 2012. Wansbeck General Hospital (hospital 1) and North Tyneside General Hospital (hospital 2) are both governed under the Northumbria Healthcare Trust and are 15 miles apart. Enhanced recovery protocols for hip fractures are a multimodal optimisation of patient care from all facets including nutrition, physiotherapy, timely surgery, and perioperative analgesia. This study looks at a single facet of care, namely, analgesia. For the sake of simplicity, the term enhanced recovery (ER) is used to describe the full analgesic protocol offered to hip fracture patients and no other interventions. We therefore acknowledge that this is not a complete enhanced recovery protocol in the full sense of the term.

The aim was to gain an accurate representation of how the ER protocol impacts on pain scores, opiate requirements, and outcomes following hip fracture. Local Caldicott approval was obtained. There are two arms to this retrospective study: control group (CG) and the ER.

It was recognised that not all patients with a hip fracture could be treated with the full ER protocol. Components and variations of the enhanced recovery (ER) protocol include the following:

(1) The full ER protocol:

    (i) including both LIA and CATH together.

(2) CATH only (analysed as a subgroup) due to

    (i) anaesthetist preference;

    (ii) recent local anaesthetic nerve block given instead.

(3) LIA only (analysed as a subgroup) due to

    (i) risk of cumulative local anesthetic toxicity;

    (ii) agitated patients at risk of pulling out CATH.

(4) Non-ER protocol group receiving no aspects of the ER due to

    (i) a risk of local anaesthetic toxicity and risk of pulling out CATH;

    (ii) these patients who were managed with only traditional oral and parenteral analgesia as an alternative;

    (iii) non-ER protocol patients receiving the same analgesia as the CG, but as they were treated at the time of the ER protocol they were not consecutive or unselected.

The CG group includes 100 consecutive patients treated immediately before the introduction of ER in April 2010. They received oral and parenteral multimodal analgesia only. Fifty consecutive patients from each of the two recruiting hospitals were selected.

Both the CG and the ER had the same protocol for admission fast-tracking to a trauma ward and were prioritised for theatre within 36 hours. Orthogeriatric input was mandatory within the first 24 hours of admission between both groups. A formal analgesia, laxative, and antiemetic protocol was equivalent between both groups. There was a large crossover in the rehabilitation facilities available to both hospitals due to their proximities. Discharge criteria were multifactorial but consistent between both hospitals during the ER and CG. Discharge was dictated by a consultant assessment of medical fitness, occupational therapy assessment of social circumstances, and physiotherapy assessment of mobility. One difference between the groups was the employment of a dedicated nutritionist for hip fracture patients in the latter half of the ER protocol data collection at both hospitals.

In both groups patients managed nonoperatively were excluded.

Data was gathered from medical notes, physiotherapy notes, medication charts, observation charts, and theatre records. Patient demographics, comorbidities, fracture pattern, and type of operative management were recorded.

Pain scores were measured according to the Numerical Rating Scale (NRS) between 0 and 10 [19]. The NRS scores were documented by nursing staff on each occasion of recording of postoperative observations. Patients with cognitive impairment who could not provide NRS for pain did not have a value recorded and were not included in the analysis of the NRS. The development of new confusion in the postoperative period was documented as it may also interfere with the quality NRS pain scores. In addition to pain scores, it was recognised that confused patients have more complex social needs, often delaying their discharge. Therefore a separate subgroup of patients without cognitive impairment were analysed to define the impact of the ER protocol on their discharge outcomes.

Nursing staff and patients were not blinded to those who received ER. Nurses provided analgesia for all patients requiring breakthrough pain relief regardless of the new ER protocol. Postoperative analgesia requirement for all patients was recorded, including "regular" and "as required" analgesia. All multimodal postoperative analgesia was recorded including paracetamol, mild opiates, and morphine.

The destination of discharge, that is, own home, residential care, or nursing home, was recorded for each patient. Direct discharge to the patients' home was considered the major endpoint in care within patient mortality and discharge to another care facility affecting this endpoint. The length of stay (on an acute ward) was also an important outcome measure. The duration of care in the rehabilitation facility was recorded when applicable. Thirty-day mortality of patients during the acute hospital admission was recorded for all patients. Data collection was undertaken exclusively by the authors.

Statistical analysis was performed using GraphPad Prism version 5.3 using the one-way ANOVA test to delineate between CG, LIA only, CATH only, and the "ER" (both LIA and CATH together). Fisher's exact test (two-tailed) was used for two-sided outcome analysis.

2.1. Enhanced Recovery (ER) Technique. Levobupivacaine (0.125%, 100 mL) (Chirocaine, Abbott Laboratories, Illinois, USA) was infiltrated (LIA) intraoperatively in a wide and layered field including joint capsule, muscle, fat, and skin. An epidural catheter (CATH) was positioned with the tip of the catheter deep to the joint capsule for an arthroplasty procedure and deep to the fascia lata for a fixation procedure. This CATH has a microbiological filter and exits away from the surgical field. 20 mL of levobupivacaine was infused through the catheter after skin closure and also for postoperative boluses (at 6, 14, and 24 hours). The AmbIT pump (Summit Medical Products, Inc., Sandy, UT) was used to deliver the boluses and the theatre and ward nursing staff received regular sessions to train and update them in using this device. After the fourth bolus, local anaesthetic was discontinued and the catheter was removed on the ward.

3. Results

There were 434 patients recorded during the ER period. Exclusions for nonoperative management were 2% ($n = 2$) during the CG period and 1.6% ($n = 7$) of patients during the ER period (see Table 1).

The outcomes of patients in the CG are compared to those in the ER period in Table 2. The decrease in 30-day mortality was significant (Fisher's exact test, $p = 0.0024$). Length of stay decreased from 15 days (CG) to 10 days (ER); however the proportion of patients being transferred to rehabilitation facilities increased, $p < 0.0001$. On subgroup analysis

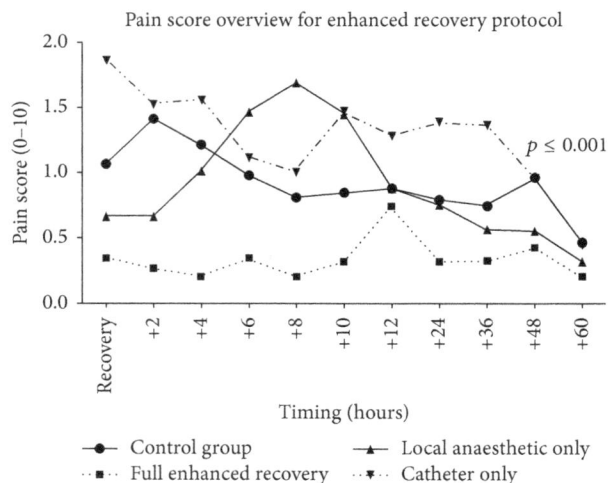

FIGURE 1: Numerical Reporting Scale (NRS) pain scores for the control group and the enhanced recovery subgroups.

of cognitively intact patients only (Table 3), significantly less CG were discharged to their own home compared to the ER ($p = 0.0031$) and reduced the requirement for further nursing care (36.7% for CG versus 27% for ER, $p = 0.1159$). All cognitively intact patients received some form of the ER protocol. Inpatient confusion was matched between the CG and the enhanced recovery group ($p = 0.087$).

Comparing all cognitively intact patients in the CG with those in the enhanced recovery period also demonstrates a decrease in 30-day mortality, a decrease in direct discharge home, and an increase in discharge to another care facility.

Figure 1 demonstrates that cognitively intact patients in the CG reported significantly higher pain over the first 3 days compared to the cognitively intact members of the full ER, $p < 0.0001$. The LIA initially reported low pains scores compared to the CG, but by 6 hours NRS pain scores were higher in the LIA. Patients with CATH had a higher level of pain compared to the CG despite equivalent regular and as required analgesia. Patterns of NRS pain scores in the subgroups of the enhanced recovery protocol matched the patterns in opiate requirement, as seen in Table 4.

There were no identified episodes of local anaesthetic toxicity in all 406 patients who received levobupivacaine via LIA and/or CATH.

Data on superficial and deep infection was not routinely recorded in our database and therefore a breakdown of infection rates for each subgroup of the ER is not available. However, data submitted to Public Health England for the Surgical Site Infection Surveillance Service was available for review for each hospital, specifically for "repair of hip fracture" and with a quarterly breakdown of cases. Within the 3 months of the CG data collection, there were zero superficial infections and one episode of deep infection (0.3% of cases). During the ER protocol in 2010 and 2011, there were no superficial infections. Over the 48 months of the ER protocol data collection, there were six deep infections in hospital 1 (0.9% of cases versus national average of 1.7%

TABLE 1: Patient demographics, mechanism of injury, fracture pattern, and management.

	Control group	Enhanced recovery period
N	100	434
Age mean	78.5 years	82.2 years
(Range)	(45–99)	(44–100)
Gender		
Male	24 (24.0%)	108 (24.8%)
Female	76 (76.0%)	326 (75.2%)
Inpatient confusion	31 (31.0%)	177 (40.1%)
Injury details		
Slip/trip	43 (43.0%)	191 (44%)
Collapse	4 (4.0%)	25 (5.8%)
Activity related	3 (3.0%)	49 (11.3%)
Slip on ice	0 (0.0%)	8 (1.8%)
Intoxicated	1 (1.0%)	7 (1.6%)
Fall in hospital	4 (4.0%)	9 (2.1%)
Assaulted	1 (1.0%)	0 (0%)
Unknown	41 (41.0%)	132 (30.4%)
Pathological	3 (3.0%)	13 (3.0%)
Fracture type		
Intracapsular	59 (59.0%)	239 (55.1%)
Extracapsular	35 (35.0%)	133 (30.6%)
Basicervical	4 (4.0%)	42 (9.7%)
Pertrochanteric	0 (0.0%)	14 (3.2%)
Subtrochanteric	2 (2.0%)	5 (1.2%)
Greater trochanter	0 (0.0%)	1 (0.2%)
Side		
Bilateral	0 (0.0%)	1 (0.2%)
Left	48 (48.0%)	217 (50%)
Right	52 (52.0%)	216 (49.8%)
FICB given?		
Yes	NA	326 (75.1%)
No	NA	108 (24.9%)
Procedure		
Nonoperative	2 (2.0%)	7 (1.6%)
Cannulated screws	7 (7.0%)	20 (4.6%)
Dynamic hip screw	26 (26.0%)	144 (33.2%)
Intramedullary fixation	16 (16.0%)	17 (3.9%)
Cemented bipolar hemiarthroplasty	2 (2.0%)	3 (0.7%)
Cemented Exeter hemiarthroplasty	11 (11.0%)	49 (11.3%)
Cemented Thompson's hemiarthroplasty	29 (29.0%)	183 (42.2%)
Uncemented Austin Moore hemiarthroplasty	1 (1.0%)	0 (0%)
Cemented Austin Moore hemiarthroplasty	3 (3.0%)	0 (0%)
Uncemented THR	1 (1.0%)	0 (0%)
Cemented THR	2 (2.0%)	15 (3.5%)
Enhanced recovery		
None	100 (100%)	28 (6.5%)
Full ER	NA	316 (72.8%)
LIA only	NA	75 (17.3%)
CATH only	NA	15 (3.5%)

TABLE 1: Continued.

	Control group	Enhanced recovery period
Reasons for partial/no enhanced recovery		
Total	NA	118 (27.2%)
Renal impairment	NA	44 (10.1%)
Catheter pulled out by patient	NA	6 (1.4%)
Catheter blocked	NA	8 (1.8%)
Femoral nerve block given	NA	27 (6.2%)
Reason not documented	NA	31 (7.1%)
Previous adverse drug reaction to local anaesthetic	NA	2 (0.4%)

TABLE 2: Patient outcomes for the control group and the enhanced recovery cohort.

	Control group	Enhanced recovery cohort
N	100	434
Length of stay, mean (range)		
Orthopaedic ward	15 (3–114) days	10 (3–44) days
Rehabilitation	15 (1–64) days	15 (1–114) days
Sum duration for a 100-patient group	1680 days	1470 days
Discharge destination		
30-day mortality	15 (15%)	24 (5.5%) $p = 0.0024$
Own home	52 (52%)	162 (37.3%) $p = 0.0090$
Rehabilitation	12 (12%)	138 (31.8%) $p < 0.0001$
Care home	21 (21%)	110 (25.3%) $p = 0.4393$

of cases) and nine deep infections in hospital 2 (1.5% versus national average of 1.7% of cases) (Public Health England for the Surgical Site Infection Surveillance Service for "Repair Neck of Femur").

Nursing staff did comment that cognitively impaired patients occasionally picked at the CATH dressing; however only 1.4% ($n = 6$) of patients had a catheter that was recorded as being removed prematurely. Similarly, 1.8% ($n = 8$) of patients with the CATH experienced intraluminal blockage of the catheter.

4. Discussion

This study has been performed over a 2-year period, in two hospitals, utilising a control group. The 100 patients retrospectively selected for the control group were identified as the most recently treated patients prior to the ER protocol in the two hospitals. This paper illustrates a working and practical model of an enhanced recovery protocol for patients with hip fractures.

The impact on the duration of inpatient stay was striking. The ER protocol provided a 5-day reduction in total length of stay ($p < 0.0001$) (Table 2). Although the discharge policy did not formally change between the CG and the ER, there may be other confounding factors which impact on this reduction. The reduction in acute stay did not extend into the mean duration of stay in further care, with both the CG and the ER having a mean stay of 15 days in rehabilitation. The reduction of 30-day mortality may have influenced the length of stay of

survivors and the significant increase of patient discharges to rehabilitation hospitals during the enhanced recovery period, 12% (CG) versus 31.8% (enhanced recovery period), Fishers exact test, $p < 0.0001$.

There were 24 deaths during the data collection of the ER protocol period, including 14 patients who did not receive LIA or CATH. There were no inpatient deaths in the 230 patients who underwent the full ER protocol. There was a significant overall reduction of 30-day mortality from 15% (CG) to 5.5% (enhanced recovery period), $p = 0.0024$ (Fisher's exact test).

The lack of deaths in patients with the full ER protocol is striking. This may simply relate to pain relief and reduced opiate use. However, the use of continuous local anaesthetic has been shown to reduce postoperative ileus [20, 21], postoperative neurocognitive decline [22], and acute lung injury [23]. There is also evidence that local anesthetic has antimicrobial properties, particularly against *Staphylococcus aureus, Enterococcus faecalis, and Escherichia coli* in wound infections [24]. The Public Health England data on local infection rates is reassuring as no excess of deep infection was attributable to the ER period. In fact, the superficial and deep infection rates for hip fracture surgery remained lower than the national average.

The use of the NRS pain scores allowed efficient data collection of a large number of patients over many different measuring points during the inpatient stay. The disadvantage is that the 40.1% ($n = 177$) of patients with cognitive impairment in the enhanced recovery period could not report an objective score of their pain. Furthermore, pain and inadequate analgesia contribute towards confusion in elderly

TABLE 3: Subgroup analysis of management options and patient outcomes. Patients with cognitive impairment are excluded.

	Control group	Enhanced recovery period		
		Full ER	LIA only	CATH only
N	79	230	49	15
Discharge destination				
30-day mortality	7 (8.8%)	0 (0%)	3 (6.1%)	4 (26.7%)
Own home	43 (54.4%)	168 (73%)	31 (63.3%)	2 (13.3%)
Care facility	29 (36.7%)	62 (27%)	15 (30.6%)	9 (60%)
Length of stay in days				
Ortho. ward (mean)	15	9	9	10
Rehab (mean)	19	17	17	18
Total	34 (3–114)	26 (3–80)	26 (3–88)	28 (3–82)

patients [25, 26] and previous studies have shown that the local anaesthetic blocks can reduce the prevalence of delirium in hip fracture patients [27, 28]. Tools exist for identifying pain levels in patients with cognitive impairment; however these are time-consuming and subjective and require a great deal of experience for the assessor [29]. The NRS pain scores in patients with normal levels of cognition were significantly lower throughout the hospital stay in the ER group than in the CG group (one-way ANOVA test, $p < 0.001$). The authors recognise that although the reduction of pain is statistically significant, it is only a reduction in the range of 0.5–1 out of 10 (Figure 1). This small change questions the clinical importance of this pain reduction; however, the combination of the demonstrable reduction in opiate requirement would support the effectiveness of the analgesic effect.

The provision of analgesia in the patients with dementia is an important humanitarian issue. Patients with cognitive impairment are often overlooked for opiate analgesia due to fluctuating consciousness and they do not express their severity of pain by the usual means [14]. The enhanced recovery protocol removes this discrimination and allows patients with cognitive impairment adequate and continued analgesia.

By using the LIA in isolation there was a clear reduction in pain over the first 4 hours, at which point there was a rise in postoperative pain (Figure 1). After this rise, the pain scores became more consistent with patients in the CG. The pattern may illustrate the half-life of the levobupivacaine at this site (approximately 2 to 2.6 hours). Despite the pattern in Figure 1, LIA has been shown to reduce wound pain sensitivity for up to three months following elective surgery [16]. In a study of 300 randomly assigned hip arthroplasty patients it is hypothesised that lower levels of acute postoperative pain impact on lower chronic pain experienced by the patient [30]. The analysis of the 15 patients (3.5% of the enhanced recovery period) who were managed with the CATH only reported a higher level of postoperative pain and however utilised less opiates than the CG. The CATH patients had a relatively high morphine requirement of 46 mg versus 31.8 mg in the ER group and also had a high mortality rate of 4 out of 15 patients (28.6%). The 30-day mortality figures in the CATH group may represent high-risk patients in whom the anaesthetist had deemed it unsafe to administer LIA.

The impact on opiate analgesia was evident in the ER group and to a lesser extent in LIA and CATH in isolation (Table 4). The reduction of morphine intake in this elderly group is important in order to decrease the potentially severe consequences of opiate toxicity. In terms of overall patient outcomes, the reduction of morphine intake may have contributed to the reduced mortality rate.

This study has limitations. Three-quarters (75.1%) of those in the ER group also received fascia iliaca compartment block (FICB) in the emergency department on admission to hospital. The FICB technique was gaining popularity in the emergency department during the time of data collection for the ER protocol. FICB was an analgesic intervention which aimed to supplement preoperative pain relief and was not considered as part of the postoperative pain relief delivered by the LIA and CATH. In 27 patients, surgery was prompt enough after a FICB that the full ER package was not delivered, to avoid local anaesthetic toxicity. There were no patients in the CG who received the FICB. As the half-life of levobupivacaine is 2–2.6 hours [31], any patient who receives a FICB and is operated on within 12 hours may receive local anaesthetic that is in addition to the ER. The FICB is therefore a confounding factor in this paper. Another limitation is that the CG and ER may not be comparable groups based on variations in treatment allocation and discharge destination. Randomising treatment groups would have provided clarity on this matter and given a clearer understanding of the impact of LIA and CATH on final outcomes. Nursing staff delivering postoperative analgesia and recording NRS pain scores were not blinded, as they needed to deliver the CATH analgesia on the wards. This may contribute to a study effect bias, as those in the ER may have been deemed not to require additional oral analgesia. However, nursing staff were encouraged to provide analgesia on an individual need basis.

Previous studies have commented on the cost effectiveness of LIA and CATH stating that the protocol is too expensive to justify in elective cases [32]. A cost analysis of local anaesthetic used in an enhanced recovery protocol for elective joint arthroplasty is awaiting publication [30]. The cost of the full ER is estimated at £138 per patient, with a breakdown of consumables of levobupivacaine at £24, the catheter at £8, and the AmbIT pump at £30 each [33]. Jones reported elective orthopaedic bed costs of £285 per

TABLE 4: Opiate requirement for the control group versus the enhanced recovery protocol. Patients with cognitive impairment are excluded.

	Control group	Enhanced recovery period		
		ER	LIA only	CATH only
N	100	230	49	15
Cumulative mean	49.2 mg	31.8 mg	37.8 mg	46 mg
(Range)	(0–80 mg)	(0–98 mg)	(0–82 mg)	(3–55 mg)

day in 2008 [34]. According to the mean reduction in acute length of stay between the enhanced recovery period and the CG (5.1 days), the estimated saving per person is £1315.50. Excluding patients with cognitive impairment, those who received ER were also more likely to return directly home ($p = 0.0031$) rather than a care facility (Table 3). This may have far-reaching cost benefits for the healthcare system that surpass the short-term costs of staff training and equipment.

This study demonstrates the effective use of an enhanced recovery programme applied to patients with a hip fracture. Local anaesthetic as part of an enhanced recovery programme for patients with a hip fracture is favorable to traditional opiate-centered analgesia in terms of pain relief, duration of inpatient stay, discharge directly to home, and 30-day mortality. Patients receiving local anaesthetic infiltration and delivery by catheter have a better outcome than either technique in isolation. No patients receiving an intra-articular catheter developed deep wound infection and there were no recorded episodes of local anaesthetic toxicity. This enhanced recovery protocol can be considered to be a safe way to improve patient outcomes. A randomised controlled trial should be undertaken and specific attention should be made to the impact on mobility, morbidity, and 30-day mortality.

Conflict of Interests

The authors declare that there is no conflict of interests regarding the publication of this paper.

References

[1] J. P. Dillon, L. Brennan, and D. Mitchell, "Local infiltration analgesia in hip and knee arthroplasty: an emerging technique," *Acta Orthopaedica Belgica*, vol. 78, no. 2, pp. 158–163, 2012.

[2] D. R. Kerr and L. Kohan, "Local infiltration analgesia: a technique for the control of acute postoperative pain following knee and hip surgery—a case study of 325 patients," *Acta Orthopaedica*, vol. 79, no. 2, pp. 174–183, 2008.

[3] A. Malviya, K. Martin, I. Harper et al., "Enhanced recovery program for hip and knee replacement reduces death rate," *Acta Orthopaedica*, vol. 82, no. 5, pp. 577–581, 2011.

[4] National Clinical Guideline Centre, *The Management of Hip Fracture in Adults*, NICE Clinical Guidelines no. 124, Royal College of Physicians, London, UK, 2011.

[5] H. Kehlet and L. Ø. Andersen, "Local infiltration analgesia in joint replacement: the evidence and recommendations for clinical practice," *Acta Anaesthesiologica Scandinavica*, vol. 55, no. 7, pp. 778–784, 2011.

[6] L. Ø. Andersen, K. S. Otte, H. Husted, L. Gaarn-Larsen, B. Kristensen, and H. Kehlet, "High-volume infiltration analgesia in bilateral hip arthroplasty. A randomized, double-blind placebo-controlled trial," *Acta Orthopaedica*, vol. 82, no. 4, pp. 423–426, 2011.

[7] D. W. Chen, P.-H. Hsieh, K.-C. Huang, C.-C. Hu, Y.-H. Chang, and M. S. Lee, "Continuous intra-articular infusion of bupivacaine for post-operative pain relief after total hip arthroplasty: a randomized, placebo-controlled, double-blind study," *European Journal of Pain*, vol. 14, no. 5, pp. 529–534, 2010.

[8] T. H. Lunn, H. Husted, S. Solgaard et al., "Intraoperative local infiltration analgesia for early analgesia after total hip arthroplasty: a randomized, double-blind, placebo-controlled trial," *Regional Anesthesia and Pain Medicine*, vol. 36, no. 5, pp. 424–429, 2011.

[9] K. Specht, J. S. Leonhardt, P. Revald et al., "No evidence of a clinically important effect of adding local infusion analgesia administered through a catheter in pain treatment after total hip arthroplasty," *Acta Orthopaedica*, vol. 82, no. 3, pp. 315–320, 2011.

[10] P. Essving, K. Axelsson, E. Åberg, H. Spännar, A. Gupta, and A. Lundin, "Local infiltration analgesia versus intrathecal morphine for postoperative pain management after total knee arthroplasty: a randomized controlled trial," *Anesthesia & Analgesia*, vol. 113, no. 4, pp. 926–933, 2011.

[11] T. P. Murphy, D. P. Byrne, P. Curtin, J. F. Baker, and K. J. Mulhall, "Can a periarticular levobupivacaine injection reduce postoperative opiate consumption during primary hip arthroplasty?" *Clinical Orthopaedics and Related Research*, vol. 470, no. 4, pp. 1151–1157, 2012.

[12] R. Rikalainen-Salmi, J. G. Förster, K. Mäkelä et al., "Local infiltration analgesia with levobupivacaine compared with intrathecal morphine in total hip arthroplasty patients," *Acta Anaesthesiologica Scandinavica*, vol. 56, no. 6, pp. 695–705, 2012.

[13] C. A. Busch, M. R. Whitehouse, B. J. Shore, S. J. MacDonald, R. W. McCalden, and R. B. Bourne, "The efficacy of periarticular multimodal drug infiltration in total hip arthroplasty," *Clinical Orthopaedics and Related Research*, vol. 468, no. 8, pp. 2152–2159, 2010.

[14] R. S. Morrison and A. L. Siu, "A comparison of pain and its treatment in advanced dementia and cognitively intact patients with hip fracture," *Journal of Pain and Symptom Management*, vol. 19, no. 4, pp. 240–248, 2000.

[15] P. Banerjee and C. McLean, "The efficacy of multimodal high-volume wound infiltration in primary total hip replacement," *Orthopedics*, vol. 34, no. 9, pp. e522–e529, 2011.

[16] J. Aguirre, B. Baulig, C. Dora et al., "Continuous epicapsular ropivacaine 0.3% infusion after minimally invasive hip arthroplasty: a prospective, randomized, double-blinded, placebo-controlled study comparing continuous wound infusion with morphine patient-controlled analgesia," *Anesthesia and Analgesia*, vol. 114, no. 2, pp. 456–461, 2012.

[17] A. M. Morin and H. Wulf, "High volume local infiltration analgesia (LIA) for total hip and knee arthroplasty: a brief review of the current status," *Anasthesiologie Intensivmedizin Notfallmedizin Schmerztherapie*, vol. 46, no. 2, pp. 84–86, 2011.

[18] I. Dobrydnjov, C. Anderberg, C. Olsson, O. Shapurova, K. Angel, and S. Bergman, "Intraarticular vs. extraarticular ropivacaine infusion following high-dose local infiltration analgesia after total knee arthroplasty: a randomized double-blind study," *Acta Orthopaedica*, vol. 82, no. 6, pp. 692–698, 2011.

[19] P. E. Bijur, C. T. Latimer, and E. J. Gallagher, "Validation of a verbally administered numerical rating scale of acute pain for use in the emergency department," *Academic Emergency Medicine*, vol. 10, no. 4, pp. 390–392, 2003.

[20] K. P. Harvey, J. D. Adair, M. Isho, and R. Robinson, "Can intravenous lidocaine decrease postsurgical ileus and shorten hospital stay in elective bowel surgery? A pilot study and literature review," *The American Journal of Surgery*, vol. 198, no. 2, pp. 231–236, 2009.

[21] S. B. Groudine, H. A. G. Fisher, R. P. Kaufman Jr. et al., "Intravenous lidocaine speeds the return of bowel function, decreases postoperative pain, and shortens hospital stay in patients undergoing radical retropubic prostatectomy," *Anesthesia and Analgesia*, vol. 86, no. 2, pp. 235–239, 1998.

[22] J. P. Mathew, G. B. Mackensen, B. Phillips-Bute et al., "Randomized, double-blinded, placebo controlled study of neuroprotection with lidocaine in cardiac surgery," *Stroke*, vol. 40, no. 3, pp. 880–887, 2009.

[23] A. Borgeat, "Non anesthetic action of local anesthetics," *Periodicum Biologorum*, vol. 115, no. 2, pp. 113–117, 2013.

[24] A. M. Parr, D. E. Zoutman, and J. S. D. Davidson, "Antimicrobial activity of lidocaine against bacteria associated with nosocomial wound infection," *Annals of Plastic Surgery*, vol. 43, no. 3, pp. 239–245, 1999.

[25] A. Adunsky, R. Levy, E. Mizrahi, and M. Arad, "Exposure to opioid analgesia in cognitively impaired and delirious elderly hip fracture patients," *Archives of Gerontology and Geriatrics*, vol. 35, no. 3, pp. 245–251, 2002.

[26] G. Ardery, K. Herr, B. J. Hannon, and M. G. Titler, "Lack of opioid administration in older hip fracture patients (CE)," *Geriatric Nursing*, vol. 24, no. 6, pp. 353–360, 2003.

[27] V. Perrier, B. Julliac, A. Lelias, N. Morel, P. Dabadie, and F. Sztark, "Influence of the fascia iliaca compartment block on postoperative cognitive status in the elderly," *Annales Françaises d'Anesthésie et de Réanimation*, vol. 29, no. 4, pp. 283–288, 2010.

[28] G. Mouzopoulos, G. Vasiliadis, N. Lasanianos, G. Nikolaras, E. Morakis, and M. Kaminaris, "Fascia iliaca block prophylaxis for hip fracture patients at risk for delirium: a randomized placebo-controlled study," *Journal of Orthopaedics and Traumatology*, vol. 10, no. 3, pp. 127–133, 2009.

[29] K. S. Feldt, "The checklist of nonverbal pain indicators (CNPI)," *Pain Management Nursing*, vol. 1, no. 1, pp. 13–21, 2000.

[30] V. Wylde, R. Gooberman-Hill, J. Horwood et al., "The effect of local anaesthetic wound infiltration on chronic pain after lower limb joint replacement: a protocol for a double-blind randomised controlled trial," *BMC Musculoskeletal Disorders*, vol. 12, article 53, 2011.

[31] R. H. Foster and A. Markham, "Levobupivacaine: a review of its pharmacology and use as a local anaesthetic," *Drugs*, vol. 59, no. 3, pp. 551–579, 2000.

[32] P. Cuvillon, J. Ripart, S. Debureaux et al., "Analgesia after hip fracture repair in elderly patients: the effect of a continuous femoral nerve block: a prospective and randomised study," *Annales Françaises d'Anesthésie et de Réanimation*, vol. 26, no. 1, pp. 2–9, 2007.

[33] T. Savaridas, I. Serrano-Pedraza, S. K. Khan, K. Martin, A. Malviya, and M. R. Reed, "Reduced medium-term mortality following primary total hip and knee arthroplasty with an enhanced recovery program. A study of 4,500 consecutive procedures," *Acta Orthopaedica*, vol. 84, no. 1, pp. 40–43, 2013.

[34] R. Jones, "Limitations of the HRG tariff: excess bed days," *British Journal of Health Care Management*, vol. 14, no. 8, pp. 354–355, 2008.

12

Factors Associated with Perforated Appendicitis in Elderly Patients in a Tertiary Care Hospital

Siripong Sirikurnpiboon and Suparat Amornpornchareon

Department of Surgery, Rajavithi Hospital, College of Medicine, Rangsit University, Phayathai Road, Rajathewee, Bangkok 10400, Thailand

Correspondence should be addressed to Siripong Sirikurnpiboon; laizan99@hotmail.com

Academic Editor: Miltiadis I. Matsagkas

Background. The incidence of perforated appendicitis in elderly patients is high and carries increased morbidity and mortality rates. The aim of this study was to identify risk factors of perforation in elderly patients who presented with clinical of acute appendicitis. *Methods.* This was a retrospective study, reviewing medical records of patients over the age of 60 years who had a confirmed diagnosis of acute appendicitis. Patients were classified into two groups: those with perforated appendicitis and those with nonperforated appendicitis. Demographic data, clinical presentations, and laboratory analysis were compared. *Results.* Of the 206 acute appendicitis patients over the age of 60 years, perforated appendicitis was found in 106 (50%) patients. The four factors which predicted appendiceal rupture were as follows: male; duration of pain in preadmission period; fever (>38°C); and anorexia. The overall complication rate was 34% in the perforation group and 12.6% in the nonperforation group. *Conclusions.* The incidence of perforated appendicitis in elderly patients was higher in males and those who had certain clinical features such as fever and anorexia. Duration of pain in the preadmission period was also an important factor in appendiceal rupture. Early diagnosis may decrease the incidence of perforated appendicitis in elderly patients.

1. Introduction

Acute appendicitis is the most common surgical disease, with an incidence of about 100 per 100,000. The life-time risk of developing appendicitis is 8.6% for males and 6.7% for females [1, 2], with 90% found in children and young adults and 10% in patients over 60 years old [3, 4].

Diagnosis of appendicitis is made mainly by history and physical examination, and laboratory study and radiologic investigation are helpful in equivocal cases. Clinical presentation has overall sensitivity and specificity of 45–81% and 36–53% [5], respectively. The possible cause is variation of appendix [6]. With regard to laboratory study, an increase in white blood cell count (WBC), predominance of polymorphonuclear leukocytes (PMN), and increased C-reactive protein (CRP) levels were associated with the risk and severity of complications in appendicitis [7]. With elderly patients, the diagnosis is more difficult, and this can lead to higher mortality and morbidity rates than in the general population.

This study aimed to analyse factors associated with rupture in elderly patients.

2. Materials and Methods

This was a retrospective study of medical records which were searched for ICD-10: K35 diagnosis codes from January 2010 to December 2014. The inclusion criteria were patients who (1) had diagnosis of acute appendicitis; (2) who were aged more than 60 years; (3) who had undergone operation in Rajvithi Hospital; and (4) whose pathological results had confirmed appendicitis. Patients who had undergone appendectomy inadvertently or whose type of appendicitis (acute appendicitis or perforated appendicitis) could not be identified from medical records or pathological reports were excluded. Each case underwent open appendectomy, and drains were placed in all patients in the perforated group. Data collected included demographic data, clinical presentation, duration of pain in the preadmission period, and

TABLE 1: Comparison of patients' characteristics in the perforated and nonperforated appendicitis groups.

	Perforated appendicitis ($n = 103$)	Nonperforated appendicitis ($n = 103$)	p value
Age (mean ± SD) (years)	68.8 ± 7.4	69.2 ± 6.8	0.989
Male sex	49 (47.6)	29 (28.2)	0.004*
Address			<0.001*
Urban	74 (71.9)	36 (35.0)	
Suburb	29 (28.1)	67 (65.0)	
Living status			<0.001*
With family	82 (86.3)	30 (29.1)	
Living alone	13 (13.7)	63 (70.9)	
Underlying disease			0.770
Diabetes mellitus	32 (31.1)	25 (24.3)	0.276
Hypertension	56 (54.4)	54 (52.4)	0.780
Myocardial infarction	10 (9.7)	11 (10.7)	0.818
Congestive heart failure	1 (1.0)	2 (1.9)	1.000
Chronic kidney disease	8 (7.8)	5 (4.9)	0.390
Chronic liver disease	0 (0)	2 (1.9)	0.498
COPD	3 (2.9)	3 (2.9)	1.000
ASA classification			0.218
I	11 (10.7)	8 (7.8)	
II	76 (73.8)	86 (83.5)	
III	16 (15.5)	9 (8.7)	
BMI (mean ± SD) (Kg)	23.8 ± 4.2	23.9 ± 3.3	0.525

*: value < 0.05 is statistically significant.

laboratory analysis. Statistical analysis was performed using univariate and multivariate logistic regression with SPSS version 17.0.

3. Results

Appendectomies were performed from 1 January 2010 to 31 December 2014 on 206 patients who were all more than 60 years old. Of these cases, 78 were males (37.9%) and 128 were females (62.1%). The mean age was 68.98 ± 7.08 years (60–91 years), and the mean BMI was 23.86 ± 3.76 (16.4–37.0). Half (103) of the appendectomies were perforated, and half (103) were nonperforated.

A total of 125 patients (60.7%) had comorbidity such as diabetes mellitus, hypertension, chronic kidney disease, chronic liver disease, cardiovascular disease, congestive heart failure, and COPD, and 71 patients had more than one comorbidity. A comparison of the basic characteristics of the groups is shown in Table 1. It was found that perforated appendicitis was associated with male sex, living in urban areas, and living alone.

With regard to clinical presentation, most patients with abdominal pain had other symptoms such as nausea, vomiting, anorexia, migratory pain from the periumbilicus to the right iliac fossa, and fever ≥38°C. Physical examination showed tenderness at the right iliac fossa, and laboratory data revealed an increase in WBC and PMN predominance. Imaging studies were done by CT (computerized tomography) scan or US (ultrasonography), and 2 patients in the perforated

group and 1 in the nonperforated group underwent both. In the perforation group, the mean time to imaging was 8.53 hours (1–24 hours) while in the nonperforated group it was 5.33 hours (2–12 hours). The clinical data of the two groups are compared in Table 2. Clinical presentation data showed that anorexia, fever of more than 38°C, and time to imaging were significantly associated with perforated appendicitis. The overall median duration of pain in the preadmission period was 24 hours (2–240 hours). Most of the patients came to the hospital 24 hours after the onset of abdominal pain. Of these, 90 (87.4%) had perforated appendicitis and 66 (64.1%) had acute appendicitis. The study showed there were statistically significant differences between the two groups. The overall median duration of pain to performance of operation was 28.5 hours (4–241.5 hours); in the perforated group the mean duration was 50 hours and in the nonperforated group it was 27 hours ($p < 0.01$), and this was a statistically significant difference. Patients who underwent imaging more than 6 hours after arriving at the hospital had a significantly higher risk of perforation. Details are shown in Table 3.

With regard to intraoperative result, 6 patients in perforated group had conversion operations: 2 to right hemicolectomy and 4 patients to ileocecectomy. Univariate analysis showed that the factors associated with perforated appendicitis were male sex, fever ≥38°C, anorexia, duration of pain in the preadmission period, and duration of pain to performance of operation. Multivariate analysis revealed that the factors significantly associated with perforated appendicitis were male sex (OR = 2.36, 95% CI, 1.25–4.44), fever ≥38°C

TABLE 2: Comparison of clinical presentation in the two groups.

Clinical presentation	Perforated appendicitis (n = 103) (%)	Acute appendicitis (n = 103) (%)	p value
Nausea and/or vomiting	67 (65)	60 (58.3)	0.316
Anorexia	65 (63.1)	50 (48.5)	0.035*
Migratory pain	60 (58.3)	58 (56.3)	0.778
Fever > 38°C	44 (42.7)	26 (25.2)	0.008*
RLQ tenderness	102 (99)	103 (100)	1.000
Rebound tenderness	91 (88.3)	83 (80.6)	0.124
WBC > 10×10^9 cell/L	87 (84.5)	89 (86.4)	0.693
Neutrophil > 75%	74 (71.8)	83 (80.6)	0.141
Alvarado score (mean ± SD)	7.58 ± 1.49	7.29 ± 1.36	0.199
Imaging study	31 (48.4)	33 (51.6)	0.763
Computerized tomography	22 (21.4)	22 (21.4)	1.000
Acute appendicitis	4 (18.2)	21 (95.5)	<0.001*
Ruptured appendicitis	18 (81.8)	1 (4.5)	
Ultrasonography	11 (10.7)	12 (11.7)	0.825
Acute appendicitis	6 (54.5)	12 (100.0)	0.024*
Ruptured appendicitis	5 (45.5)	0 (0.0)	
Time to imaging (mean ± SD)	8.53 ± 3.57	5.33 ± 2.33	<0.001*

*: value < 0.05 is statistically significant.

TABLE 3: Duration of time in perforated and acute appendicitis groups.

	Perforated appendicitis n = 103	Acute appendicitis (n = 103)	p value
Duration of pain in admission period	48 (6–240)	24 (2–96)	
<24 hours	13 (12.6%)	37 (35.9%)	<0.001*
≥24 hours	90 (87.4%)	66 (64.1%)	
Duration from pain to operation	50 (8–241)	27 (4–104)	
<24 hours	11 (10.7%)	35 (34.0%)	<0.001*
≥24 hours	37 (89.3%)	46 (66.1%)	
Duration from admission to operation	6 (1–8)	10 (9–12)	
>8 hours	16 (15.5%)	12 (11.7%)	0.416
≤8 hours	87 (84.5%)	91 (88.3%)	
Duration from arrival to imaging	8 (1–24)	6 (2–12)	
>6 hours	78 (75.7)	30 (29.1)	<0.001*
≤6 hours	25 (24.3)	73 (70.9)	

Value s are represented as numbers (percentages) and median (minimum-maximum).
*: value < 0.05 is statistically significant.

(OR = 2.17, 95% CI, 1.10–4.27), anorexia (OR = 1.92, 95% CI, 1.03–3.57), and duration of pain in the preadmission period (OR = 1.02, 95% CI, 1.01–1.04). Details are shown in Table 4.

The total number of complications was 34 (33%) in the perforated appendicitis group compared with 13 (12%) in the acute appendicitis patients ($p < 0.001$). Significant complications were pneumonia ($p = 0.046$) and surgical wound infection ($p = 0.001$). Median length of hospital stay in the perforation group was 8 days (3–48 days) and 4 days (2–136 days) in the nonperforation group, and this was statistically significant ($p < 0.001$). Of the 103 patients in the perforated appendicitis group, there were 92 cases (89.3%) of complete

recovery and two mortalities (1.9%): one patient died from septic shock 10 days after the onset of abdominal pain due to delayed diagnosis, and the other one died from congestive heart failure due to multiple comorbidities and underlying valvular heart disease. In contrast, complete recovery was observed in all nonperforated patients, and there were no mortalities. A comparison of morbidity and mortality in the two groups is shown in Table 5.

An analysis of scores for predicting ruptured appendicitis is shown in Table 6. Validation scores using cut-off value 6 in this data showed sensitivity of 56% with specificity of 83% and accuracy of 69.4% as shown in Table 7.

TABLE 4: Factors associated with perforated appendicitis by multivariate analysis.

Factor	Adjusted odds ratio	95% confidence interval	p value
Male sex	2.47	1.31–4.63	0.008
Fever > 38°C	1.97	1.03–3.78	0.024
Anorexia	1.90	1.03–3.52	0.040
Duration of pain in preadmission period	4.21	2.22–7.98	<0.001

TABLE 5: Outcomes, complications, and length of hospital stay.

Results	Perforated appendicitis ($n = 103$)	Acute appendicitis ($n = 103$)	p value
Operation conversion n (%)	8 (7.8)	0	0.003*
Complication n (%)	34 (33)	13 (12.6)	<0.001*
Pneumonia	16 (15.5)	7 (6.8)	0.046*
Respiratory failure	4 (3.9)	1 (1.0)	0.174
Gastrointestinal bleeding	2 (1.9)	0 (0)	0.498
Surgical wound infection	19 (18.4)	4 (3.9)	0.001*
Length of hospital stay			
Median (min-max)	8 (3–48)	4 (2–136)	<0.001
Discharge status n (%)			0.005*
Complete recovery	92 (89.3)	102 (99)	
Morbidity	9 (8.7)	1 (1)	
Death	2 (1.9)	0 (0)	

*: value < 0.05 is statistically significant.

TABLE 6: Scores for predicting ruptured appendicitis in elderly patients.

Factor	Adjusted OR	Score
Male	2.47	2
Fever ($T > 38$°C)	1.97	2
Anorexia	1.90	2
Pain > 24 hrs	4.21	4
Total score		10

4. Discussion

The incidence of acute appendicitis in elderly patients aged more than 60 years was about 5–10% [3, 8] with good postoperative outcome after appendectomy, but, in the case of perforated appendicitis, there were instances of mortality and higher rates of morbidity postoperatively. The incidence of perforated appendicitis was 32%–72% [9–14] mostly due to delayed diagnosis caused by equivocal history and physical examination [14–17]. In the present study, perforated appendicitis was found in 50% of cases which is comparable to the findings of previous research. The risk factors associated with perforated appendicitis were male sex, fever ≥38°C, anorexia, and duration of pain in the preadmission period.

In relation to risk factors, this research found that being of male sex was significantly related to perforation, and this is in line with the results of previous reports [18–20]. A possible explanation for this is elderly males' culture of reluctance to go to hospital, as found in a report by Sheu et al. [18].

With regard to social factors, living in metropolitan areas and living alone were risks for delaying seeking medical services. The author did not attempt to delve into this factor in detail, but possible explanations are changes in family structure, an increase in living away from one's family, and less real social participation.

With regard to clinical presentation, fever ≥38°C and anorexia were factors affecting the likelihood of having a perforated appendix. Previous studies have shown the same significance of fever [18, 21, 22]. A recent report by Shimizu et al. [23] confirmed the relationship between severity of fever and appendicitis and proposed that the neutrophil to lymphocyte ratio (NLR) was useful for predicting the severity of inflammation because pooled neutrophils in bone marrow are able to respond more rapidly to infectious disease compared to acute inflammation-related proteins that are produced by the liver such as C-reactive protein. In relation to the Alvarado score, the mean in the perforation group was 7.58 ± 1.49 and 7.29 ± 1.36 in the nonperforation group. An Alvarado score of more than 7 had sensitivity and specificity for diagnosing appendicitis, but high Alvarado scores did not correlate with severity of disease and could not discriminate between perforated and acute appendicitis [24]. In this study, the median duration of pain in the preadmission period in the perforated appendicitis patients was 48 hours. The results confirmed the findings of previous reports about the risk of perforation from delaying seeking medical attention [8, 11, 13, 21, 25–28]. A recent study by Augustin et al. [29] showed that the risk of perforation increased 36 hours after onset of pain. Similarly, in a report about another age group, Singh et al. [30] showed

TABLE 7: Validation scores for predicting ruptured appendicitis.

| | Perforation | | Total | Sensitivity | Specificity | PPV | NPV | Accuracy |
	Yes	No						
Score								
≥6	58	18	76					
<6	45	85	130	58/103 = 56%	85/103 = 83%	58/7 = 76%	85/130 = 65%	143/206 = 69.4%
Total	103	103						

a significant association between perforated appendicitis in pediatric patients and a duration of pain to admission of longer than 72 hours. With regard to time to imaging, this was significantly longer in the perforated group compared to the nonperforated one. Generally, clinical examination is more important than investigation, but the latter can be helpful where the clinical picture is equivocal in patients of extreme age. A study from Gardner et al. [31] showed imaging influenced elderly patient management in 36% of cases and affected diagnosis; however, the impact of duration from admission to operation is still a controversial issue. A report by Eko et al. [32] suggested that it should not exceed 18 hours in order to reduce postoperative morbidities and length of stay. Busch et al. [33] showed that a delay of more than 12 hours was associated with a significant increase in the rates of perforation. In contrast, another study did not show any significant difference: Partelli et al. [34] reported that delays in performing appendicitis operations did not increase postoperative complications. Similarly, Abou-Nukta et al. [17] reported that delaying appendectomy by 12–24 hours after presentation did not significantly increase the rate of perforation, operative times, or length of stay; furthermore, a recent report by Teixeira et al. [35] found that delays in the time from diagnosis to operation did not increase perforation rates.

The mortality rate of perforated appendicitis in elderly patients was about 2.3% to 10% and most commonly correlated with infection and underlying comorbid disease [8, 11–13]. In our study, there were 2 deaths (1.9%) from sepsis and underlying comorbid disease, similar to the results of other studies.

One limitation of this study was that it was a retrospective one, so that we were unable to collect some significant data which could possibly have affected the outcomes, such as patient race, economic status, type of appendicitis, and CRP level.

5. Conclusion

Male sex, fever ≥38°C, anorexia, and duration of pain in the preadmission period were the significant factors associated with perforated appendicitis in elderly patients in this study.

Conflict of Interests

The authors declare that there is no conflict of interests regarding the publication of this paper.

References

[1] S. I. Schwartz, G. T. Shires, F. C. Spencer, J. M. Daly, J. E. Fisher, and A. C. Galloway, *Principles of Surgery*, McGraw-Hill, New York, NY, USA, 7th edition, 1999.

[2] C. D. Liu and D. W. McFadden, "Acute abdomen and appendix," in *Surgery: Scientific Principles and Practice*, L. J. Greenfield, M. W. Mulholland, K. T. Oldham et al., Eds., pp. 1246–1261, Lippincott-Raven, Philadelphia, Pa, USA, 2nd edition, 1997.

[3] D. G. Addiss, N. Shaffer, B. S. Fowler, and R. V. Tauxe, "The epidemiology of appendicitis and appendectomy in the United States," *The American Journal of Epidemiology*, vol. 132, no. 5, pp. 910–925, 1990.

[4] C. L. Temple, S. A. Huchcroft, and W. J. Temple, "The natural history of appendicitis in adults: a prospective study," *Annals of Surgery*, vol. 221, no. 3, pp. 278–281, 1995.

[5] J. M. Wagner, W. P. McKinney, and J. L. Carpenter, "Does this patient have appendicitis?" *The Journal of the American Medical Association*, vol. 276, no. 19, pp. 1589–1594, 1996.

[6] J. Berry Jr. and R. A. Malt, "Appendicitis near its centenary," *Annals of Surgery*, vol. 200, no. 5, pp. 567–575, 1984.

[7] J. M. Grönroos and P. Grönroos, "Leucocyte count and C-reactive protein in the diagnosis of acute appendicitis," *British Journal of Surgery*, vol. 86, no. 4, pp. 501–504, 1999.

[8] M. G. Franz, J. Norman, and P. J. Fabri, "Increased morbidity of appendicitis with advancing age," *American Surgeon*, vol. 61, no. 1, pp. 40–44, 1995.

[9] S. Luncǎ, G. Bouras, and N. S. Romedea, "Acute appendicitis in the elderly patient: diagnostic problems, prognostic factors and outcomes," *Romanian Journal of Gastroenterology*, vol. 13, no. 4, pp. 299–303, 2004.

[10] R. Rub, D. Margel, D. Soffer, and Y. Kluger, "Appendicitis in the elderly: what has changed?" *Israel Medical Association Journal*, vol. 2, no. 3, pp. 220–223, 2000.

[11] J. F. Y. Lee, C. K. Leow, and W. Y. Lau, "Appendicitis in the elderly," *Australian and New Zealand Journal of Surgery*, vol. 70, no. 8, pp. 593–596, 2000.

[12] P. G. Blomqvist, R. E. B. Andersson, F. Granath, M. P. Lambe, and A. R. Ekbom, "Mortality after appendectomy in Sweden, 1987–1996," *Annals of Surgery*, vol. 233, no. 4, pp. 455–460, 2001.

[13] D. J. Sherlock, "Acute appendicitis in the over-sixty age group," *British Journal of Surgery*, vol. 72, no. 3, pp. 245–246, 1985.

[14] R. Pieper, L. Kager, and P. Nasman, "Acute appendicitis: a clinical study of 1018 cases of emergency appendectomy," *Acta Chirurgica Scandinavica*, vol. 148, no. 1, pp. 51–62, 1982.

[15] D. J. FitzGerald and A. M. Pancioli, "Acute appendicitis," in *Emergency Medicine—A Comprehensive Study Guide*, J. E. Tintinalli, G. D. Kelen, and J. S. Stapczynski, Eds., pp. 520–523, McGraw-Hill, Columbus, Ohio, USA, 2003.

[16] D. R. Flum, A. Morris, T. Koepsell, and E. P. Dellinger, "Has misdiagnosis of appendicitis decreased over time? A

population-based analysis," *The Journal of the American Medical Association*, vol. 286, no. 14, pp. 1748–1753, 2001.

[17] F. Abou-Nukta, C. Bakhos, K. Arroyo et al., "Effects of delaying appendectomy for acute appendicitis for 12 to 24 hours," *Archives of Surgery*, vol. 141, no. 5, pp. 504–507, 2006.

[18] B.-F. Sheu, T.-F. Chiu, J.-C. Chen, M.-S. Tung, M.-W. Chang, and Y.-R. Young, "Risk factors associated with perforated appendicitis in elderly patients presenting with signs and symptoms of acute appendicitis," *ANZ Journal of Surgery*, vol. 77, no. 8, pp. 662–666, 2007.

[19] T. L. Storm-Dickerson and M. C. Horattas, "What have we learned over the past 20 years about appendicitis in the elderly?" *American Journal of Surgery*, vol. 185, no. 3, pp. 198–201, 2003.

[20] A. H. Omari, M. R. Khammash, G. R. Qasaimeh, A. K. Shammari, M. K. B. Yaseen, and S. K. Hammori, "Acute appendicitis in the elderly: risk factors for perforation," *World Journal of Emergency Surgery*, vol. 9, article 6, 2014.

[21] D. Oliak, D. Yamini, V. M. Udani et al., "Can perforated appendicitis be diagnosed preoperatively based on admission factors?" *Journal of Gastrointestinal Surgery*, vol. 4, no. 5, pp. 470–474, 2000.

[22] P. Pruekprasert, A. Geater, P. Ksuntigij, T. Maipang, and N. Apakupakul, "Accuracy in diagnosis of acute appendicitis by comparing serum C-reactive protein measurements, Alvarado score and clinical impression of surgeons," *Journal of the Medical Association of Thailand*, vol. 87, no. 3, pp. 296–303, 2004.

[23] T. Shimizu, M. Ishizuka, and K. Kubota, "A lower neutrophil to lymphocyte ratio is closely associated with catarrhal appendicitis versus severe appendicitis," *Surgery Today*, 2015.

[24] R. Ohle, F. O'Reilly, K. K. O'Brien, T. Fahey, and B. D. Dimitrov, "The Alvarado score for predicting acute appendicitis: a systematic review," *BMC Medicine*, vol. 9, article 139, 2011.

[25] W. B. Smithy, S. D. Wexner, and T. H. Dailey, "The diagnosis and treatment of acute appendicitis in the aged," *Diseases of the Colon and Rectum*, vol. 29, no. 3, pp. 170–173, 1986.

[26] C. I. Ryden, T. Grunditz, and L. Janzon, "Acute appendicitis in patients above and below 60 years of age. Incidence rate and clinical course," *Acta Chirurgica Scandinavica*, vol. 149, no. 2, pp. 165–170, 1983.

[27] S. Eldar, E. Nash, E. Sabo et al., "Delay of surgery in acute appendicitis," *American Journal of Surgery*, vol. 173, no. 3, pp. 194–198, 1997.

[28] H. Körner, K. Söndenaa, J. A. Söreide et al., "Incidence of acute nonperforated and perforated appendicitis: age-specific and sex-specific analysis," *World Journal of Surgery*, vol. 21, no. 3, pp. 313–317, 1997.

[29] T. Augustin, B. Cagir, and T. J. VanderMeer, "Characteristics of perforated appendicitis effect of delay is confounded by age and gender," *Journal of Gastrointestinal Surgery*, vol. 15, no. 7, pp. 1223–1231, 2011.

[30] M. Singh, Y. Kadian, K. Rattan, and B. Jangra, "Complicated appendicitis: analysis of risk factors in children," *African Journal of Paediatric Surgery*, vol. 11, no. 2, pp. 109–113, 2014.

[31] C. S. Gardner, T. A. Jaffe, and R. C. Nelson, "Impact of CT in elderly patients presenting to the emergency department with acute abdominal pain," *Abdominal Imaging*, 2015.

[32] F. N. Eko, G. E. Ryb, L. Drager, E. Goldwater, J. J. Wu, and T. C. Counihan, "Ideal timing of surgery for acute uncomplicated appendicitis," *North American Journal of Medical Sciences*, vol. 5, no. 1, pp. 22–27, 2013.

[33] M. Busch, F. S. Gutzwiller, S. Aellig, R. Kuettel, U. Metzger, and U. Zingg, "In-hospital delay increases the risk of perforation in adults with appendicitis," *World Journal of Surgery*, vol. 35, no. 7, pp. 1626–1633, 2011.

[34] S. Partelli, S. Beg, J. Brown, S. Vyas, and H. M. Kocher, "Alteration in emergency theatre prioritisation does not alter outcome for acute appendicitis: comparative cohort study," *World Journal of Emergency Surgery*, vol. 4, no. 1, article 22, 2009.

[35] P. G. Teixeira, E. Sivrikoz, K. Inaba, P. Talving, L. Lam, and D. Demetriades, "Appendectomy timing: waiting until the next morning increases the risk of surgical site infections," *Annals of Surgery*, vol. 256, no. 3, pp. 538–543, 2012.

13

An Assessment of the Clinical and Economic Impact of Establishing Ileocolic Anastomoses in Right-Colon Resection Surgeries Using Mechanical Staplers Compared to Hand-Sewn Technique

S. Roy,[1] S. Ghosh,[2] and A. Yoo[3]

[1]Global Health Economics and Market Access, Ethicon, Somerville, NJ 08876, USA
[2]Global Health Economics and Market Access, Ethicon, Cincinnati, OH 45242, USA
[3]Medical Devices Epidemiology, Johnson & Johnson, New Brunswick, NJ 08901, USA

Correspondence should be addressed to S. Roy; sanjroy@gmail.com

Academic Editor: Pramateftakis Manousos-Georgios

Purpose. To estimate and compare clinical outcomes and costs associated with mechanical stapling versus hand-sewn sutured technique in creation of ileocolic anastomoses after right sided colon surgery. *Methods.* A previously conducted meta-analysis was updated for estimates of anastomotic leak rates and other clinical outcomes. A value analysis model was developed to estimate cost savings due to improved outcomes in a hypothetical cohort of 100 patients who underwent right colon surgery involving either mechanical stapling or hand-sewn anastomoses. Cost data were obtained from publicly available literature. *Results.* Findings from the updated meta-analysis reported that the mechanical stapling group had lower anastomotic leaks 2.4% ($n = 11/457$) compared to the hand-sewn group 6.1% leaks ($n = 44/715$). Utilizing this data, the value analysis model estimated total potential cost savings for a hospital to be around $1,130,656 for the 100-patient cohort using mechanical stapling instead of hand-sewn suturing, after accounting for incremental supplies cost of $49,400. These savings were attributed to lower index surgery costs, reduced OR time costs, and reduced reoperation costs driven by lower anastomotic leak rates associated with mechanical stapling. *Conclusion.* Mechanical stapling can be considered as a clinically and economically favorable option compared to suturing for establishing anastomoses in patients undergoing right colon surgery.

1. Introduction

Ileocolic resection is the most frequently performed surgical procedure for the treatment of right-sided colorectal cancer and Crohn's disease [1]. Surgical treatment for these conditions includes resection of the diseased bowel and formation of an ileocolic anastomosis. Anastomotic leak is one of the most dreaded postoperative complications in patients particularly after resection of the colon and the rectum. Further, reoperations and complications such as leaks are considered a quality indicator in colorectal surgery [2]. The prevalence of anastomotic leaks after colon and rectal resection varies by anatomic location with lower frequencies in right sided anastomoses. The reported range

for radiologically identified leaks is between 0.5% and 21% while the incidence of clinically significant anastomotic leaks after colorectal surgeries is between 1% and 12% and up to 10% to 14% in low colorectal resections [2]. Overall, patients with anastomotic leaks after colorectal surgery have significantly greater chances of morbidity (56%) and mortality rates of up to 32 % [3]. In addition to the clinical complications there is a significant economic burden to be considered as multiple reoperations, radiologic interventions, and stoma creation are often necessary to control leaks, and hospital length of stay for these patients is reported to be longer thus resulting in an increase in health care cost compared to patients with no leaks. Therefore, anastomotic leaks can impose a significant burden on patients and health care providers.

TABLE 1: Study inclusion criteria for the systematic review and meta-analysis.

Criterion	Included
Population	Age: ≥18 years
	Race: any
	Gender: male or female
	Studies conducted in humans only
	Patients receiving elective or emergency stapled and hand-sewn ileocolic anastomoses
Type of studies	RCTs comparing mechanical stapling and hand-sewn suturing related to colon resection and colonic anastomosis, meta-analysis, systematic reviews, comparative prospective nonrandomized observational studies, and comparative retrospective reviews
Language	English only
Country	Any
Sample size	Any
Intervention	Mechanical stapling versus hand-sewn suturing
Primary outcome	Overall anastomotic leak rates

Over the years, various techniques of colorectal anastomosis have been developed in search of one with lower rate of postoperative complications [4]. The introduction of stapling devices has helped to revolutionize the technical aspects of surgery that has allowed minimally invasive procedures to be developed and performed more quickly than manual sutures. Findings from a recent Cochrane systematic review and meta-analysis reported that stapled colorectal anastomosis resulted in significant reduction in anastomotic leaks compared to hand-sewn technique in right colon resections. Leak rates after colorectal surgery using stapled and hand-sewn anastomosis have been reported in the literature to be around 8% and 27%, respectively [5]. In addition, stapled ileocolic anastomoses took on an average 8.7 minutes compared to 22.4 minutes for hand-sewn technique [1].

A number of benefits conferred by the use of stapling techniques include uniformity of surgical technique, minimal tissue manipulation and trauma, less bleeding and edema at the site of anastomosis, a quicker return of gastrointestinal functions, and more rapid patient recovery which together have made the technique a desirable alternative for anastomosis compared to hand-sewing with sutures [6]. Conversely, stapling techniques have also been criticized on the grounds of expense and low improvements in anastomotic outcomes. Despite comparable results in terms of mortality, anastomotic leaks, and wound infection, the rate of stricture at the anastomotic site has been reported as considerably higher with staples than with sutures: around 8% versus 2%, respectively, for colorectal anastomosis [7].

Therefore, there is an ongoing search for an ideal method of establishing an anastomosis that will not only lower the incidence of dangerous complications but also avoid the need for reoperations. Additionally, there is limited evidence in the literature outlining the economic value of using one technique over the other for ileocolic anastomosis.

The main objectives of this study were (1) to update earlier estimates of anastomotic leak rates following ileocolic anastomosis performed using mechanical stapling and hand-sewn techniques and (2) to develop a value analysis model to estimate and compare the treatment costs associated with the two surgical options for patients undergoing elective or emergency ileocolic anastomosis from a hospital perspective.

2. Methods

2.1. Literature Review and Meta-Analysis. A comprehensive systematic search of literature was conducted using MED-LINE, EMBASE, Scopus, Cochrane library, and trial registry databases to identify studies from a period of January 1990 to December 2013 comparing clinical outcomes associated with mechanical stapling and hand-sewn suturing for ileocolic anastomosis in adults. Studies that used mechanical stapler (side-to-side or functional end-to-end) or manual suturing (hand-sewn) for ileocolic anastomosis were reviewed. The primary outcome of interest was overall anastomotic leak rates for each technique while some of the secondary outcomes of interest were rates of reoperation, anastomosis time, and length of hospital stay. The review was conducted and reported according to QUORUM guidelines. The titles and abstracts of articles found in the original search were screened by two independent reviewers. Following that, full texts of eligible studies were obtained and another reviewer independently determined the eligibility of each publication by applying a set of criteria described in Table 1. Cited references from included trials and reviews of similar trials were also searched. All studies that met the inclusion criteria were included in the review. Two independent reviewers extracted study characteristics, baseline, and outcomes data. The methodological quality of publications was assessed using the criteria previously reported in an earlier Cochrane review [1]. A third reviewer checked the resulting extractions and resolved any discrepancies. Parameters that were extracted from each study included study type, country, procedure, reason for right colon resection surgery, anastomosis location, sample size, number of patients with anastomotic leaks in each group, methods of anastomotic leak diagnosis, time required for anastomosis, nonleak complication rate, and overall complication rate. Meta-analysis was conducted

TABLE 2: Cost inputs included in value analysis model.

Parameters	Base case	Source	Scenario analysis	Source
Cost per linear stapler	$300.00	Assumption		
Cost per stapler reload	$100.00	Assumption		
Cost per 15-minute block of anesthesia time [10]	$71.62	Byrd and Singh, 2010	$35.81	
Incremental index hospitalization costs for patients with leaks [9]	$24,129.00	Hammond et al., 2014	$12,064.50	50% reduction; assumption
Average cost of a colorectal surgery without a leak [9]	$44,308.00	Hammond et al., 2014	$22,154.00	
Number of stapler reloads used per anastomosis	2	Assumption		
Cost per suture strand	$3.00	Assumption		
Charge per minute of OR time [8]	$62.19	Shippert, 2005	$31.10	
Incremental readmission costs for patients with leaks [9]	$6,409.00	Hammond et al., 2014	$3,204.50	50% reduction; assumption
Number of sutures used per anastomosis	2	Assumption		

to pool results for the outcomes of interest using the RevMan 5 software. Outcomes were summarized as odds ratios (OR) using the Mantel-Haenszel fixed-effects modeling with Chisquare test for heterogeneity.

2.2. Value Analysis. A cohort approach was used to develop a value analysis model to understand the financial implications for a hospital utilizing mechanical stapling versus hand-sewn sutured anastomoses. The model focused on estimating cost savings due to reduced leak rates, lower number of reoperations/readmission rates, and reduced operating room time associated with each technique using a hospital perspective. The target population evaluated in the model consisted of patients who underwent elective or emergency open right colon surgery using either mechanical stapling or hand-sewn sutured anastomosis. The model leveraged the leak rates data from the review and meta-analysis described above and utilized those rates to calculate differences in incidence and costs related to leaks, both in the index procedure and for readmission. In addition, for other outcomes, such as risk of reoperation and anastomosis time, the model included data from the literature that were identified during the review but not included in the meta-analysis, primarily as they were not randomized controlled trials.

All cost data were obtained from publicly available literature. Table 2 lists the cost inputs used for calculating costs related to ileocolic anastomoses in a hypothetical cohort of 100 patients compared between mechanical stapling with manual suturing. The cost of colorectal surgery with and without leaks was based on the findings of a recent retrospective analysis conducted in 6,174 patients in the United States, where anastomoses were established using mechanical stapling or hand-sewn suturing [8]. An average cost of $44,308 for a colorectal surgery without a leak was used in the model. Furthermore, as patients with anastomotic leaks had 1.3 times higher 30-day readmission risk, the incremental cost of readmissions of $6,409 was used in the analysis [9]. Direct cost for anesthetic services (i.e., cost per 15-minute block of

anesthesia time) was obtained from published results of the American Society of Anesthesiologists survey [10].

As mechanical stapling was expected to result in a more favorable cost outcome, a scenario analysis was conducted by forcing model inputs to be significantly less favorable to the mechanical stapling option in order to examine the level of robustness of the data.

3. Results

The literature review identified four new studies in addition to those that were already included in an earlier Cochrane review. Overall twelve studies that met the study inclusion criteria were identified for the review, of which eight were randomized control trials (RCTs), three were retrospective assessments, and one was a prospective study. There were no significant differences between most of the patient baseline characteristics. Follow-up duration ranged from 30 days after discharge to a median of 87 months [13, 15].

Eight RCTs with a total of 1,172 patients with ileocolic anastomosis were included in the pooled meta-analysis. Details of the RCTs included in the analysis are presented in Table 3. Of the RCTs included, 2 studies were from Germany, 2 were from Scotland, 1 was from France, 1 was from Japan, 1 was from US, and 1 was a global study with patients from US, UK, and Canada. The nonrandomized studies were conducted in UK and Italy. The main findings from the study demonstrated that the mechanical stapling group had lower (2.4%) anastomotic leaks ($n = 11/457$) compared to 6.1% leaks reported ($n = 44/715$) in the hand-sewn group (Table 4). Overall, the mechanical stapling group had significantly lower odds (0.46; 95% CI = 0.24–0.89; $P = 0.02$) of anastomotic leaks compared with the hand-sewn anastomosis group (Figure 1).

The rate of reoperation, when reported, was also lower for the mechanical stapling group compared to the hand-sutured group, with the difference ranging from 4.3% to 26.1% in one study [18]. Furthermore, mechanical stapling was faster

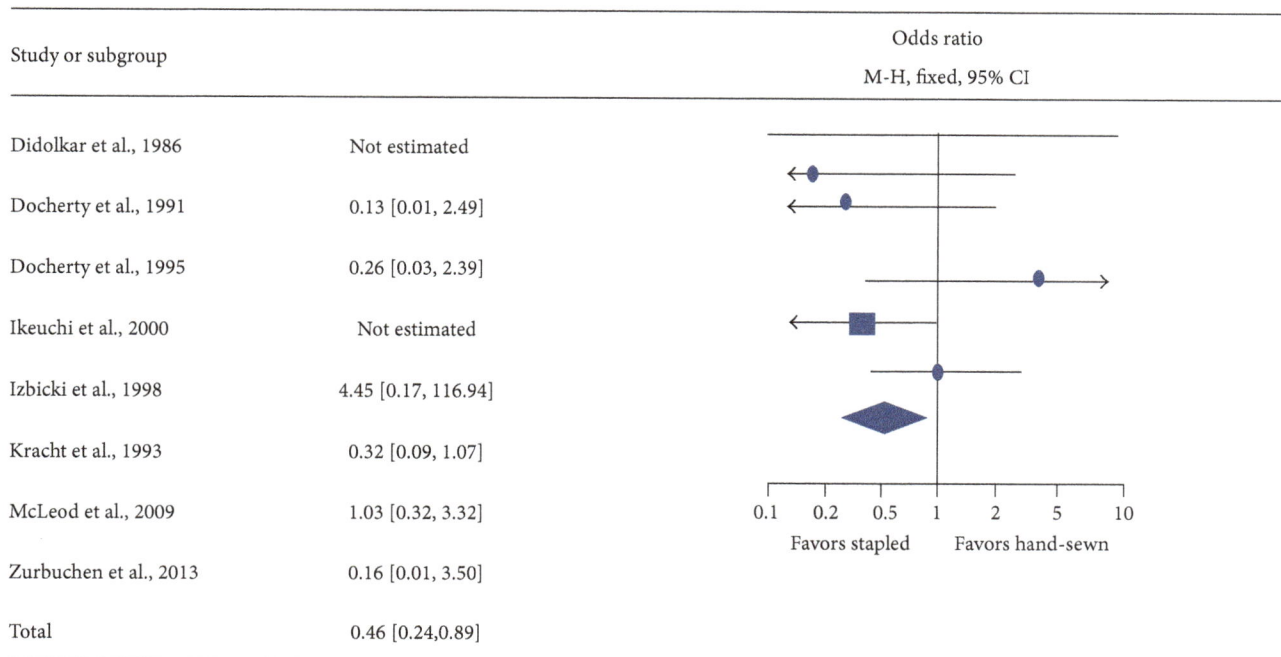

Study or subgroup		Odds ratio M-H, fixed, 95% CI
Didolkar et al., 1986	Not estimated	
Docherty et al., 1991	0.13 [0.01, 2.49]	
Docherty et al., 1995	0.26 [0.03, 2.39]	
Ikeuchi et al., 2000	Not estimated	
Izbicki et al., 1998	4.45 [0.17, 116.94]	
Kracht et al., 1993	0.32 [0.09, 1.07]	
McLeod et al., 2009	1.03 [0.32, 3.32]	
Zurbuchen et al., 2013	0.16 [0.01, 3.50]	
Total	0.46 [0.24, 0.89]	

FIGURE 1: Forrest plot of comparison using data from all studies for anastomotic leak rates.

TABLE 3: Clinical trials included in the meta-analysis.

Study or subgroup	Year	Stapled		Hand-sewn		Weight	Odds ratio
		Events	Total N	Events	Total N		M-H, fixed, 95% CI
Didolkar et al. [11]	1986	0	22	0	16		Not estimated
Docherty et al. [12]	1991	0	70	4	87	13.6%	0.13 [0.01, 2.49]
Kracht et al. [13]	1993	3	106	26	334	44.5%	0.32 [0.09, 1.07]
Docherty et al. [6]	1995	1	133	4	122	12.9%	0.26 [0.03, 2.39]
Izbicki et al. [14]	1998	1	15	0	21	1.3%	4.45 [0.17, 116.94]
Ikeuchi et al [15]	2000	0	11	0	18		Not estimated
McLeod et al. [16]	2009	6	84	6	86	18.7%	1.03 [0.32, 3.32]
Zurbuchen et al. [17]	2013	0	36	2	31	9.0%	0.16 [0.01, 3.50]

TABLE 4: Postoperative anastomotic leak rates between the two groups as reported in the articles included in the review.

Study or subgroup	Stapled		Hand-sewn		Weight	Odds ratio
	Events	Total N	Events	Total N		M-H, fixed, 95% CI
Total (95% CI)	—	457	—	715	100%	0.46 [0.24, 0.89]
Total events	11	—	44	—		—

Heterogenecity Chi^2 = 5.39, df = 5 (P = 0.37), and I^2 = 7%.
Test for overall effect: Z = 2.31 (P = 0.02).

and saved on average 13.6 minutes per patient compared to hand-sewn technique in a study that captured and reported anastomosis time [6]. Tables 2 and 5 report economic and clinical estimates from the meta-analysis and from other pieces of published literature that were included in the value analysis. Inputs used in the scenario analysis are described in Tables 2 and 5.

Findings from the value analysis model demonstrated that with the included inputs and assumptions ileocolic anastomosis established in a cohort of 100 patients using mechanical stapling instead of hand-sewn suturing could result in significant savings for a hospital. The savings were estimated at around $1,130,656 for the cohort of 100 patients or about $11,000 per patient procedure. The savings were net of incremental supplies cost of about $50,000 that reduced the overall savings by about 4%. The cost savings were primarily realized through avoidance of incremental costs, both in the index procedure [$96,516 (9%)] and in

TABLE 5: Clinical inputs included in value analysis model.

Parameters	Base case		Scenario analysis		
	Stapled	Hand-sewn	Stapled	Hand-sewn	Source
Overall leak rate [1]	2.49%	6.14%	2.49%	3.07%	50% reduction for hand-sewn
Reoperation rate [15]	4.3%	26.1%	4.3%	13.1%	
Average time for anastomosis [1]	8.72 min	22.36 min	13.84 min	10.82 min	Most difference found in the literature

TABLE 6: Potential cost savings using mechanical staplers.

Parameters	Base case results	% contribution to savings	Scenario analyses results
Total number of patients using open mechanical staplers	100		100
Potential OR time savings	23 hours		−5 hours
Supplies cost for open mechanical staplers	$50,000	−4%	$50,000
Supplies cost for sutures	$600		$600
Potential savings in OR time cost	$84,827	8%	$ −9,391
Potential savings in anesthesia cost	$7,162	1%	$3,581
Potential savings in index surgery costs through avoided anastomotic leaks	$96,516	9%	$12,065
Potential savings in readmission costs through avoided anastomotic leaks	$25,636	2%	$3,205
Potential savings in reoperation costs	$965,914	85%	$193,848
Net savings using open mechanical staplers	$1,130,656	100%	$153,907
Net savings per patient using open mechanical staplers	$11,307		$1,539

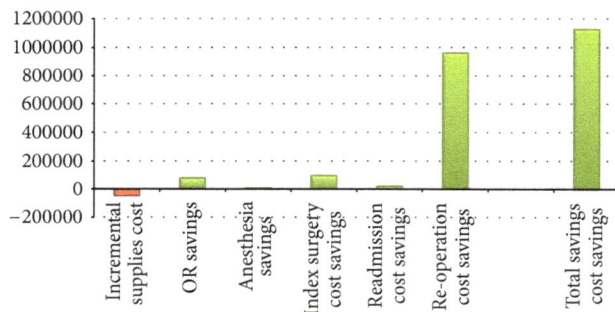

FIGURE 2: Potential cost savings using mechanical staplers.

readmissions [$25,636 (2%)] that were made possible with reduced anastomotic leak rates with mechanical stapling compared to hand suturing. Large savings of $965,914 (85%) could be achieved due to lower rates of reoperations/readmissions for patients who had mechanical stapling. Furthermore, from a hospital perspective, as mechanical stapling is faster compared to hand-sewn suturing, the requirement for anesthetic services and OR time was substantially lower, leading to cost savings of about $7,162 (1%) and $84,827 (8%), respectively (Figure 2). In addition, owing to the shorter time taken for the anastomosis, the collective gain in operating room time could be close to 23 hours for the cohort of 100 procedures, thus freeing up the operating room for potential additional patient care utilization. Table 6 represents key results from the value analysis model.

Results of the model were robust to the effect of conservative assumptions employed in a scenario analysis. Table 6 presents the corresponding results which show that in spite of enforcing significant reductions in potentially better outcomes with stapling the hypothetical hospital could retain an overall net saving of about $153,907 which translates to a saving of about $1,539 per person.

4. Discussion

Anastomotic leaks are among the most prevalent and detrimental complications that occur after colorectal surgery. Postoperative anastomotic leaks remain a significant complication and are associated with high morbidity, mortality, reoperation, and duration of hospitalization [19–23]. In cases of surgery for malignant pathology, anastomotic leakage is related to diminished five-year disease-specific survival and higher local recurrence rates [11, 21, 24]. It is therefore imperative for health care providers to find optimal techniques to prevent postoperative anastomotic leaks which can possibly help to ease the associated clinical and economic burden. It has been documented that anastomotic leaks are the strongest indicators of hospital costs in colorectal surgeries and impose a significant economic burden on patients and health care providers due to additional readmission rates, reoperations, postoperative infections, and longer durations of hospital stay [25]. Patients with anastomotic leaks have a 1.3-fold greater chance of readmission within a 30-day period compared to those without leaks which leads to a significant increase in the overall cost of care. It has been reported that patients with leaks spend approximately 7 days more in a hospital with average incremental costs of $24,129 compared to those without leaks [9]. The total burden of leaks in terms of length of stay per 1,000 patients was 16,800 and 26,300 days for patients with no leaks and with leaks, respectively [9]. Furthermore, the total cost burden per 1,000 patients was reported to be $44.3 million in patients with no leaks as compared to $72.9 million for those with leaks, which further highlights the negative impact of anastomotic leaks and underscores the importance of cost reductions for patients and hospitals using appropriate anastomotic techniques [9].

In recent years, to inform decision-making by surgeons, evidence has been generated to show how certain anastomotic techniques, such as the stapled side-to-side technique, are more advantageous while considering treatment for specific conditions such as cancer and Crohn's disease as they are simple, uniform, reliable, and safe to perform [24, 26]. This is also supported by results from the meta analysis conducted in the current study which suggests the possibility of clinical benefit from the use of mechanical stapling following a right colon resection due to lower anastomotic leaks compared to hand-sewn technique especially if the operation is performed in patients with colon cancer. The study also estimates potential cost savings from a hospital perspective that can be availed using mechanical stapling technique, where appropriate.

While the present study outlines the advantages of mechanical stapling, there are few potential limitations that need to be considered. The study modeled net cost savings of using mechanical stapling for ileocolic resections by making certain assumptions and utilizing data from published literature for key parameters which makes the findings subject to all general limitations applicable for such assessments. The model arguably presents a conservative assessment of potential benefit of the lesser risk of anastomotic leaks as it does not consider costs associated with mortality. While anastomotic leak rates were found to be lower with stapling, it is also important to mention for fair balance that studies included in the review reported additional outcomes, some of which were better in the hand-sutured group of patients. While these outcomes may or may not have had any direct impact on leak rates, they could potentially somewhat reduce expected savings from reduction in leak rates.

One important consideration relevant to the effectiveness of device use and surgical technique is the level of skill a surgeon possesses. This study does not account for the potential impact of surgeon skills and learning curve upon the surgical outcome. As this is one of the first studies to quantify the financial benefits of mechanical stapling compared to suturing in the establishment of an ileocolic anastomosis using a model built on evidence from literature, future research needs to focus on conducting real-world studies to support this finding.

5. Conclusion

In conclusion, the results of this study underscore the potential clinical and economic benefits of mechanical stapling compared to hand-sutured anastomosis in right colon surgery. Such benefits are attributed to cost reduction owing to a meaningful reduction in the risk of anastomotic leaks which likely results in reduced length of inpatient stay, lower rate of readmission and reoperation postdischarge, and shortened anastomosis time.

Conflict of Interests

All authors are employees and stock holders of Johnson & Johnson who are among several companies that manufacture and sell medical devices included in the analyses presented in this paper.

Acknowledgments

The authors are indebted to Saurabh (Rob) Aggarwal of Novel Health Strategies LLC, Columbia, MD, for his technical assistance in executing the meta-analysis and the development of the value analysis model, and to Shalaka Marfatia of pharmEDGE, Syosset, NY, for her assistance with the writing of the paper.

References

[1] P. Y. G. Choy, I. P. Bisset, J. G. Docherty et al., "Stapled versus handsewn methods for ileocolic anastomosis," *Cochrane Database of Systematic Reviews*, no. 9, Article ID CD004320, 2011.

[2] A. M. Morris, L.-M. Baldwin, B. Matthews et al., "Reoperation as a quality indicator in colorectal surgery: a population-based analysis," *Annals of Surgery*, vol. 245, no. 1, pp. 73–79, 2007.

[3] H.-K. Choi, W.-L. Law, and J. W. C. Ho, "Leakage after resection and intraperitoneal anastomosis for colorectal malignancy: analysis of risk factors," *Diseases of the Colon & Rectum*, vol. 49, no. 11, pp. 1719–1725, 2006.

[4] E. Fouda, A. El Nakeeb, A. Magdy, E. A. Hammad, G. Othman, and M. Farid, "Early detection of anastomotic leakage after elective low anterior Resection," *Journal of Gastrointestinal Surgery*, vol. 15, no. 1, pp. 137–144, 2011.

[5] A. Gajda and K. Bielecki, *The Causes and Prevention of Anastomotic Leak After Colorectal Surgery*, Department of General Surgery, Orbowski hospital, Warsaw, Poland, 1999.

[6] J. G. Docherty, J. R. McGregor, A. M. Akyol, G. D. Murray, and D. J. Galloway, "Comparison of manually constructed and stapled anastomoses in colorectal surgery," *Annals of Surgery*, vol. 221, no. 2, pp. 176–184, 1995.

[7] S. A. Lustosa, D. Matos, A. N. Atallah, and A. A. Castro, "Stapled versus handsewn methods for colorectal anastomosis surgery," *Cochrane Database of Systematic Reviews*, Article ID CD003144, 2001.

[8] R. Shippert, "A study of time-dependent operating room fees and how to save $100000 by using time-saving products," *American Journal of Cosmetic Surgery*, vol. 22, no. 1, pp. 25–33, 2005.

[9] J. Hammond, S. Lim, Y. Wan, X. Gao, and A. Patkar, "The burden of gastrointestinal anastomotic leaks: an evaluation of clinical and economic outcomes," *Journal of Gastrointestinal Surgery*, vol. 18, no. 6, pp. 1176–1185, 2014.

[10] J. R. Byrd and L. Singh, "ASA survey results for commercial fees paid for anesthesia services—2010," *American Society of Anesthesiologists*, vol. 74, no. 10, pp. 44–47, 2010.

[11] M. S. Didolkar, W. P. Reed, E. G. Elias, L. A. Schnaper, S. D. Brown, and S. M. Chaudhary, "A prospective randomized study of sutured versus stapled bowel anastomoses in patients with cancer," *Cancer*, vol. 57, no. 3, pp. 456–460, 1986.

[12] J. G. Docherty, E. Rankin, and D. J. Galloway, "Anastomotic integrity and local recurrence after colorectal cancersurgery," Personal communication: J. G. Docherty, 1991.

[13] M. Kracht, J.-M. Hay, P.-L. Fagniez, and A. Fingerhut, "Ileocolonic anastomosis after right hemicolectomy for carcinoma: stapled or hand-sewn?" *International Journal of Colorectal Disease*, vol. 8, no. 1, pp. 29–33, 1993.

[14] J. R. Izbicki, K. A. Gawad, S. Quirrenbach et al., "Can stapled anastomosis in visceral surgery still be justified? A prospective controlled randomized study of the cost-effectiveness of hand-sewn and stapled anastomoses," *Chirurg*, vol. 69, no. 7, pp. 725–734, 1998.

[15] H. Ikeuchi, M. Kusunoki, and T. Yamamura, "Long-term results of stapled and hand-sewn anastomoses in patients with Crohn's disease," *Digestive Surgery*, vol. 17, no. 5, pp. 493–496, 2000.

[16] R. S. McLeod, B. G. Wolff, S. Ross, R. Parkes, and M. McKenzie, "Recurrence of Crohn's disease after ileocolic resection is not affected by anastomotic type: results of a multicenter, randomized, controlled trial," *Diseases of the Colon and Rectum*, vol. 52, no. 5, pp. 919–927, 2009.

[17] U. Zurbuchen, A. J. Kroesen, P. Knebel et al., "Complications after end-to-end vs. side-to-side anastomosis in ileocecal Crohn's disease—early postoperative results from a randomized controlled multi-center trial (ISRCTN-45665492)," *Langenbeck's Archives of Surgery*, vol. 398, no. 3, pp. 467–474, 2013.

[18] M. Muñoz-Juárez, T. Yamamoto, B. G. Wolff, M. R. B. Keighley, and N. Mortensen, "Wide-lumen stapled anastomosis vs. conventional end-to-end anastomosis in the treatment of Crohn's disease," *Diseases of the Colon and Rectum*, vol. 44, no. 1, pp. 20–25, 2001.

[19] J. T. Mäkelä, H. Kiviniemi, and S. Laitinen, "Risk factors for anastomotic leakage after left-sided colorectal resection with rectal anastomosis," *Diseases of the Colon & Rectum*, vol. 46, no. 5, pp. 653–660, 2003.

[20] H. S. Snijders, M. W. J. M. Wouters, N. J. van Leersum et al., "Meta-analysis of the risk for anastomotic leakage, the postoperative mortality caused by leakage in relation to the overall postoperative mortality," *European Journal of Surgical Oncology*, vol. 38, no. 11, pp. 1013–1019, 2012.

[21] K. G. Walker, S. W. Bell, M. J. F. X. Rickard et al., "Anastomotic leakage is predictive of diminished survival after potentially curative resection for colorectal cancer," *Annals of Surgery*, vol. 240, no. 2, pp. 255–259, 2004.

[22] R. Golub, R. W. Golub, R. Cantu Jr., and H. D. Stein, "A multivariate analysis of factors contributing to leakage of intestinal anastomoses," *Journal of the American College of Surgeons*, vol. 184, no. 4, pp. 364–372, 1997.

[23] I. Kanellos, K. Blouhos, H. Demetriades et al., "The failed intraperitoneal colon anastomosis after colon resection," *Techniques in Coloproctology*, vol. 8, no. 1, supplement, pp. S53–S55, 2004.

[24] C. Simillis, S. Purkayastha, T. Yamamoto, S. A. Strong, A. W. Darzi, and P. P. Tekkis, "A meta-analysis comparing conventional end-to-end anastomosis vs. other anastomotic configurations after resection in Crohn's disease," *Diseases of the Colon & Rectum*, vol. 50, no. 10, pp. 1674–1687, 2007.

[25] R. Vonlanthen, K. Slankamenac, S. Breitenstein et al., "The impact of complications on costs of major surgical procedures: a cost analysis of 1200 patients," *Annals of Surgery*, vol. 254, no. 6, pp. 907–913, 2011.

[26] J. Ruiz-Tovar, J. Santos, A. Arroyo et al., "Microbiological spectrum of the intraperitoneal surface after elective right-sided colon cancer: are there differences in the peritoneal contamination after performing a stapled or a handsewn anastomosis," *International Journal of Colorectal Disease*, vol. 27, no. 11, pp. 1515–1519, 2012.

Knowledge, Practice, and Associated Factors towards Prevention of Surgical Site Infection among Nurses Working in Amhara Regional State Referral Hospitals, Northwest Ethiopia

Freahiywot Aklew Teshager,[1] Eshetu Haileselassie Engeda,[2] and Workie Zemene Worku[2]

[1]*Gondar University Referral Hospital, University of Gondar, P.O. Box 196, Gondar, Ethiopia*
[2]*Department of Nursing, College of Medicine and Health Sciences, University of Gondar, P.O. Box 196, Gondar, Ethiopia*

Correspondence should be addressed to Eshetu Haileselassie Engeda; eshet143@gmail.com

Academic Editor: Thomas Strecker

Knowledge and practice of nurses about surgical site infections (SSIs) are not well studied in Ethiopia. This paper contains findings about Northwest Ethiopian nurses' knowledge and practice regarding the prevention of SSIs. The main objective of the study was to assess knowledge, practice, and associated factors of nurses towards the prevention of SSIs. The study was done using a questionnaire survey on randomly selected 423 nurses who were working in referral hospitals during the study period. The study showed that more than half of the nurses who participated in the survey had inadequate knowledge about the prevention of SSIs. Moreover, more than half of them were practicing inappropriately. The most important associated factors include lack of training on evidence based guidelines and sociodemographic variables (age, year of service, educational status, etc.). Training of nurses with the up-to-date SSIs guidelines is recommended.

1. Background

Worldwide, healthcare associated infections (HAIs) constitute a major public health problem affecting millions of people every year [1]. Estimates of recent studies in developed countries indicated that at least 5% of hospitalized patients acquire infection [2]. Although the burden of HAIs in Africa is not well studied, a systematic review in the region reported that it is frequently much higher than in the developed nations [1, 3]. Most literatures revealed that surgical site infections (SSIs) were the most common healthcare associated infections accounting for more than 30% of cases of HAIs [4, 5].

Surgical site infections are defined as infections that occur within 30 days of the operation if no implant is left in place or within 1 year of operation if an implant is left in place and the infection appears to be related to the operation in general surgery [6]. A systematic review in Korea reported up to 9.7% incidence rate of SSIs [7] and an Ethiopian study on patients following obstetric surgery revealed a higher rate of 11.4% [8]. Throughout the literature, SSIs were associated with intrinsic factors including advanced age, malnutrition, metabolic diseases, smoking, obesity, hypoxia, immune-suppression, and length of preoperative stay [9]. Moreover, extrinsic factors like application of skin antiseptics, preoperative shaving, antibiotic prophylaxis, preoperative skin preparation, inadequate sterilization of instruments, surgical drains, surgical hand scrubs, and dressing techniques were among the most frequently reported risk factors [10, 11].

Nurses, working around the clock, are in an ideal position to participate or play a leading role in taking initiatives that aimed to ensure quality of care and thus to enhance patient safety which includes prevention of SSIs [12]. However, a significant number of studies indicated that most nurses lacked the required knowledge about prevention of SSIs and the majority of them did not practice properly according to evidence-based guidelines and recommendations [13, 14].

According to the literature, factors associated with knowledge and practice of nurses towards the prevention of SSIs include but are not limited to work experience, level of nursing education, work load, training on infection prevention mechanisms, and nonadherence in infection prevention and patient safety guidelines [15, 16]. In some studies, insufficient utilization of available evidences was also observed [17].

The World Health Organization (WHO), in its guideline for safe surgery, has set a number of recommendations regarding the prevention of SSIs. According to this guideline, highly recommended practices to prevent SSIs include routine use of prophylactic antibiotic within 60 minutes prior to skin incision, the use of sterility indicators during sterilization of surgical instruments, presurgical skin disinfection, and the implementation of surgical safety checklist [18].

Despite the availability of some studies in the developed countries, evidences regarding the level of knowledge and practice towards prevention of SSIs and associated factors are very limited in Africa. A systematic review on SSIs in the region has also revealed that there is a critical shortage of evidences particularly in Sub-Saharan Africa including Ethiopia [3]. Therefore, this study was aimed at assessing knowledge, practice, and associated factors regarding prevention of surgical site infection among nurses working in two selected hospitals in Amhara Regional State, Northwest Ethiopia.

2. Materials and Methods

Institution-based cross-sectional study was conducted from March 10 to 25, 2015, in two randomly selected referral hospitals (Gondar University Referral Hospital and Debre Markos Referral Hospital) of Amhara regional State, Ethiopia. Gondar University Referral Hospital is found in Gondar Town 748 km far from Addis Ababa to the Northwest of Ethiopia. It is a teaching hospital which acts as a referral center for the nearby general hospitals. Having more than 500 inpatient beds, it provides referral services for over 5 million inhabitants in the northwest region of Ethiopia. Debre Markos Referral Hospital is also among the study sites, which is found in Debre Markos Town 305 km far from Addis Ababa to the Northwest of Ethiopia. This hospital has 400 inpatient beds and acts as a referral center for general hospitals in the area and serves 5 million inhabitants.

Sample size was determined by using single population proportion formula by considering the following assumptions: 95% confidence interval (CI), 50% proportion (since there was no previous study in the study areas), and 5% marginal error. By adding 10% nonresponse rate, the final sample size was 423. Since the study hospitals followed a yearly rotation policy (interdepartmental rotation), all nurses of the two hospitals were included in the study regardless of their working area. Simple random sampling technique was used to select the study participants. The samples were proportionally allocated to each hospital and respondents were selected using computer generated random number.

The outcome measures of this study were knowledge (knowledgeable/not knowledgeable) and practice (good practice/not good practice) of nurses regarding prevention of surgical site infection. The independent variables included sociodemographic characteristics (age, sex, marital status, religion, ethnicity, level of education, and work experience) and institutional factors (training about infection prevention, availability of antiseptic solution, availability of antibiotic prophylaxis, and availability of personal protective equipment).

English version of structured and pretested self-administered questionnaire was used to collect the data (English is the medium of instruction in all Ethiopian nursing schools). Nurse's knowledge regarding the prevention of SSIs was measured by 12 multiple choice questions in which only one correct answer was found. The questions addressed the most important recommendations by the national infection prevention and patient safety guideline (about correct time of prophylactic antibiotics, presurgical skin preparation, techniques of surgical wound dressing, etc.). On the other hand, nurses' practice in the prevention of SSIs was measured by 12 items in which responses were answered in a 3-point Likert scale (never practice, sometimes practice, and always practice).

Four diploma holders for data collection (two for each hospital) and two B.S. holders for supervision (one for each hospital) were recruited during the data collection period (both the data collectors and the supervisors were not from the same hospitals). At each hospital the aim of the study was clearly explained to the study participants before they filled the questionnaire. The data collectors and supervisors were trained for one day on how to facilitate the data collection process and prevent errors. Questionnaires were reviewed and checked for completeness, accuracy, and consistency by supervisors and the research team every day during the data collection period.

The data were coded, entered into Epi Info version 3.5.3 statistical package, and exported to SPSS version 20 software for analysis. At the beginning of the analysis, summation of the practice scale was made. Then, the variable was recoded and dichotomized. Descriptive statistics were used to illustrate the means, standard deviations, medians, and frequencies of the study variables. Bivariate analysis was computed and those variables whose P values are less than or equal to 0.2 were fitted into the backward stepwise multivariate logistic regression model. Odds ratios with 95% confidence interval were used to determine the strength of association between dependent and independent variables. P values less than or equal to 0.05 were considered as statistically significant.

Ethical clearance was obtained from University of Gondar Ethical Review Board. The aim of the study was clearly explained to participants and respected hospital officials. The data collection was begun after obtaining consent from each participant. Confidentiality was maintained by excluding the name of participants from questionnaires. No other person except the data collection facilitators and the research team members had access to filled questionnaires.

3. Results

3.1. Sociodemographic Characteristics of the Study Participants. A total of 423 nurses, 317 (74.9%) from University

TABLE 1: Sociodemographic characteristics of the study participants, Gondar and Debre Markos Referral Hospitals, Northwest Ethiopia, 2015 (*n* = 423).

Variable	Frequency	Percent
Age		
20–29 years	340	80.4
≥30 years	83	19.6
Sex		
Male	239	56.5
Female	184	43.5
Marital status		
Single	244	57.7
Married	179	42.3
Educational level		
Diploma	36	8.5
B.S. degree	379	89.6
Master's degree	8	1.9
Ward		
Surgical	157	37.1
OB/GYN*	74	17.5
Medical	83	19.6
Pediatrics	63	15.0
OPD**	46	10.8
Ever took infection prevention training		
Yes	188	44.4
No	235	55.6

*OB/GYN: obstetrics and gynecology; **OPD: outpatient department.

of Gondar Hospital and 106 (25.1%) from Debre Markos Hospital, participated in this study which made the response rate 100%. Two hundred thirty-nine (56.5%) of them were males. The median age of the study participants was 27 years with interquartile range (IQR) of 25–29 years. The majority of them (89.4%) were followers of Orthodox Christianity and B.S. degree holders (89.6%). More than half of the participants (57.8%) were singles (Table 1).

3.2. Knowledge about Prevention of Surgical Site Infection. The mean score of the knowledge questions was 6.19 (SD = 1.3). In this study, only 172 (40.7%) [95% CI: 36.3, 45.7] of the respondents were found to be knowledgeable about prevention of surgical site infection.

3.3. Factors Associated with Knowledge of Nurses about Prevention of SSI. In the bivariate analysis, age, service year, sex of the participants, and ever taking training on infection prevention methods were factors which were significantly associated with knowledge about prevention of surgical site infection. However, only service year, sex of the participants, and ever taking training on infection prevention were found to be significantly associated in the multivariate analysis.

Male nurses were about 3 times more likely to be knowledgeable about prevention of surgical site infection than

female participants (AOR = 3.22, 95% CI: 2.09, 4.95). Those nurses who have served for more than 5 years were about 2 times more likely to be knowledgeable about prevention of surgical site infection than those whose service years are 5 years or less (AOR = 1.81, 95% CI: 1.12, 2.94). Those nurses who have ever taken training on infection prevention methods were about 2 times more likely to be knowledgeable about prevention of surgical site infection than those who have not (AOR = 1.95, 95% CI: 1.27, 2.99) (Table 2).

3.4. Practice of Nurses on Prevention of SSI. In this study, the proportion of nurses who had good practice of surgical site infection prevention activities was found to be 206 (48.7%).

3.5. Factors Associated with Practice of SSI Prevention Activities. In the bivariate analysis, age, service years, sex of the participants, ever taking training on infection prevention methods, and educational level were found to be significantly associated with practice of surgical site infection prevention activities. However, only age, sex, and educational level of the participants were found to be significantly associated in the multivariate analysis.

Female nurses were about 2 times more likely to practice surgical site infection prevention activities as compared to male nurses (AOR = 2.35, 95% CI: 1.58, 3.50). Those nurses who are 30 years or older were about 2 times more likely to practice surgical site infection prevention actives as compared to those who are less than 30 years old (AOR = 1.79, 95% CI: 1.08, 2.97). Nurses who have diploma were about 2 times more likely to practice surgical site infection prevention activities as compared to those who have B.S. degree or higher (AOR = 2.26, 95% CI: 1.08, 4.76) (Table 3).

4. Discussion

Prevention of SSIs is one of the most important challenges in delivering optimum nursing care. Although all health professionals involved in patient care are responsible for ensuring patient safety in this regard, nurses play a major role since they are usually involved in each step around the clock [19]. According to literature, nurses' role in the prevention of SSIs is very crucial [20]. Therefore, nurses must have adequate knowledge and good practice regarding the prevention of SSIs.

In this study, the proportion of nurses who were knowledgeable about prevention of surgical site infection was found to be 40.7% with a mean score of 56.3%. This finding indicated that more than half of the nurses working in the two referral hospitals demonstrated inadequate knowledge on prevention of surgical site infections, a finding in line with many of similar and related studies in Africa and western countries [13, 21, 22]. Similarly, this finding is in agreement with a Nigerian study in that only 40% of the participants had adequate knowledge regarding prevention of SSIs [16]. In the Nigerian study, the majority of nurses (66%) had adequate knowledge on general infection control mechanisms in contrast with the low proportion in the same participants regarding prevention of SSIs (40%). The implication of the Nigerian finding is that prevention of SSIs needs additional

TABLE 2: Multivariate logistic regression of factors associated with knowledge about surgical site infection prevention activities among nurses working in Gondar and Debre Markos Referral Hospitals, Northwest Ethiopia, 2015 (n = 423).

Variables	Knowledgeable		OR (95% CI)	
	Yes	No	COR (95% CI)	AOR (95% CI)
Sex				
Male	123 (51.5%)	116 (48.5%)	2.92 (1.93, 4.42)	**3.22 (2.09, 4.95)**
Female	49 (26.6%)	135 (73.4%)	1	1
Age				
≥30 years	43 (51.8%)	40 (48.2%)	1.76 (1.09, 2.85)	*
<30 years	129 (37.9%)	211 (62.1%)	1	
Service years				
More than 5 years	58 (52.7%)	52 (47.3%)	1.95 (1.25, 3.02)	**1.81 (1.12, 2.94)**
Five years or less	114 (36.4%)	199 (63.6%)	1	1
Ever took IP training				
Yes	95 (50.5%)	93 (49.5%)	2.10 (1.41, 3.11)	**1.95 (1.27, 2.99)**
No	77 (32.8%)	158 (67.2%)	1	1

*Not significant.

TABLE 3: Multivariate logistic regression of factors associated with practice of nurses in surgical site infection prevention activities in Gondar and Debre Markos Referral Hospitals, Northwest Ethiopia, 2015 (n = 423).

Variables	Good practice		OR (95% CI)	
	Yes	No	COR (95% CI)	AOR (95% CI)
Sex				
Female	111	73	2.31 (1.56, 3.41)	**2.35 (1.58, 3.50)**
Male	95	144	1	1
Age				
≥30 years	51	32	1.90 (1.16, 3.11)	**1.79 (1.08, 2.97)**
<30 years	155	185	1	1
Service years				
More than 5 years	60	50	1.37 (0.09, 2.12)	*
Five years or less	146	167	1	
Ever took IP training				
Yes	99	89	1.33 (0.91, 1.96)	*
No	107	128	1	
Educational level				
Diploma	24	12	2.25 (1.10, 4.63)	**2.25 (1.08, 4.76)**
B.S. degree + M.S.	182	205	1	1

*Not significant.

evidence-based knowledge apart from general information on infection control which might be acquired during college study. Therefore, since the knowledge-based questions were designed based on up-to-date guidelines, the possible reason for lower finding in the current Ethiopian study might be lack of in-service refreshment trainings on evidence-based SSIs prevention guidelines and recommendations.

This study revealed that sex of the study participants was significantly associated with knowledge about prevention of surgical site infection. Male nurses were found to be three times more likely to be knowledgeable about prevention of surgical site infection when compared with female nurses. The possible explanation of this finding might be linked with

the educational level of male nurses in that in this study the majority of the B.S. or M.S. holders were male nurses. Therefore, the difference in knowledge score could be due to the difference in educational level as those participants who had B.S. or M.S. degree are more likely to have better knowledge than diploma holders.

Year of service was another sociodemographic factor which was significantly associated with knowledge about prevention of surgical site infection. Those study participants who have served for more than five years were about two times more likely to be knowledgeable about prevention of surgical site infection than those whose service years are five years or less. This finding is in line with findings from

European and African studies in which year of experience was positively associated with knowledge regarding infection prevention [16, 21]. The positive association from this study could be due to the fact that as the number of years of practice increases, health workers are more likely to be exposed to surgical departments repeatedly and became more experienced through working with senior medical staff.

In this study, knowledge about prevention of surgical site infection was significantly associated with ever taking training on infection prevention methods. Those nurses who have ever taken training on infection prevention methods were about two times more likely to be knowledgeable about prevention of surgical site infection than those who do not. This finding is comparable with a result across the literature where training of staffs on safe practices was positively associated with the knowledge about health care associated infections [13, 19]. This could be due to the fact that updating the knowledge of the health workers about prevention of infection could have changed the older understanding of the health workers and could have resulted in good score on knowledge questions. Moreover, since the current infection prevention and patient safety national guideline of Ethiopia incorporated detailed information and evidence-based recommendations about prevention of surgical site infection, nurses who have taken this training could have better knowledge regarding prevention of SSIs.

This study has also tried to identify the level of practice of the nurses in the study areas regarding prevention of surgical site infection. In this study, the proportion of nurses who were practicing proper surgical site infection prevention activities was 48.7% (95% CI: 43.9, 53.5). This result is lower than the result from a study done in an Egyptian hospital where 57.1% of the health workers were found to practice infection prevention activities satisfactorily. However, it is higher than findings from studies done in Italy where only 38% of the nurses practice use of all infection prevention methods. This could be due to difference in attitude of the health workers towards applying infection prevention methods. It could also be due to the difference in the operational definition of the satisfactory practice from study to study. Difference in knowledge of the health workers concerning prevention of surgical site infection could also be another factor for this discrepancy.

Findings from this study showed that age of the study participants was one of the sociodemographic factors which were significantly associated with the practice of activities of prevention of surgical site infection. This study showed that nurses who are 30 years or older were about two times more likely to practice surgical site infection prevention activities properly when compared with those who are less than 30 years old. Positive association of year of service with practice of infection prevention activities can be explained by the fact that practice makes perfect, which means they might have improved their practice from year to year.

Sex of the nurses was another factor which was significantly associated with good practice of activities of surgical site infection. Female nurses were about two times more likely to practice surgical site infection prevention activities when compared with male nurses.

The other factor which was significantly associated with the good practice of surgical site infection prevention activities is educational status of the study participants. In contrast to many other studies, diploma nurses were about two times more likely to practice surgical site infection prevention activities when compared to those with B.S. degree or higher. This negative finding might be partly due to the educational system of the nursing schools where in all three-year diploma nursing programs the percentage of practical courses is 70% with 30% theoretical supplement; however, in a four-year degree program the percentage of practical courses is below 50%.

5. Conclusion

Knowledge and practice of surgical site infection prevention activities among nurses working in Gondar and Debre Markos Referral Hospitals were found to be low. Being male, serving for more than five years, and taking training on infection prevention activities were factors which were significantly associated with knowledge of prevention of surgical site infection. On the other hand, being thirty years or older, being female, and being of diploma level were factors which were significantly associated with good practice of surgical site infection prevention activities. Therefore, efforts have to be made to update the knowledge of nurses regarding surgical site infection prevention activities. Moreover, hospital administrators should encourage highly educated nurses to focus on implementing their knowledge into practice.

Conflict of Interests

The authors declare that they have no competing interests.

Authors' Contribution

Freahiywot Aklew Teshager, Eshetu Haileselassie Engeda, and Workie Zemene Worku participated in all steps of the study from its commencement to writing. They have reviewed and approved the submission of the paper.

Acknowledgments

The authors would like to acknowledge the University of Gondar for financial support. The authors' deepest gratitude also goes to those who participated in this study.

References

[1] S. Bagheri Nejad, B. Allegranzi, S. B. Syed, B. Ellisc, and D. Pittetd, "Health-care-associated infection in Africa: a systematic review," *Bulletin of the World Health Organization*, vol. 89, no. 10, pp. 757–765, 2011.

[2] M. G. Menegueti, S. R. Canini, F. Bellissimo-Rodrigues, and A. M. Laus, "Evaluation of Nosocomial Infection Control Programs in health services," *Revista Latino-Americana de Enfermagem*, vol. 23, no. 1, pp. 98–105, 2015.

[3] A. M. Aiken, D. M. Karuri, A. K. Wanyoro, and J. Macleod, "Interventional studies for preventing surgical site infections in sub-Saharan Africa—a systematic review," *International Journal of Surgery*, vol. 10, no. 5, pp. 242–249, 2012.

[4] L. Danzmann, P. Gastmeier, F. Schwab, and R.-P. Vonberg, "Health care workers causing large nosocomial outbreaks: a systematic review," *BMC Infectious Diseases*, vol. 13, no. 1, article 98, 2013.

[5] E. Ott, S. Saathoff, K. Graf, F. Schwab, and I. F. Chaberny, "The prevalence of nosocomial and community acquired infections in a university hospital: an observational study," *Deutsches Arzteblatt International*, vol. 110, no. 31-32, pp. 533–540, 2013.

[6] M. A. Smith and N. R. Dahlen, "Clinical practice guideline surgical site infection prevention," *Orthopaedic Nursing*, vol. 32, no. 5, pp. 242–248, 2013.

[7] K. Y. Lee, K. Coleman, D. Paech, S. Norris, and J. T. Tan, "The epidemiology and cost of surgical site infections in Korea: a systematic review," *Journal of the Korean Surgical Society*, vol. 81, no. 5, pp. 295–307, 2011.

[8] D. Amenu, T. Belachew, and F. Araya, "Surgical site infection rate and risk factors among obstetric cases of Jimma University Specialized Hospital, Southwest Ethiopia," *Ethiopian Journal of Health Sciences*, vol. 21, no. 2, pp. 91–100, 2011.

[9] E. Korol, K. Johnston, N. Waser et al., "A systematic review of risk factors associated with surgical site infections among surgical patients," *PLoS ONE*, vol. 8, no. 12, Article ID e83743, 2013.

[10] N. Petrosillo, C. M. J. Drapeau, E. Nicastri et al., "Surgical site infections in Italian Hospitals: a prospective multicenter study," *BMC Infectious Diseases*, vol. 8, article 34, 2008.

[11] K.-S. Cha, O.-H. Cho, and S.-Y. Yoo, "Risk factors for surgical site infections in patients undergoing craniotomy," *Journal of Korean Academy of Nursing*, vol. 40, no. 2, pp. 298–305, 2010.

[12] M. D. McHugh and A. W. Stimpfel, "Nurse reported quality of care: a measure of hospital quality," *Research in Nursing & Health*, vol. 35, no. 6, pp. 566–575, 2012.

[13] S. F. A. Brisibe, B. Ordinioha, and P. K. Gbeneolol, "Knowledge, attitude, and infection control practices of two tertiary hospitals in Port-Harcourt, Nigeria," *Nigerian Journal of Clinical Practice*, vol. 17, no. 6, pp. 691–695, 2014.

[14] B. G. Mitchell, R. Say, A. Wells, F. Wilson, L. Cloete, and L. Matheson, "Australian graduating nurses' knowledge, intentions and beliefs on infection prevention and control: a cross-sectional study," *BMC Nursing*, vol. 13, no. 1, article 43, 2014.

[15] R. M. Daud-Gallotti, S. F. Costa, T. Guimarães et al., "Nursing workload as a risk factor for healthcare associated infections in ICU: a prospective study," *PLoS ONE*, vol. 7, no. 12, Article ID e52342, 2012.

[16] T. T. Famakinwa, B. G. Bello, Y. A. Oyeniran, O. Okhiah, and R. N. Nwadike, "Knowledge and practice of post-operative wound infection prevention among nurses in the surgical unit of a teaching hospital in Nigeria," *International Journal of Basic, Applied and Innovative Research*, vol. 3, no. 1, pp. 23–28, 2014.

[17] A. E. Andersson, I. Bergh, J. Karlsson, B. I. Eriksson, and K. Nilsson, "The application of evidence-based measures to reduce surgical site infections during orthopedic surgery—report of a single-center experience in Sweden," *Patient Safety in Surgery*, vol. 6, article 11, 2012.

[18] World Health Organization (WHO), "WHO guidelines for safe surgery: 2009: safe surgery saves lives," November 2015, http://apps.who.int/iris/bitstream/10665/44185/1/9789241598552_eng.pdf.

[19] D. E. Fry and R. V. Fry, "Surgical site infection: the host factor," *AORN Journal*, vol. 86, no. 5, pp. 801–814, 2007.

[20] S. O. Labeau, S. S. Witdouck, D. M. Vandijck et al., "Nurses' knowledge of evidence-based guidelines for the prevention of surgical site infection," *Worldviews on Evidence-Based Nursing*, vol. 7, no. 1, pp. 16–24, 2010.

[21] I. Fashafsheh, A. Ayed, F. Eqtait, and L. Harazneh, "Knowledge and practice of nursing staff towards infection control measures in the Palestinian hospitals," *Journal of Education and Practice*, vol. 6, no. 4, pp. 79–90, 2015.

[22] N. Y. A. El-Enein and H. M. El Mahdy, "Standard precautions: a KAP study among nurses in the dialysis unit in a University Hospital in Alexandria, Egypt," *Journal of the Egyptian Public Health Association*, vol. 86, no. 1-2, pp. 3–10, 2011.

15

Audit of Orthopaedic Surgical Documentation

Fionn Coughlan, Prasad Ellanti, Cliodhna Ní Fhoghlu, Andrew Moriarity, and Niall Hogan

St. James's Hospital, Dublin, Ireland

Correspondence should be addressed to Fionn Coughlan; fionn3@gmail.com

Academic Editor: Atul Goel

Introduction. The Royal College of Surgeons in England published guidelines in 2008 outlining the information that should be documented at each surgery. St. James's Hospital uses a standard operation sheet for all surgical procedures and these were examined to assess documentation standards. *Objectives.* To retrospectively audit the hand written orthopaedic operative notes according to established guidelines. *Methods.* A total of 63 operation notes over seven months were audited in terms of date and time of surgery, surgeon, procedure, elective or emergency indication, operative diagnosis, incision details, signature, closure details, tourniquet time, postop instructions, complications, prosthesis, and serial numbers. *Results.* A consultant performed 71.4% of procedures; however, 85.7% of the operative notes were written by the registrar. The date and time of surgery, name of surgeon, procedure name, and signature were documented in all cases. The operative diagnosis and postoperative instructions were frequently not documented in the designated location. Incision details were included in 81.7% and prosthesis details in only 30% while the tourniquet time was not documented in any. *Conclusion.* Completion and documentation of operative procedures were excellent in some areas; improvement is needed in documenting tourniquet time, prosthesis and incision details, and the location of operative diagnosis and postoperative instructions.

1. Introduction

Accurate and detailed operation notes are of great importance in all surgical specialities not only for safe patient care but also for providing information for research, audit, and medicolegal purposes [1]. The Royal College of Surgeons Good Surgical Practice guidelines published in 2008 set the standard for all practicing surgeons. These have been updated in 2014 [2]. Operative notes are often presented in legal malpractice cases, and studies have shown that up to 45 percent of operative notes are indefensible medicolegally. Incomplete and illegible notes are a potential source of weakness in a surgeon's defence [3].

Clear, concise, and legible notes are therefore crucial following all surgical procedures. This is difficult to achieve with handwritten notes, especially in the context of legibility. Sweed et al. found that 20 percent of their orthopaedic operation notes contained illegible parts [4]. The new 2104 guidelines now suggest that all notes should "preferably" be "typed."

St. James's Hospital uses a standard operation sheet for all surgical procedures. The orthopaedic operation notes were examined to assess documentation standards. There are 3 studies which audited operation notes for elective total knee replacements in accordance with the British Orthopaedic Association guidelines [5–7]. Our study examined our operation notes based on the recommendations found in the Royal College of Surgeons of England Good Surgical Practice Guide (2008) [2]. Only 1 previous study has used these same guidelines to audit its orthopaedic operation notes [4].

2. Objectives

To retrospectively audit 63 operation notes of inpatients under the care of the orthopaedic service in St. James's Hospital from 9 April 2014 to 21 October 2014 according to the Royal College of Surgeons of England Good Surgical Practice guidelines in February 2008.

3. Methods

A total of 63 operation notes were audited by one single reviewer. The operation notes all were based on the standard template (Figure 1) found in St. James's Hospital for all

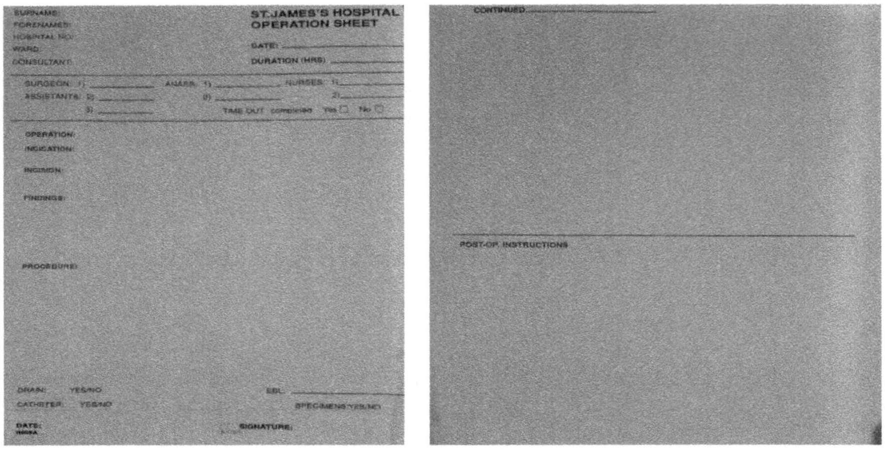

(a)   (b)

FIGURE 1: St. James's Hospital operation proforma: front and back.

surgical procedures. St. James's operation sheet contains headings for patient details, time and date, duration (hours), surgeon, assistants, anaesthetists, nurses, timeout completed (yes/no), operation, indication, incision, findings, procedure, drain (yes/no), catheter (yes/no), specimen (yes/no), and post-op instructions. The notes were audited in accordance with the College of Surgeons guidelines in terms of date and time of surgery, surgeon, procedure, elective or emergency indication, operative diagnosis, incision details, signature, closure details, tourniquet time, post-op instructions, complications, prostheses, and serial numbers.

4. Results

All 63 notes were handwritten on St. James's Hospital standard operation sheet. 71.4% ($n = 45$) of the 63 operations were performed by a consultant surgeon versus 28.6% ($n = 18$) that were performed by trainee registrars. The majority of the operative notes were written by the registrar (85.7%; $n = 54$), followed by the consultant (11.1%; $n = 7$) and the senior house officer (3.17%; $n = 2$). A total of 38.1% ($n = 24$) of all operative notes were written by the lead surgeon, with 61.9% ($n = 39$) written by an assistant. Of the 24 operative notes written by the lead surgeon, 29.1% ($n = 7$) were done by a consultant versus 71% ($n = 17$) by the registrar. All 63 operative notes were handwritten on St. James's Hospital operation sheets. All of the operative notes included date and time of surgery, name of lead surgeon (and any assistants if present), procedure name, and signature. Operative diagnosis was present in 74.6% of the operation notes; however, it was only found in the designated location 63.8% of the time. Incision details were included in 81.7% of the sheets; however, 3 procedures were closed and did not require an incision. Tourniquets were applied in 23.8% of the procedures with none having a documented tourniquet time (0%). Closure details were documented in all but one procedure (98.3%). Postoperative instructions were included in 96.3% of the operative notes, but 41% were located in

the incorrect location on the operative sheet. 50 procedures involved the use of prosthetic equipment; however, only 30% of these had documented or attached serial number adhesives to the operation sheet. None of the operative sheets stated whether it was an elective or emergency procedure.

5. Discussion

The Royal College of Surgeons of England Good Surgical Practice guidelines help the surgeon create concise, clear, and informative operation notes. This not only allows for better patient care postoperatively but also protects the surgeon medicolegally. Having the proforma operation sheet ensures that the minimum information required is present in all notes and it has been shown to be effective in improving the standard of operation notes [7]. There is only 1 operation sheet template shared among all specialties in St. James's Hospital and therefore it does not allow for the specifics pertaining to different specialities. In orthopaedic surgery, documentation of operation details could be improved with the addition of specific headings for tourniquet application and time, as well as antibiotics used at induction. These were included in the Sheffield proforma and led to better completion of detailed notes [7]. The benefits of proforma have been documented with other specialities such as pediatric surgery [8] and maxillofacial surgery [9].

Singh et al. have shown that audits such as these can significantly improve the quality of the operative notes by simply highlighting the deficient areas [10]. Others have suggested the use of a checklist as an additional tool to improve the quality of the operative notes [5].

A similar study to ours was conducted by Sweed et al. in their orthopaedic department which demonstrated similar deficient areas of operative note documentation, in particular the poor documentation of tourniquet time [4].

The important issue of legibility exists within all handwritten notes. It has been shown that using computer templates/proforma along with typed notes proves to be superior to handwritten notes [11]. However, when other staff members were asked to read notes, the problem of legibility arose. The use of electronic operation notes is currently being piloted by other surgical specialities in St. James's Hospital, with the aim that this will be available to orthopaedic surgery in the near future.

Electronic notes are beneficial in many ways. They can be accessed repeatedly and remotely from any hospital computer system. This eliminates the possibility of an operative note being lost or destroyed and markedly improves the notes in terms of detail and legibility [12]. The headings used in the notes not only can be standardised, but also can be edited to suit individual specialities, with specific headings and sections, as there is no need to print out standard proforma sheets. Electronic operation notes will become easier to audit and review for research purposes, as they are easier to access and will save the reviewer considerable time. Templates can also be added for common procedures so as to save time in the writing of an operation note and to guide trainees as to how a particular surgeon approaches a case or how they prefer their operation notes to be written and what information each note should contain.

A study conducted by the Centre for Disease Control and Prevention looked at the use of electronic patient records and showed that 74% of physicians highlighted the ability to access patient information as a benefit, along with 74% believing that electronic records had improved overall patient care [13].

Ghani et al. undertook a study piloting their "smart" electronic operation note system for orthopaedic trauma operation notes. They showed a marked improvement in the quality of documentation, both in terms of information detail and readability. The "smart" electronic notes were deemed to be completely legible (100%) compared with only 66% of the handwritten notes [12].

The 2014 Royal College of Surgeons Good Surgical Practice guidelines now state that all operation notes are "preferably typed." This recommendation was not present in the 2008 guidelines and certainly favours a move towards electronic notes so as to be compliant with best surgical practice and patient care.

One issue remains is that some surgeons create illustrations in their operative notes to help explain certain complex issues. While this would be currently limited to electronic notes, the use of touch screen technology could provide a solution to this issue.

Limitations of this study included the small amount of operation notes collected between the allotted time periods. Ideally, a larger number of operation notes would have been collected. At the time of publication, the electronic operation notes are not available to the orthopaedic department, so a follow-up evaluation of the new electronic template was not possible. This would have allowed for a reaudit to assess any improvement in documentation with the electronic notes. While a standardised proforma exists in St. James's Hospital for all surgical procedures, an orthopaedic-specific proforma was not available. The operative notes audited were limited to those of inpatients in the orthopaedic ward during the specified time. This eliminated the day-case procedures

and their operation notes, which would have increased the numbers of notes reviewed in the audit. Allowing for these limitations, the date collected shows areas of strength and weakness in St. James's Hospital orthopaedic operation note proforma and in the documentation of orthopaedic surgeries.

This data will allow for improvements to be made in documentation by the orthopaedic surgeons in the future. It highlighted the poor tourniquet time documentation, which can be improved upon, and also the need for prosthesis serial numbers to be documented, given the potential for future revisions or surgeries on the same patient.

6. Conclusions

The completion and documentation of surgical procedures on our standard St. James's Hospital operation sheets were excellent in terms of recording date, time, surgeon, closure details, procedure name, and signatures. Improvement is needed in documenting tourniquet time, prosthesis serial numbers, correct use of the template headings, incision, and operative diagnosis. These improvements could be made with the introduction of an orthopaedic-specific proforma with headings for tourniquet time, antibiotics, and prosthesis serial numbers.

Given the new RCSE guidelines recommendation for 2014, it is recommended that electronic notes be introduced in the orthopaedic department. As the electronic notes will be piloted in St. James's Hospital in the near future, it is our plan to audit those notes and compare them with the results we have obtained from the proforma sheets.

Conflict of Interests

The authors declare that there is no conflict of interests regarding the publication of this paper.

References

[1] General Medical Council, *Good Medical Practice*, 2006.

[2] The Royal College of Surgeons, *Good Surgical Practice*, The Royal College of Surgeons of England, London, UK, 2008.

[3] L. P. Lefter, S. R. Walker, F. Dewhurst, and R. W. L. Turner, "An audit of operative notes: facts and ways to improve," *ANZ Journal of Surgery*, vol. 78, no. 9, pp. 800–802, 2008.

[4] T. A. Sweed, A. A. Bonajmah, M. A. Mussa et al., "Audit of operation notes in an Orthopaedic unit," *Journal of Orthopaedic Surgery*, vol. 22, no. 2, pp. 218–220, 2014.

[5] D. Morgan, N. Fisher, A. Ahmad, and F. Alam, "Improving operation notes to meet British Orthopaedic Association guidelines," *Annals of The Royal College of Surgeons of England*, vol. 91, pp. 217–219, 2009.

[6] R. Din, D. Jena, B. N. Muddu, and D. Jennna, "The use of an aide-memoire to improve the quality of operation notes in an orthopaedic unit," *Annals of The Royal College of Surgeons of England*, vol. 83, no. 5, pp. 319–320, 2001.

[7] H. Al Hussainy, F. Ali, S. Jones, J. C. McGregor-Riley, and S. Sukumar, "Improving the standard of operation notes in orthopaedic and trauma surgery: the value of a proforma," *Injury*, vol. 35, no. 11, pp. 1102–1106, 2004.

[8] B. K. Y. Chan, K. Exarchou, H. J. Corbett, and R. R. Turnock, "The impact of an operative note proforma at a paediatric surgical centre," *Journal of Evaluation in Clinical Practice*, vol. 21, no. 1, pp. 74–78, 2015.

[9] K. Payne, K. Jones, and A. Dickenson, "Improving the standard of operative notes within an oral and maxillofacial surgery department, using an operative note proforma," *Journal of Maxillofacial and Oral Surgery*, vol. 10, no. 3, pp. 203–208, 2011.

[10] R. Singh, R. Chauhan, and S. Anwar, "Improving the quality of general surgical operation notes in accordance with the Royal College of Surgeons guidelines: a prospective completed audit loop study," *Journal of Evaluation in Clinical Practice*, vol. 18, no. 3, pp. 578–580, 2012.

[11] A. O'Bichere and D. Sellu, "The quality of operation notes: can simple word processors help?" *Annals of the Royal College of Surgeons of England*, vol. 79, no. 5, supplement, pp. 204–209, 1997.

[12] Y. Ghani, R. Thakrar, D. Kosuge, and P. Bates, "'Smart' electronic operation notes in surgery: an innovative way to improve patient care," *International Journal of Surgery*, vol. 12, no. 1, pp. 30–32, 2014.

[13] E. Jamoom, P. Beatty, A. Bercovitz, D. Woodwell, K. Palso, and E. Rechtsteiner, *Physician Adoption of Electronic Health Record Systems: United States, 2011*, Centers for Disease Control and Prevention, Atlanta, Ga, USA, 2012.

16

Panniculectomy Combined with Bariatric Surgery by Laparotomy: An Analysis of 325 Cases

Vincenzo Colabianchi,[1] Giancarlo de Bernardinis,[2] Matteo Giovannini,[3] and Marika Langella[1]

[1]*Plastic Surgery Unit, Casa di Cura Villa Alba, Bologna Medical Center, 40136 Bologna, Italy*
[2]*General Surgery Unit, Presidio Ospedaliero Villa Letizia, 67100 L'Aquila, Italy*
[3]*General Surgery Unit, Casa di Cura Villa Alba, Bologna Medical Center, 40136 Bologna, Italy*

Correspondence should be addressed to Marika Langella; marikalangella@yahoo.it

Academic Editor: Ramón Vilallonga

Surgical treatment of obese patients is much debated in the literature because of the significant intraoperative risks related to comorbidities presented by this type of patients. Recent literature suggests that panniculectomy should follow bariatric surgery after the patient's weight loss has been stabilized. However, when performed by laparotomy, bariatric surgery can be combined with panniculectomy. This paper presents the analysis of 325 cases of patients undergoing abdominal panniculectomy combined with bariatric surgery. The study highlights the risks, complications, and benefits of the combined procedure and describes a standardized technique for excision of a large abdominal panniculus in a short operating time.

1. Introduction

Obesity and overweight are recognized as one of the most important public health problems. In recent years, bariatric surgery has become increasingly popular and a valid alternative to dieting for patients with morbid obesity [1, 2]. Patients who are candidates for obesity surgery often exhibit a moderate to large panniculus (grades 1 to 5), according to the classification by Igwe Jr. et al. [3, 4]. A large pendulous abdomen can affect mobility, limits physical activity, affects personal hygiene, and has a negative impact on the professional life of patients [5]. A sagging abdomen, which is exacerbated after marked postbariatric weight loss, also may cause lymphedema of the abdominal wall, which may limit the social and sexual life of the patient and lead to negative psychological consequences and depression [6]. Moreover, after bariatric surgery by laparotomy, patients are left with an unsightly permanent scar from the xiphoid process to the umbilicus, which may be distressing, especially for younger women.

Recent literature suggests that panniculectomy should be performed separately from bariatric surgery and only after the weight loss of the patient has been stabilized [2, 7, 8]. However, to prevent these conditions during the weight-loss period, bariatric surgery can be combined with abdominal panniculectomy if prolonged operating time and excessive blood loss are avoided [4, 5, 9].

The authors report a detailed description of the results of 325 patients treated by combining bariatric surgery with immediate panniculectomy.

2. Patients and Methods

Between January 2008 and February 2014, 325 patients (171 women and 154 men), with morbid obesity, underwent bariatric surgery combined with abdominal panniculectomy. The patients were operated on at the Plastic Surgery Unit of the Casa di Cura Villa Alba (Bologna, Italy) and at the General Surgery Unit of the San Pierdamiano Hospital (Faenza Ravenna, Italy), by the same surgical team. The study was performed in accordance with the ethical standards of the 1964 Declaration of Helsinki and its subsequent amendments.

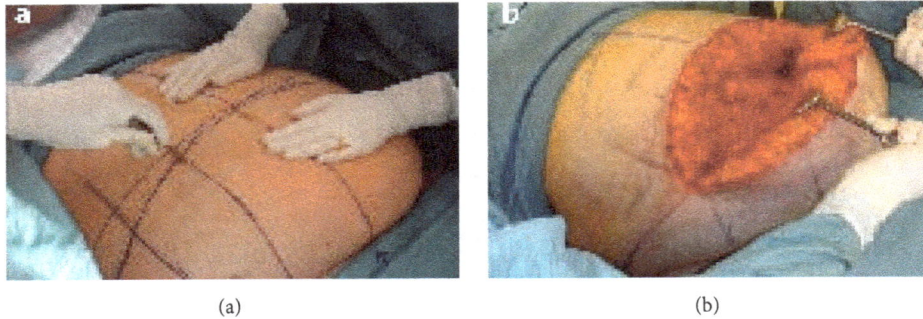

(a)

(b)

FIGURE 1: (a) Incision made in the medial two-thirds of the upper horizontal line. (b) Operative field. Mobilization of the dermal-fat flap from top to bottom.

TABLE 1: Body mass index (BMI) distribution among the study cohort.

BMI (Kg/m²)	Woman (n)	Men (n)	Total (n)
38.9–50	7	5	12
50.1–55	10	9	19
55.1–60	84	59	143
60.1–65	60	56	116
65.1–70	10	25	35
Total	**171**	**154**	**325**

Written informed consent was obtained from all patients prior to their inclusion in the study.

The patients had a mean age of 41.5 ± 9.1 years (range: 18 to 65 years) and mean body mass index (BMI) of 59.3 ± 10.4 kg/m (range: 52.7 to 69.4 kg/m), with a mean overweight of 243%. BMI distribution among the study cohort is shown (Table 1).

The severity of the pendulous abdomen was classified into five grades, according to Van Hout et al. [6]. Most patients (69%, n = 225) had panniculus grades 2 and 3 (Table 2). Eighteen patients (5.5%) had pendulous abdomen complicated by lymphedema. The following comorbidities, obtained directly from the medical record and the patient's history, were recorded: hypertension (65%); diabetes (45%), obstructive sleep apnea syndrome (OSAS) (36%); hypercholesterolemia (31%); chronic obstructive pulmonary disease (COPD) (25%), depression (24%); asthmatic bronchitis (18%); arthralgia (16%); gastroesophageal reflux disease (GERD) (15%); and chronic ischemic heart disease (12%) (Table 3).

All patients included in this study were initially evaluated by a multidisciplinary team before undergoing bariatric surgery by laparotomy combined with abdominal panniculectomy.

Patients with central obesity, BMI greater than 70 kg/m, severe cardiorespiratory disease, and incisional hernias in subcostal or xiphopubic scars, and those in whom an excessive stress on the final suture line was predicted with the pinch test were excluded from the study.

The complications arising from the combination of bariatric surgery with panniculectomy were grouped into two three-year periods. This distinction in two periods has been made to take into account the experience of the surgical team.

2.1. Preoperative Marking and Management. The amount of tissue to be resected was assessed by the pinch test with the patient standing up and then in a semiflexed position (30°) on a bed. A vertical line extending from the xiphoid process to the symphysis pubis and passing over the umbilicus was marked. The lateral limits of the diamond-shaped area of skin and adipose tissue to be resected were marked with the patient in a sitting position. Horizontal lines were marked, using the abdominal fold as the lower limit and the upper edge of the umbilicus as the upper limit of the lateral marks. If the skin was irritated or infected, the inferior line was moved distally to the healthy skin. Finally, two vertical paramedian lines were marked bilaterally to the xiphopubic line to ensure symmetrical resection of the adipose tissue, and a line defining the position of the costal arches was traced. Before surgery, all patients received antithromboembolic prophylaxis, including the wearing of compression stockings and administration of dalteparin sodium, combined with antibiotic prophylaxis with third-generation cephalosporins.

2.2. Surgical Procedures. The operation was performed by the same surgical team and with the aid of mechanical means for lifting adipose tissue.

An incision was made in the medial two-thirds of the upper horizontal line with a cold blade scalpel (Figure 1(a)). The subcutaneous tissue was dissected with an electrocautery in spray mode at 35% intensity to limit heat damage to the adipose tissue. The incision was deepened until Scarpa's fascia was exposed and extended laterally to the muscle fascia on the midline. Special attention was given to the umbilical stump, which was usually buried. This maneuver allows direct access to the periumbilical perforators, which have a considerably large caliber in obese patients, permitting meticulous hemostasis and reduction of blood loss. The dermal-fat flap was elevated with limited undermining of the supraumbilical and epigastric regions and extended superiorly to the xiphoid process. The lateral undermining of the abdominal flap toward the costal arch should be avoided as much as possible to minimize dead space and prevent damage to the

TABLE 2: Distribution of panniculus grading [9] in the study cohort ($n = 325$).

Grades	Description	N
Grade 1	Panniculus covers pubic hairline but not the entire mons pubis	31
Grade 2	Panniculus extends to cover the entire mons pubis	101
Grade 3	Panniculus extends to cover the upper thigh	124
Grade 4	Panniculus extends to mid-thigh	61
Grade 5	Panniculus extends to the knee and beyond	8

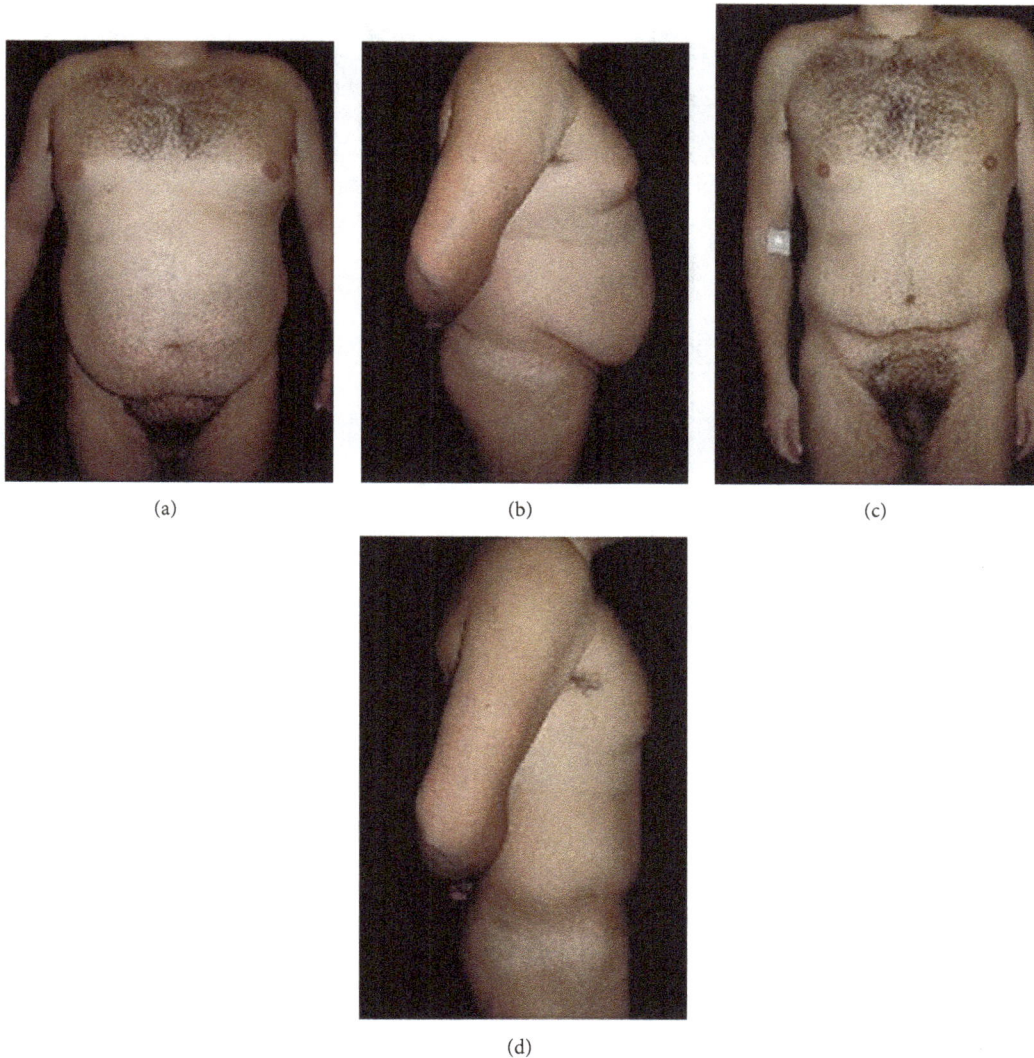

(a)   (b)   (c)

(d)

FIGURE 2: (a) Preoperative frontal view and (b) lateral view of a male patient (BMI = 44 kg/m^2; body weight = 136 kg). (c) Postoperative frontal view and (d) lateral view five years after surgery (body weight = 73 kg).

abdominal vasculature. The described dissection, although limited, allows the creation of an operative field sufficient to perform the entire procedure.

Proceeding cautiously, the panniculus adiposus was undermined from the muscle fascia up to the suprapubic line. In order not to skeletonize the muscle fascia, a layer of adipose tissue was left, so that part of the lymphatic system was preserved, thus reducing the risk of seroma formation.

This maneuver can be facilitated by placing the patient in the anti-Trendelenburg position, rotating the operating table by 180°, and mobilizing the flap from top to bottom (Figure 1(b)). Then, the patient was placed in the semirecumbent position (30° between the trunk and legs), allowing the evaluation and better control of the exact amount of tissue to be diathermied to ensure that the incision is closed without excessive tension on the suture line. The skin incisions were

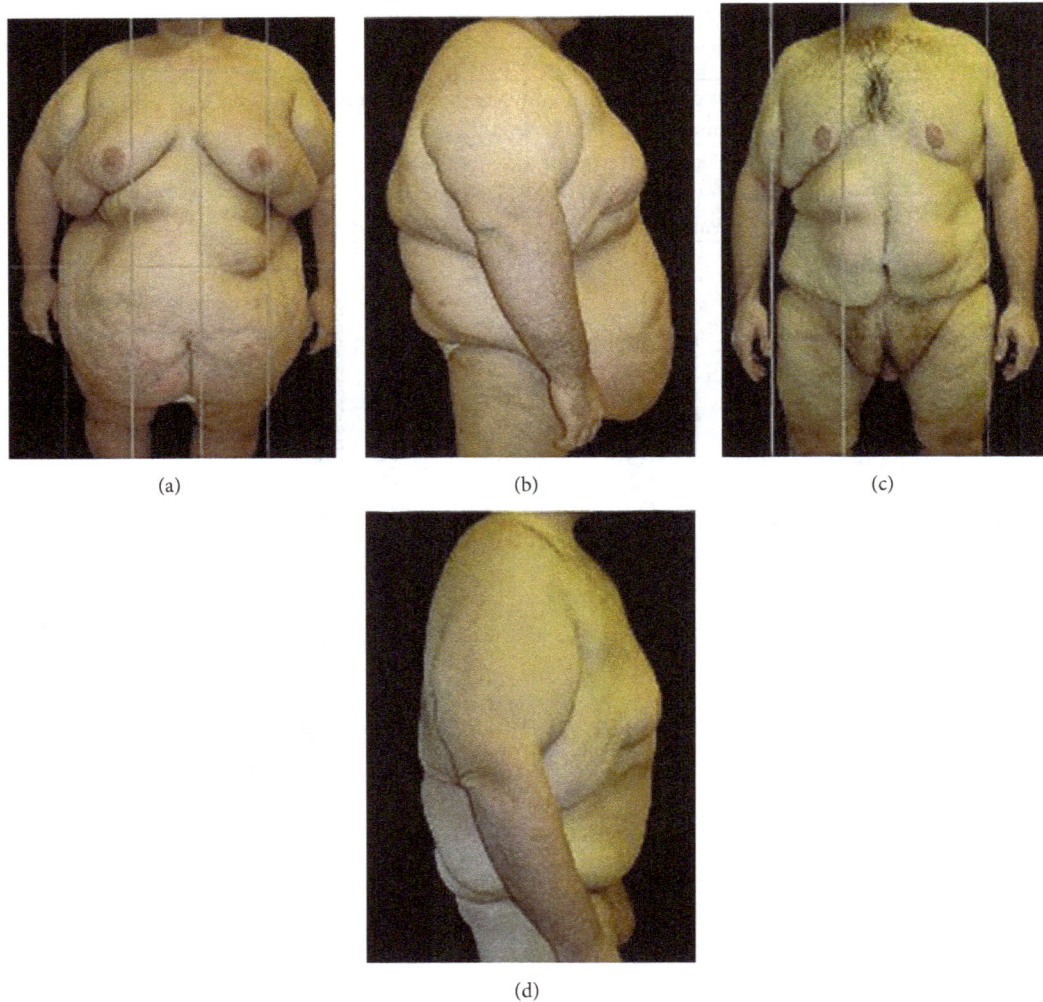

FIGURE 3: (a) Preoperative frontal view and (b) lateral view of a male patient (BMI = 69.9 kg/m^2; body weight = 220 kg). (c) Postoperative frontal view and (d) lateral view five years after surgery (body weight = 110 kg).

TABLE 3: Comorbidities of patients (n = 325).

Comorbidities	
OSAS	36%
Depression	24%
GERD	15%
NIDDM	38% (84% severe diabetes)
IDDM	7% (16% severe diabetes)
COPD	25%
Arthralgia	16%
CV pathologies	12%
Hypertension	65%
Hypercholesterolemia	31%
Asthmatic bronchitis	18%

OSAS: obstructive sleep apnea syndrome; GERD: gastroesophageal reflux disease; NIDDM: non-insulin-dependent diabetes mellitus; IDDM: insulin-dependent diabetes mellitus; COPD: chronic obstructive pulmonary disease; CV pathologies: cardiovascular pathologies.

completed bilaterally on the upper horizontal line and along the entire length of the lower horizontal line. Next, the subcutaneous tissue was dissected down to near the fascia, starting from the sides of flap and proceeding medially. In the suprapubic region, a 2 to 3 cm thick layer of adipose tissue was not removed to prevent scar contracture or formation of atrophic scars. The abdominal panniculus was removed and weighed (to make the necessary adjustments to correct for postoperative infusion therapy).

The median laparotomy between the xiphoid process and the umbilicus allows biliary-intestinal bypass to be performed. Closure of abdominal wall was carried out in two layers: one for the parietal peritoneum and one for the fascia. Hemostasis was accurately controlled, the abdominal wall was washed with antibiotic solution, and one suction drain (caliber 21) was placed on each side.

Umbilical reconstruction involved a double-Y incision of the abdominal skin. The umbilicus was sutured with

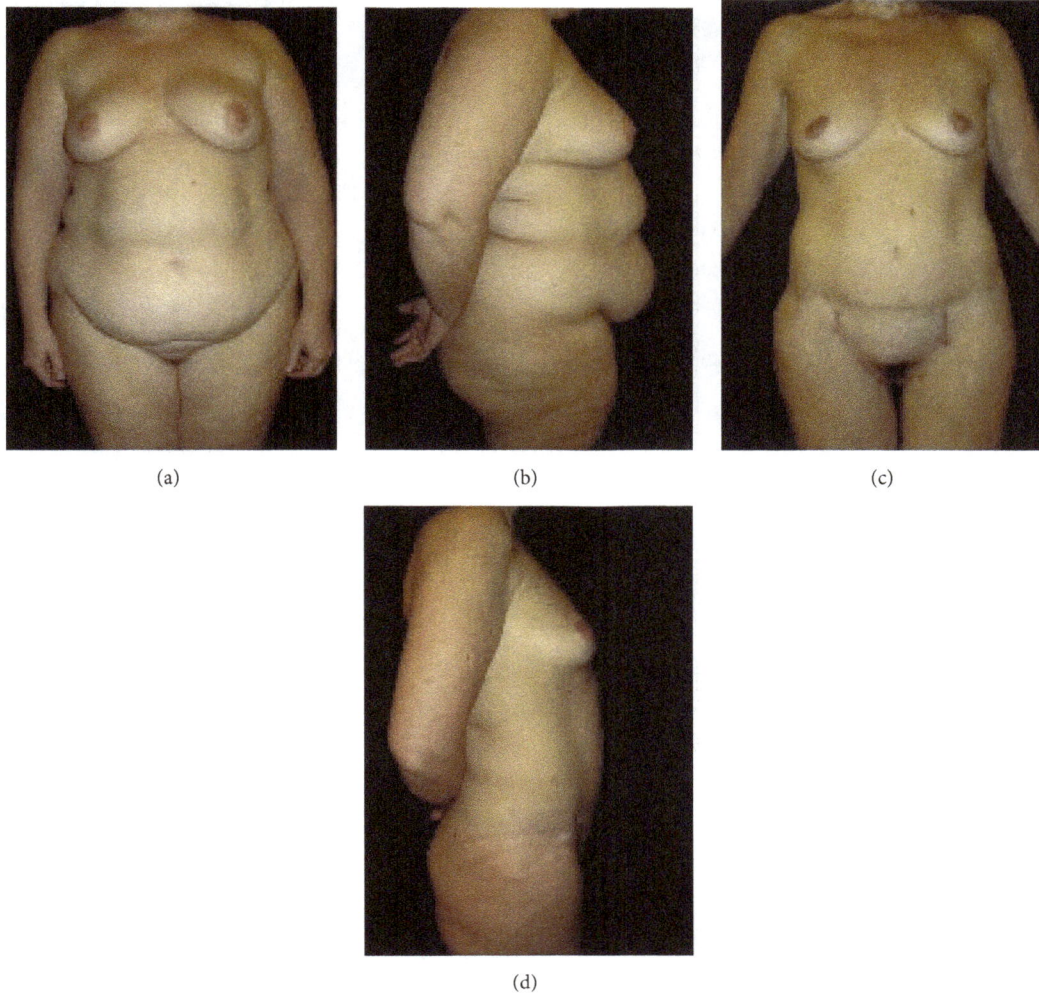

FIGURE 4: (a) Preoperative frontal view and (b) lateral view of a female patient (BMI = 50 kg/m^2; body weight = 135 kg). (c) Postoperative frontal view and (d) lateral view three years after surgery (body weight = 65 kg).

Gillies stitches using 4-0 nylon suture (avoiding its fixation to the muscle fascia), leaving a stump of length similar to the thickness of the dermal-fat flap. This preventive measure is useful to reduce the mechanical stress on the umbilicus, which is already burdened by the partial devascularization caused by the undermining of the skin.

Eight to ten stitches were placed fixing the Scarpa's fascia to the muscle aponeurosis to close the dead space. The subcutaneous tissue was closed in three layers with absorbable 2-0 and 3-0 vicryl suture. Closure of the skin was then performed with intradermal sutures for patients with panniculus grade 1 or 2 and metal staples for patients with panniculus grade 3, 4, or 5. A compressive dressing was then applied and maintained in place for 60 days.

The mean operating time for the different steps of abdominal panniculectomy combined with bariatric surgery was 45 minutes for tissue dissection, 75 minutes for bariatric procedures, and 1 hour for abdominal closure, for a total of 3 hours.

3. Results

The mean redundant panniculus excised was 6.5 kg (range: 3.2–16.5 kg).

Patients who had panniculus grade 1 or 2 had the drains removed before hospital discharge on postoperative day 7, and for those who had panniculus grade 3, 4, or 5, the drains were removed on postoperative day 14.

The mean hospital stay was 8 days (range: 5–13 days). Complications associated with panniculectomy (Table 4) and those associated with bariatric surgery (Table 5) were grouped into two three-year periods. A marked decrease in the incidence of complications occurred during the second period of 3 years as shown in Figures 2 and 3. This result shows how the practical experience of the team in the management of this type of patients is essential.

It was observed that 23.5% of patients had hernias or incisional hernias; 78% of these hernias were repaired with direct suture and 22% with surgical mesh. Two patients

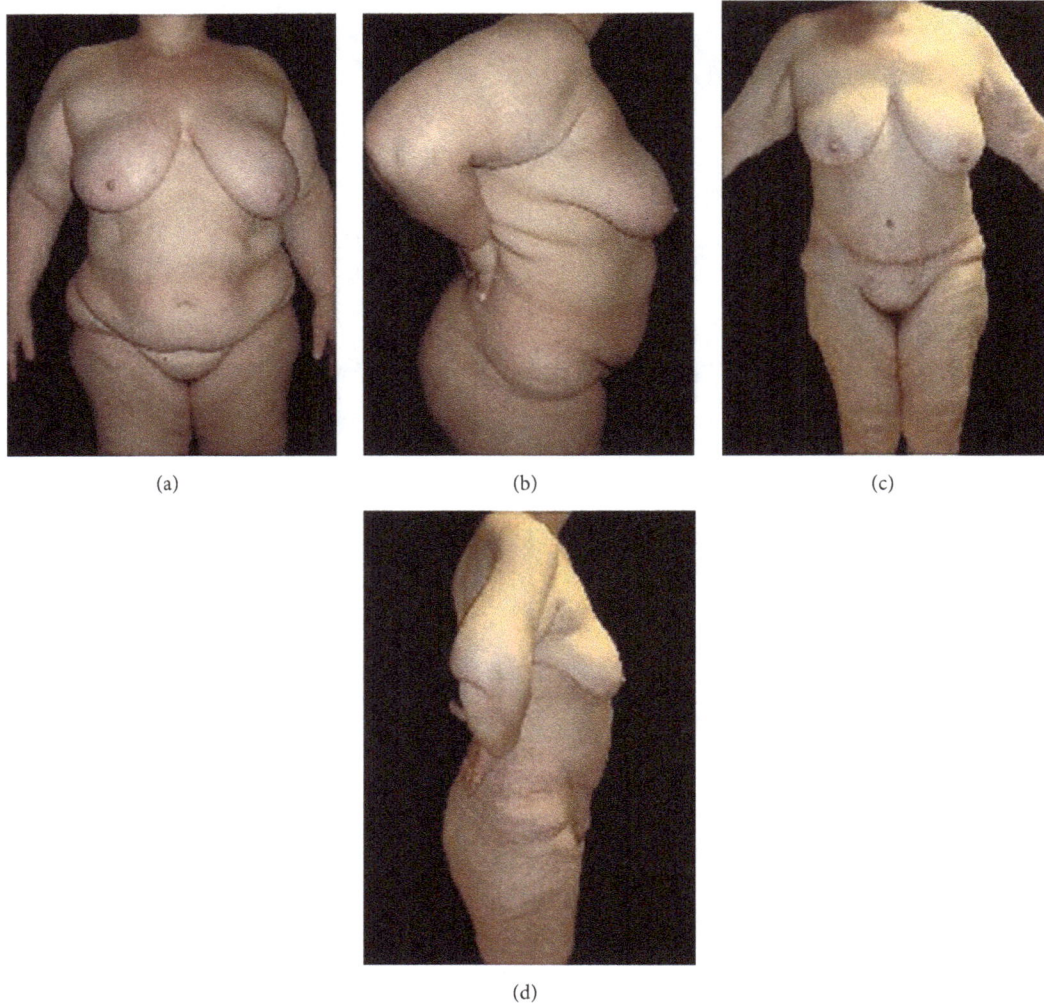

FIGURE 5: (a) Preoperative frontal view and (b) lateral view of a female patient (BMI = 39 kg/m²; body weight = 106 kg). (c) Postoperative frontal view and (d) lateral view 11 months after surgery (body weight = 71 kg).

TABLE 4: Postoperative complications for the 325 patients during the study period associated with panniculectomy.

Postoperative complications, n (%)	2007–2013 (N = 325)	2007–2010 (N = 164)	2010–2013 (N = 161)
Seroma	59 (18.2)	51 (31.1)	8 (5.0)
Dehiscence	44 (13.5)	31 (18.9)	13 (8.1)
Dysesthesia/anesthesia	33 (10.2)	17 (10.4)	16 (9.9)
Liponecrosis	29 (8.9)	19 (11.6)	10 (6.2)
Superficial edema	19 (5.8)	13 (7.9)	6 (3.7)
Hemorrhage	17 (5.2)	12 (7.3)	5 (3.1)
Cardiorespiratory complications	16 (4.9)	11 (6.7)	5 (3.1)
Skin necrosis	13 (4.0)	10 (6.1)	3 (1.9)
Loss of the umbilicus	1 (0.3)	1 (0.6)	0 (0)

(0.61%) died of acute myocardial infarction and one (0.31%) due to septicemia, caused by anastomotic dehiscence.

Apart from a few exceptional cases, patients who underwent panniculectomy did not require further aesthetic and nonsurgical procedures. Seromas were treated with antibiotics and fluid collection drainage on an outpatient basis.

Typical examples of patients treated with bariatric surgery combined with panniculectomy are shown (Figures 2–8).

4. Discussion

This study, conducted on 325 patients, applying a combined approach of bariatric surgery and panniculectomy, shows that benefits, including immediate reduction of the abdominal apron and prevention of the worsening of this condition during weight loss; no visible scarring; improved personal hygiene and resolution of dermatological problems; prevention of lymphedema of the abdominal wall during the weight loss period, as the exacerbation of the abdominal ptosis may lead to lymphatic and venous stasis; improved quality of life and self-esteem and weight loss, can be achieved. Also, one

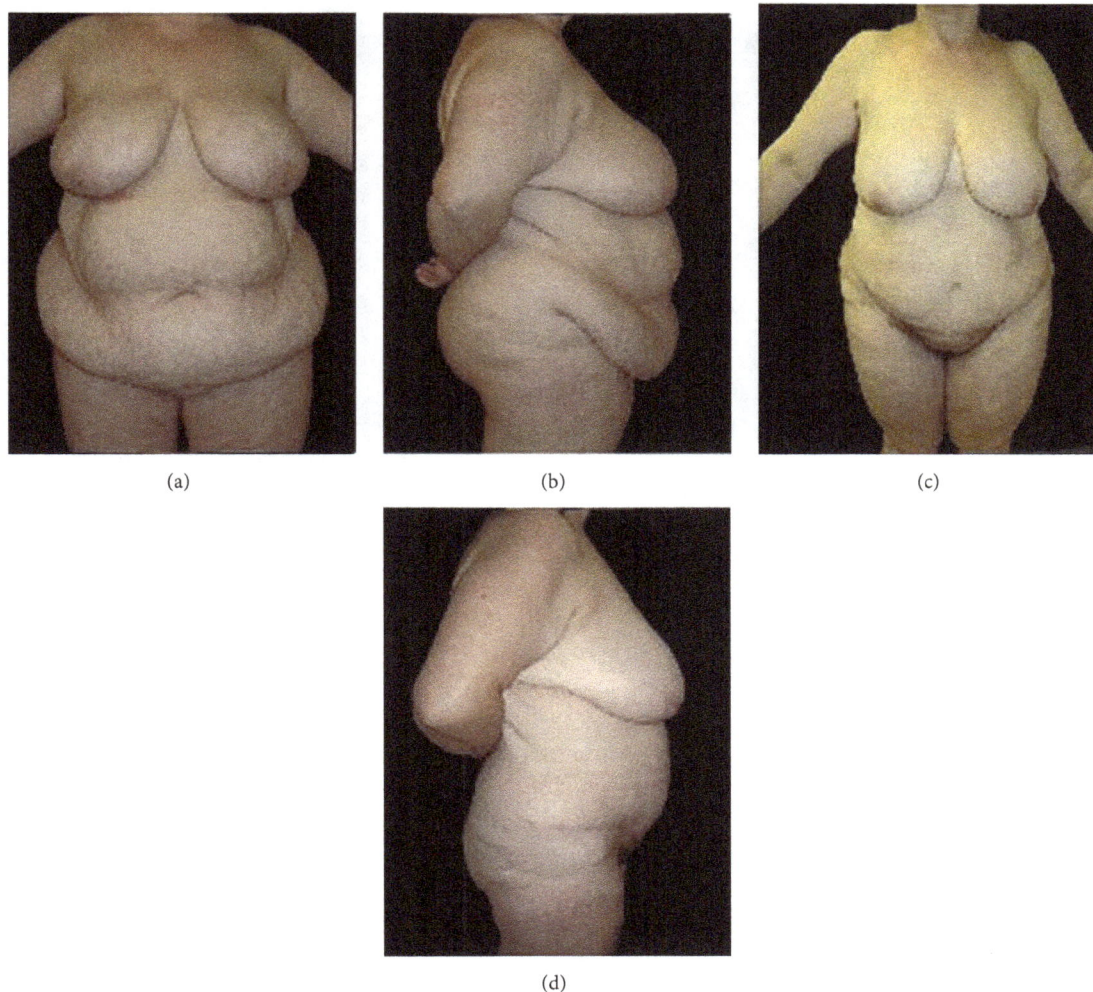

FIGURE 6: (a) Preoperative frontal view and (b) lateral view of a female patient (BMI = 46 kg/m^2; body weight = 129 kg). (c) Postoperative frontal view and (d) lateral view five years after surgery (body weight = 82 kg).

TABLE 5: Postoperative complications for the 325 patients during the study period associated with the bariatric surgery.

Postoperative complications, n (%)	2007–2013 (N = 325)	2007–2010 (N = 164)	2010–2013 (N = 161)
Incisional hernia	59 (18.2)	38 (23.2)	
Respiratory insufficiency	44 (13.5)	31 (18.90)	13 (8.07)
DVT/PE	33 (10.2)	25 (15,24)	8 (4.9)
Surgical infection	29 (8.9)	24 (14,63)	5 (3.1)
Intestinal occlusion	19 (5.8)	16 (9.7)	3 (1.8)
Hemoperitoneum	17 (5.2)	11 (6.7)	6 (3.7)
Anastomotic dehiscence	16 (4.9)	12 (7.3)	4 (2.4)
Renal failure	13 (4.0)	9 (5.4)	4 (2.4)
Intraoperative death	1 (0.3)	1 (0.6)	0 (0)

DVT/PE: deep vein thrombosis and pulmonary embolism.

of our main concerns was to develop a surgical strategy for elimination of postlaparotomy scars, especially in younger women.

The correction of the resection plane of the diamond-shaped panniculus, meticulous hemostasis, adequate compression during the postoperative period, and use of subcutaneous drains during an appropriate period of time resulted in a marked reduction of specific immediate complications, including bleeding, seroma formation, infection, and wound dehiscence. The postoperative complications of this large sample of 325 patients were evaluated in two successive 3-year periods to assess the practical effects of increasing surgical experience over time. At the first 3 years, the present study was characterized by large incidence rates of postoperative complications, which gradually decreased (Figures 2 and 3). The incidence rates of postoperative complications in the second 3-year period of the study were similar to those

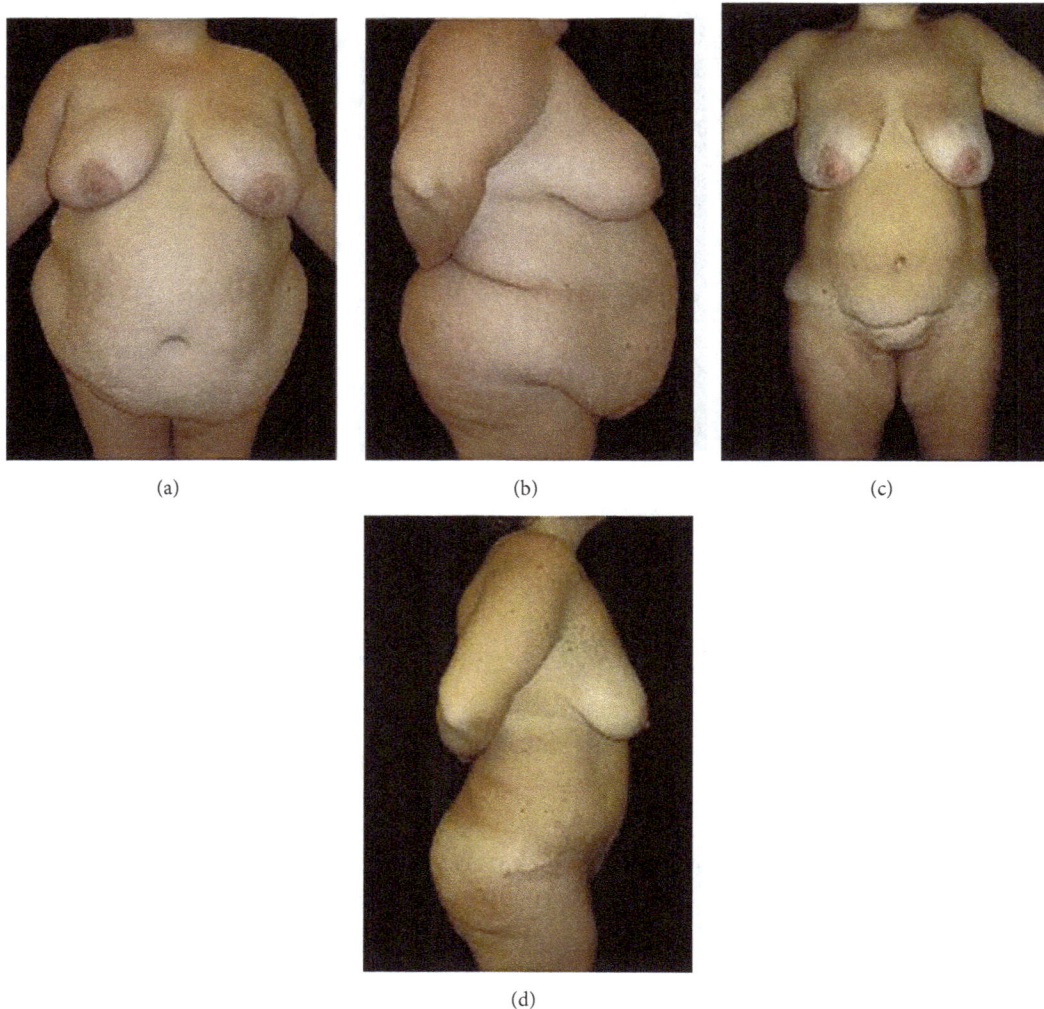

FIGURE 7: (a) Preoperative frontal view and (b) lateral view of a female patient (BMI = 55 kg/m^2; body weight = 147 kg). (c) Postoperative frontal view and (d) lateral view five years after surgery (body weight = 67 kg).

reported by Igwe Jr. et al. [4] for both combined and post-bariatric panniculectomy (Table 6). Therefore, the surgical experience acquired during the study period decreased operating time and hospital stay, motivating us to extend the indications of panniculectomy combined with bariatric surgery by laparotomy.

At present, the literature suggests that abdominal lipectomy should be performed at a later stage to bariatric surgery, after weight loss has been stabilized. It has been reported that abdominoplasty should be conducted up to two years after the bariatric surgery [2, 7, 8]. In our country, as in other countries, the time between the two operations can be much longer because of economic reasons, and this long wait may lead to depression, stress, and poor quality of life of the patient [6].

Some patients who did not undergo panniculectomy combined with bariatric surgery (because they were excluded from the study due to severe comorbidities) had abdominal lymphedema during the weight loss period after bariatric surgery with involvement of the lower limbs. There was a particular case in which absorption of a lymphedema (which reached extraordinary dimensions and weighed about 70 kg) after bariatric surgery required a long outpatient treatment with diuretics before the panniculus could be successfully removed.

The bariatric technique used in this study falls into the category of malabsorptive procedures. This technique led to a stable weight reduction without dietary restrictions in this large case series. Advances in laparoscopic techniques and instrumentation have enabled surgeons to perform bariatric operations for morbid obesity laparoscopically [2]. The laparoscopic approach reduces postoperative pain, decreases complications, shortens length of hospital stay, and allows an early return of the patient to work [10]. Laparoscopy provides benefits, such as reduced operative trauma and decreased risk of incisional hernia and postoperative wound infection

TABLE 6: Comparison of postoperative complications found in this study in the first and second 3-year periods with those reported in a previous study [9].

Postoperative complications	First 3 years ($N = 164$)	Second 3 years ($N = 161$)	Combined treatment ($N = 428$)	Postbariatric panniculectomy ($N = 149$)
Dehiscence	18.9%	8.1%	9.8%	7.4%
Seroma	31.1%	5.0%	4.2%	4.7%
Hemorrhage	7.3%	3.1%	1.9%	1.3%
DVT/PE	4.9%	0.6%	—	—
Incisional hernia	23.2%	6.8%	—	—
Skin necrosis	6.1%	1.9%	—	—
Death	0.6%	0%	—	—

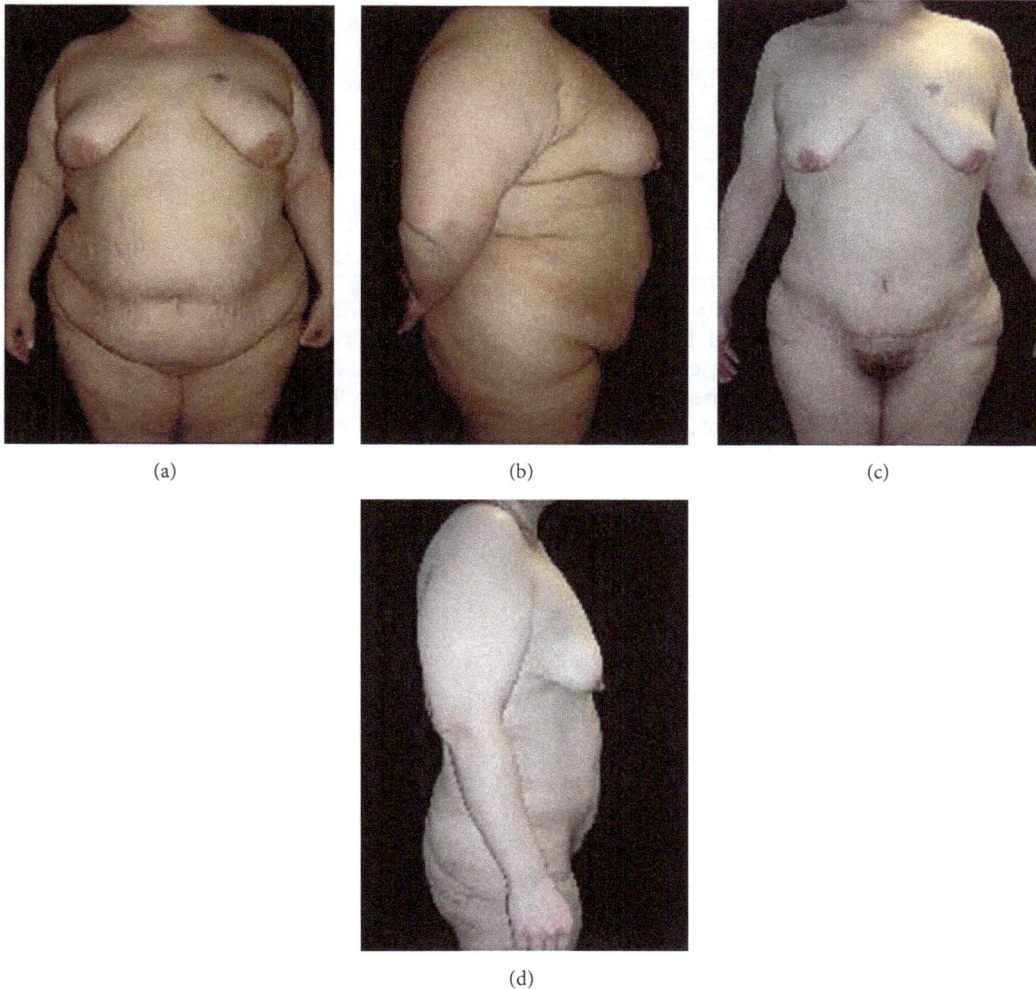

(a) (b) (c)

(d)

FIGURE 8: (a) Preoperative frontal view and (b) lateral view of a female patient (BMI = 45 kg/m^2; body weight = 133 kg). (c) Postoperative frontal view and (d) lateral view 18 months after surgery (body weight = 72 kg).

[11]. Bariatric surgery combined with panniculectomy may be performed using a laparoscopic approach. Further studies combining panniculectomy with laparoscopic bariatric surgery are necessary for comparison of results obtained by the different techniques.

Over the years we have performed this procedure in patients with pendulous abdomen of different grades [4]. Based on the feedback from surgeons, we hypothesized that there are other anthropometric and physiological parameters that are also important to be evaluated during surgery and postoperative period, including the frontal projection of the abdominal apron on the thoracoabdominal wall; the lateral projections of the abdominal apron on the anterior axillary lines (2 measuring points); plicometry under the midline and midclavicular line (3 measuring points); and the degree of absorption of the abdominal panniculus. The use of these seven parameters, which complement the classification by Igwe Jr. et al. [4], allows the creation of a scoring system that can anticipate the difficulty of the surgical procedures and risks of early postoperative complications.

The patients who participated in this study, except in few exceptional cases, did not require aesthetic and nonrevision surgeries because of the subsequent weight loss. In addition, the patient is hospitalized and undergoes general anesthesia only once.

The development of the described technique combining panniculectomy with bariatric surgery allowed us to significantly extend the indications of this treatment, with very good results both in the short and long terms.

5. Conclusions

The retrospective study of 325 patients with morbid obesity who underwent panniculectomy combined with bariatric surgery between 2008 and 2014 indicated that removal of adipose tissue improves the patient's quality of life during the weight-loss period and prevents all the disabling complications, including lymphedema. These complications would make postbariatric panniculectomy necessary, with increased risks to the patient. Incidence rates of postoperative complications associated with the combined surgical treatment were similar to those of postbariatric panniculectomy. With adequate preparation, the combined treatment can be extended to patients with morbid obesity and pendulous abdomen complicated by lymphatic stasis. The patients who participated in this study, except in few exceptional cases, did not require revision surgeries. Accordingly, we believe that the combined technique described in this paper is not only a suitable alternative treatment for economic reasons, but also a sound choice that improves postoperative aesthetic and functional outcome.

Disclosure

Level of evidence is Level IV, case series.

Conflict of Interests

The authors declare that they have no conflict of interests.

References

[1] J. M. Cooper, K. T. Paige, K. M. Beshlian, D. L. Downey, and R. C. Thirlby, "Abdominal panniculectomies high patient satisfaction despite significant complication rates," *Annals of Plastic Surgery*, vol. 61, no. 2, pp. 188–196, 2008.

[2] J. L. Sebastian, "Bariatric surgery and work-up of the massive weight loss patient," *Clinics in Plastic Surgery*, vol. 35, no. 1, pp. 11–26, 2008.

[3] M. Bueter, A. Ahmed, H. Ashrafian, and C. W. le Roux, "Bariatric surgery and hypertension," *Surgery for Obesity and Related Diseases*, vol. 5, no. 5, pp. 615–620, 2009.

[4] D. Igwe Jr., M. Stanczyk, H. Lee, B. Felahy, J. Tambi, and M. A. Fobi, "Panniculectomy adjuvant to obesity surgery," *Obesity Surgery*, vol. 10, no. 6, pp. 530–539, 2000.

[5] T. O. Acarturk, G. Wachtman, B. Heil, A. Landecker, A. P. Courcoulas, and E. K. Manders, "Panniculectomy as an adjuvant to bariatric surgery," *Annals of Plastic Surgery*, vol. 53, no. 4, pp. 360–366, 2004.

[6] G. C. M. Van Hout, S. K. M. Verschure, and G. L. Van Heck, "Psychosocial predictors of success following bariatric surgery," *Obesity Surgery*, vol. 15, no. 4, pp. 552–560, 2005.

[7] M. M. McMahon, M. G. Sarr, M. M. Clark et al., "Clinical management after bariatric surgery: value of a multidisciplinary approach," *Mayo Clinic Proceedings*, vol. 81, no. 10, supplement, pp. S34–S45, 2006.

[8] A. M. Wolf and H. W. Kuhlmann, "Reconstructive procedures after massive weight loss," *Obesity Surgery*, vol. 17, no. 3, pp. 355–360, 2007.

[9] R. U. Gmür, A. Banic, and D. Erni, "Is it safe to combine abdominoplasty with other dermolipectomy procedures to correct skin excess after weight loss?" *Annals of Plastic Surgery*, vol. 51, no. 4, pp. 353–357, 2003.

[10] N. Balagué, C. Combescure, O. Huber, B. Pittet-Cuénod, and A. Modarressi, "Plastic surgery improves long-term weight control after bariatric surgery," *Plastic and Reconstructive Surgery*, vol. 132, no. 4, pp. 826–833, 2013.

[11] D. Leslie, T. A. Kellogg, and S. Ikramuddin, "Bariatric surgery primer for the internist: keys to the surgical consultation," *Medical Clinics of North America*, vol. 91, no. 3, pp. 353–381, 2007.

17

The Use of Tutomesh for a Tension-Free and Tridimensional Repair of Uterovaginal and Vaginal Vault Prolapse: Preliminary Report

Danilo Dodero[1] **and Luca Bernardini**[2]

[1]*Divisione di Ostetricia e Ginecologia, ASL 4 Chiavarese, Ospedale Rivoli, 16033 Lavagna, Italy*
[2]*Dipartimento Materno Infantile, Ostetricia e Ginecologia, ASL 5 Spezzino, 19100 La Spezia, Italy*

Correspondence should be addressed to Danilo Dodero; ddodero@asl4.liguria.it

Academic Editor: Eelco de Bree

Objective. To evaluate efficacy in terms of vaginal capacity, coital function, and recurrence prevention of a new biological mesh of bovine pericardium (Tutomesh) in the repair of severe POP. *Methods.* Thirty cases of patients suffering from stage III uterine or apical prolapse undergone surgical repair by means of a modified sacrospinous ligament suspension combined with mesh attachment to both the cardinal ligaments, posterior and anterior colporrhaphy, and perineal body fixation. The mesh was replaced inside the pelvis with the goal of reconstructing the tridimensional fascial disposition of the structures sustaining the correct axis of vagina. Follow-up was done at 12 months with POPIQ analysis. *Results.* One total mesh failure occurred early after surgery due to marked deficiency of anatomy. Two cystoceles were observed at 12 months in two patients treated for apical prolapse where anterior repair was not performed. Two other patients developed a de novo SUI at 12 months. No reported abnormalities of coital function or dyspareunia were ever found after surgery. *Conclusions.* It is possible that the utilization of a tension-free and tridimensional placement of Tutomesh might favor a more physiologic reconstruction of the vaginal axis as compared with traditional sacrospinous ligament suspension.

1. Introduction

Pelvic organ prolapse (POP) refers to loss of support of the anterior or posterior vaginal wall or the vaginal apex leading to protrusion into or out the vaginal canal of the bladder, rectum, small bowel, and uterus. In most cases POP is a collection of different support defects [1]. Among studies of ambulatory women the prevalence of POP is estimated to vary from 30% to 93% and the number of women seeking care for disorders of the pelvic floor is predicted to increase, looking at the population aging trends, by 45% in the near future [2]. The risk of POP increases with parity and advancing age but previous surgery to correct prolapse which almost always includes hysterectomy is the single greatest factor. In women whose initial hysterectomy was for genital prolapse the risk of repeating surgical correction has been estimated to recur in 20–43% of the cases [3]. Goals of surgery are many including relief of symptoms, correction of the anterior and posterior vaginal wall defects, prevention of new bladder or sexual problems, avoiding iatrogenic pelvic support defects, and achievement of long term success with no need for future pelvic surgery. Nevertheless because the success rate of initial surgery is depending on the capacity to restore normal pelvic floor anatomy, failure to address support defects at all levels is believed to predispose to recurrence of prolapse at the weakest point [1]. It is here briefly stated that the fibromuscular tissue of the vagina is enveloped by the endopelvic fascia which creates an anatomic and functional continuum with other ligaments including the cardinal/uterosacral ligaments (upper suspension level or level 1 DeLancey), lateral attachments to the arcus tendinous fascia and pubo-ileo-coccygeus fascia (middle suspension level or level 2 DeLancey), and at lower level the urogenital diaphragm anteriorly and perineal body posteriorly (lower suspension level or level 3 DeLancey) [4]. In addition to this the endopelvic fascia of the vagina also fuses anteriorly with the pubocervical fascia (Halban's fascia) and posteriorly with the rectovaginal fascia (Denonvilliers' fascia) [5, 6]. The pathophysiology of POP is multifactorial. It can result from genetic predisposition followed by defects of the connective tissue or muscular support or a combination. Tears in the endopelvic fascia permit the opposing soft tissues to bulge through the vaginal wall. Loss of muscular support places the endopelvic fascia under constant strain that results in damage to the connective tissue [1]. Tears in the endopelvic fascia can also cause stretch injury to the innervation of the muscular support. The insertion of the cardinal/uterosacral ligaments into the pericervical ring occurs at the level of the ischial spines and it is the detachment at this level that provides the anatomic rationale for development of posthysterectomy vaginal descent and enterocele (apical prolapse) [7, 8]. Surgery is limited to correction of connective tissue tears or breaks and overcorrection needs to be avoided because it can lead to new support problems. Although the uterus itself does not contribute to POP, most surgeons feel that removing the uterus maximizes the opportunity to correct apical support. There are many different surgical approaches to POP. They can be performed either abdominally or laparoscopically or vaginally [9–11]. Also they may imply the surgical employment of native tissue only or that of different sling or meshes grafts. Choice for best surgical correction of POP should be made on individual bases according to a number of different variables such as patient age, health conditions, and sexual activity as well as type of tissues defects [1]. For this reason different categories of operations exist best suited for various clinical indications having alternatively either obliterative or restorative or even compensatory finalities [1]. Here we describe a mixed restorative/compensatory surgical approach as a novel form of severe uterovaginal prolapse and vaginal vault descent treatment. The procedure involves the utilization of a new biological mesh of bovine pericardium (Tutomesh) for apical, lateral, and posterior fascial repair at the same time. For our purpose the xenograft mesh is precisely arranged and remodeled in our hands for multiple surgical landmarks sites affixation. These include deep and inward suspension to the right sacrospinous ligament, bilateral attachment to the cardinal ligaments remnants (paracervix and vaginal chorion), and forward anterior augmentation of native rectovaginal fascia (previously repaired) by means of final mesh attachment to the perineal body. By adopting such a technique an attempt is here made to ideally reproduce a tridimensional mesh replacement according to internal distribution of fascia and suspensory ligaments inside the pelvis (integral theory of Petros) [12]. Because of this tension-free mesh collocation, a lesser posterolateral deviation of the vaginal axis and also reduced apex narrowing are expected as compared to the traditional methods of sacrospinous ligament fixation. Although infections, when meshes are introduced vaginally, are always a possibility, the biological properties of such new mesh and the peculiar modality of its placement inside the pelvic floor may be of advantage to respect normal function of the surrounding tissues, reduce risk of tape erosion and dyspareunia, and at the same time maintain a lasting valid mechanical support of the pelvic organs.

TABLE 1: Patients characteristics: sample means and SDs.

Number of patients	30
Number of cases with uterine prolapse stage III or IV	20
Number of cases with apical prolapse	10
After vaginal hysterectomy for prolapse	7
After vaginal hysterectomy	2
After abdominal hysterectomy	1
Age (SD)	68.41 (9.22)
Body mass index (SD)	28.11 (3.9)
Parity (SD)	2.5 (0.50)

2. Material and Methods

2.1. Patients. From October 2013 up to October 2014, thirty ($n = 30$) consecutive patients referred to our division for marked uterovaginal prolapse or posthysterectomy vaginal vault prolapse were treated. Informed consent was obtained from all patients scheduled for surgery for stage III or greater uterine prolapse ($n = 20$ patients) and stage II or greater vaginal cuff prolapse ($n = 10$ patients). Baseline assessments before surgery included a history and physical examination including POP-Q examinations on maximum Valsalva effort in the lithotomy position and urodynamic testing (Table 1). The POP-Q uses the hymen as a fixed point of reference and describes six specific topographic points on the vaginal wall (Aa, Ba, C, D, Bp, and Ap) and 3 distances (genital hiatus, perineal body, and total vaginal length). The prolapse of each segment is measured in centimeters during Valsalva relative to the hymenal ring with points inside the vagina reported as negative numbers and outside as positive [13]. The numeric values are then translated to a stage. Stage 3 refers to the lowest point > 1 cm below hymenal ring when the vagina is not completely prolapse. Also, condition-specific QoL and the effect of complications (i.e., protruding vaginal wall, dyspareunia, pain, voiding, and bowel dysfunction) were assessed using validated QoL questionnaires. Sexual life satisfaction and harmful effects of prolapse on QoL were determined by Prolapse Impact Sexual Questionnaire (PISQ-short form), the Urinary Impact Questionnaire (UIQ), the Colon Rectoanal Impact Questionnaire (CRAIQ), and the Pelvic Organs Prolapse Impact Questionnaire (POPIQ), respectively [14, 15]. The QoL instruments and the physical examination were repeated at 3 and 12 months after surgery. Standardized guidelines based on the literature and mesh manufacturer's recommendations for this specific surgical procedure were provided to all the surgical team participants. Only two surgeons have been involved in this study both of them with experience in pelvic surgery.

2.2. Mesh (Tutomesh): "Butterfly 3D" (Kit Patented). Tutomesh© is an avital, acellular, xenogeneic collagen membrane made from bovine pericardium meeting the standards of safety and quality, for instance, according to the German Medical Device Act (MPG) or according to the European Directives (93/42/EEC and 2003/32/EC). The raw material exclusively originates from BSE-free countries

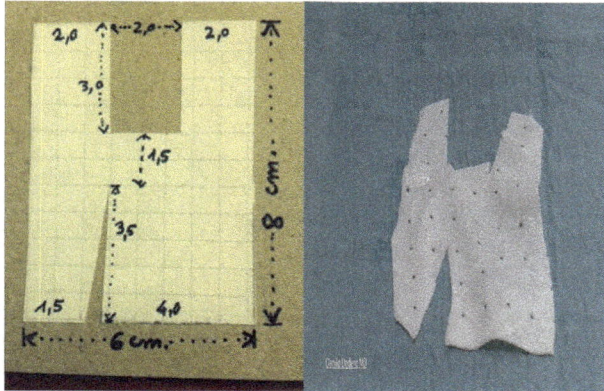

FIGURE 1

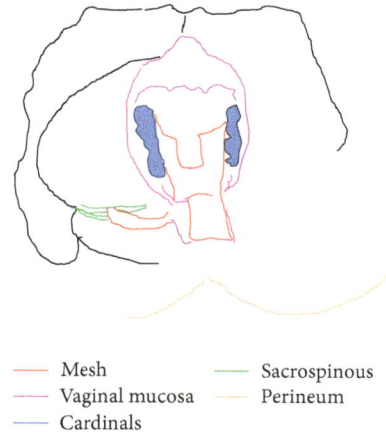

FIGURE 2

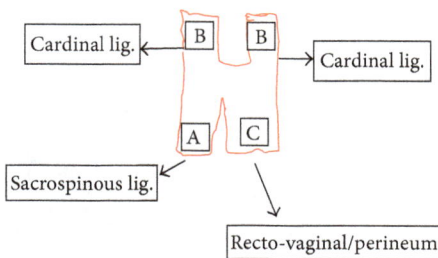

FIGURE 3

and is subjected to the proven Tutoplast process. Tutomesh consists of 92% native collagen type I, which is maintained in its three-dimensional structure and for its biomechanical properties. This renders the transplant extremely resistant to tensile forces without impeding the remodeling process after implantation. Tutomesh is a natural collagen membrane without further treatment for cross-linking. If handled and placed appropriately the mesh acts as a scaffold which allows the in-growth of vessels and fibroblasts with their deposition of site-specific collagen. In this way Tutomesh is gradually replaced by the patient's own tissue which will transform into the site-specific tissue by time. For the fixation of Tutomesh monofilament and not resorbable suturing material is recommended. In order to prevent the suture from cutting the mesh, the edge of the Tutomesh should be folded in for approximately 1 cm [16, 17]. Clinical practice suggests that the mesh is perfectly positioned by fixing it at multiple points with interrupted sutures. For our purposes Tutomesh is retailed in H shaped form in order to be attached to multiple surgical landmarks, avoiding direct tension and deviation of the vaginal axis at the same time: A, sacrospinous ligament; B, cardinal ligaments; C, perineal body (Figures 1, 2, and 3).

2.3. Surgical Procedure. At our division vaginal hysterectomy is performed from a long time based on classic principles of vaginal surgery with recent modifications due to the employment of modern surgical instruments and precious teachings personally received at the Emory University Hospital (USA) by Professor Kovac [18]. A number of almost 200 vaginal hysterectomies are performed annually most for grade I or

II uterine-vaginal prolapse frequently coupled to anterior and/or posterior colporrhaphy. In general when vaginal hysterectomy is performed for mild uterovaginal prolapse, our routine practice is to add a prophylactic modified McCall culdoplasty at the end of hysterectomy [19–21]. To this end the vaginal vault is closed by executing a ligamentous form of colpopexy as follows: one end of a suture previously inserted in the anterior flap of peritoneum is used for taking successive bites in the peritoneum on the right side until the suture reaches the right broad ligament where it is passed through the tuboovarian stump. The suture picks up the peritoneum and the broad ligament in successive bites and includes the stumps of the uterine vessels and uterosacral ligament. Care is taken to insert the needle distal to the ligatures. The suture is then passed through the right edge of the posterior peritoneal flap, through the posterior vaginal wall and out into the right side of the posterior vaginal fornix. A similar suture begun on the anterior portion of the peritoneum is placed on the left side to close the left half of the open vaginal vault. These sutures are then separately tied. These sutures anchor the broad and uterosacral ligaments to the vaginal vault, take care of peritonization, and close the vaginal vault. The anterior and posterior vaginal walls are approximated with interrupted or continuous sutures (Vicryl 0, Ethicon, Johnson & Johnson, USA). A cystocele or rectocele is repaired at this time.

In cases of worse uterovaginal prolapse we have always traditionally recurred to restorative (sacrospinous ligament suspension) or even compensatory (total vaginal wall mesh repair) forms of surgical repair according to Amreich-Richter or Prolift (Gynecare Prolift, Ethicon, Johnson & Johnson, USA) recommendations, respectively. Sometimes the two approaches have been also variably combined. Despite the overall good results achieved in most cases with both these approaches, our anecdotal experience of some complications and recurrences (in the percentage commonly reported for these techniques) prompted us toward the research for a possibly better way of repair as here described in detail.

(A) Vaginal Hysterectomy for Grade III Uterine-Vaginal Prolapse. First an infiltration of the anterior, lateral, and posterior

vaginal fornix is made by using a modified physiologic solution (100 cc of saline solution + 30 IU of Oxytocin + 2 ampules of Naropin 2 mg/mL). With a scalpel a transverse incision is made through the anterior vaginal mucosa below the attachment of the bladder and prosecuted by less deep lateral incision on each side of the cervix toward the posterior vaginal fornix which is incised at a considerable distance from the external os. The anterior wall of the vagina with the attached bladder is then separated from the uterus with bipolar scissors. Afterwards the incised posterior mucosa is pushed down and back to expose the peritoneum. The posterior cul-de-sac peritoneum is opened with scissors and a narrow retractor inserted into the peritoneal cavity. The description of the vaginal hysterectomy is familiar to every surgeon and it is not further described here because it is outside of the study scope. Anterior colporrhaphy has been always executed in all cases ($n = 20$). A vertical incision of the vagina is made in the midline. The vaginal muscularis is plicated using 2-0 absorbable suture in an interrupted fashion (Vicryl 2-0, Ethicon, Johnson & Johnson, USA). Care is taken to ensure that the vaginal muscularis is not removed from the underlying detrusor muscle. If there is loss of the urethrovesical angle a plicating suture at the urethrovesical junction is placed to restore anatomy (the Kelly plication). Sometimes one bridge suture passing through the pubourethral ligaments on each side (Nichols suspension) or a transobturator mesh urethroplasty (TOT) is alternatively performed to correct urethral mobility and prevent de novo IUS occurrence [16]. The redundant vaginal wall is then resected and the vaginal edges are reopposed using 2-0 absorbable suture in a continuous crossed fashion while being careful to pick up underlying vaginal muscularis to close the dead space (Vicryl 2-0, Ethicon, Johnson & Johnson, USA).

(B) *Vaginal Vault Prolapse*. Two Allis clamps are placed at the recognizable angles of the vaginal scar. The saline solution is similarly injected under the vaginal mucosa followed by a vertical or transverse incision of the mucosa. Using scissors and toothed pickups the vaginal epithelium including the muscularis is dissected with caution from the underlying peritoneum (enterocele) and bladder or rectum mucosa. Care is taken to respect integrity of the fragile peritoneal folds below the dissection. Anterior colporrhaphy to reduce the protrusion of the bladder and vagina in order to prevent cystocele recurrence is generally performed. However, in the series here studied this was done only in 8 out 10 patients.

(C) *Posterior Compartment Repair (Same for A and B)*. Posterior colporrhaphy includes the plication of the pararectal and rectovaginal fascia over the rectal wall. In the past, levator ani plications used to be more frequently done for the treatment of rectocele but because of dyspareunia we moved toward a fascial plication only according to Kovac [18]. Posterior compartment repair is similar, done either after vaginal hysterectomy or in presence of apical vault prolapse: after injecting the saline solution under the vaginal mucosa, a longitudinal posterior colpotomy is performed in the midline after a diamond-shaped incision of the perineum. Once again the vaginal epithelium is carefully dissected from the

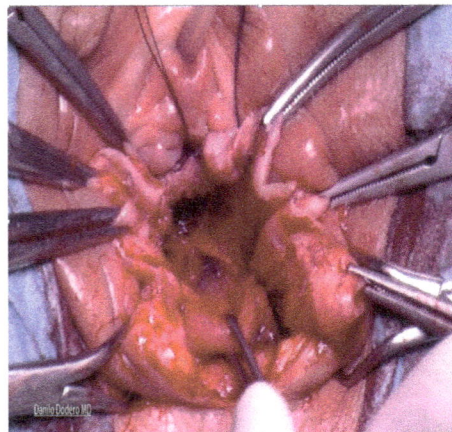

FIGURE 4

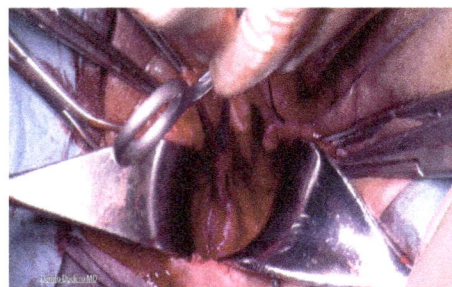

FIGURE 5

muscularis (rectovaginal fascia) and left apart along with the rectum wall. The pararectal space is bilaterally prepared with mobilization of the rectum from its lateral connections by blunt finger dissection. After introducing one finger into the rectum it is possible to better evaluate size and level of fascial defect and provide best fascial repair. After clamping with Allis the rectovaginal fascia (Figure 4), interrupted sutures to close the defect and anchor the rectovaginal fascia to the perineal body are given. During this suture a finger inside the rectum allows checking for eventual mistaken bites of the rectal mucosa into the suture.

The procedure used for sacrospinous fixation is basically done according to the technique originally described by Amreich-Richter [22, 23] although having here a different rationale. The technique comprises dissection into the right paravaginal space, identification of the right ischial spine, and clear visualization of the right sacrospinous ligament (Figure 5).

Using one single no absorbable 2-0 thread a double stitched suture (Ethibond Excel 2-0, Ethicon, Johnson & Johnson, USA) is placed through the ligament one and half fingerbreadths from the tip of the ischial spine. Both ends of the suture are left untied and kept for later transfixion of the inferior right arm of the H shaped Tutomesh ("Butterfly 3D" kit patented). In our technique whatsoever direct attachment of the vaginal vault to the ligament is intentionally avoided. Next step implies the recognition of the cardinal ligaments

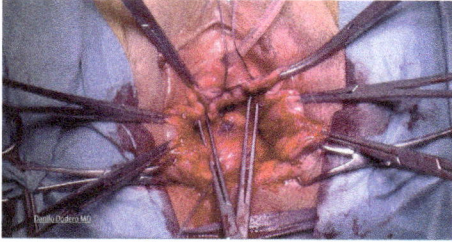

FIGURE 6

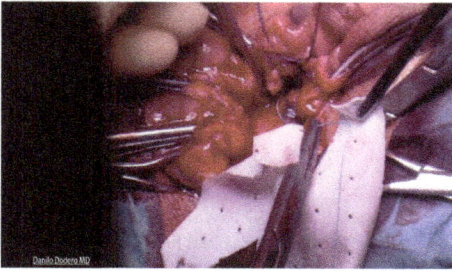

FIGURE 7

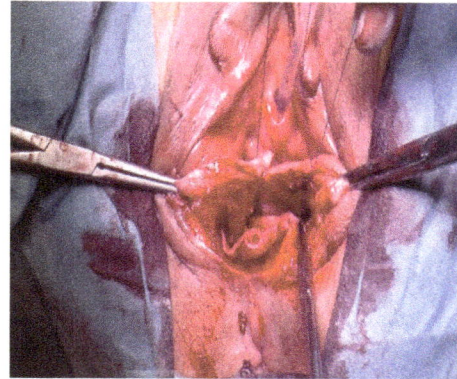

FIGURE 8

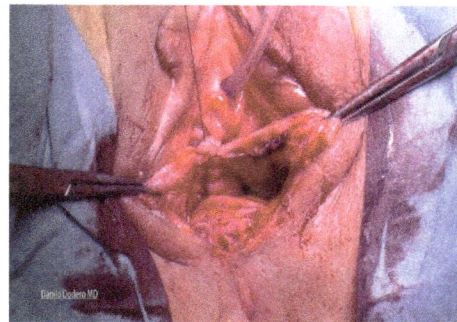

FIGURE 9

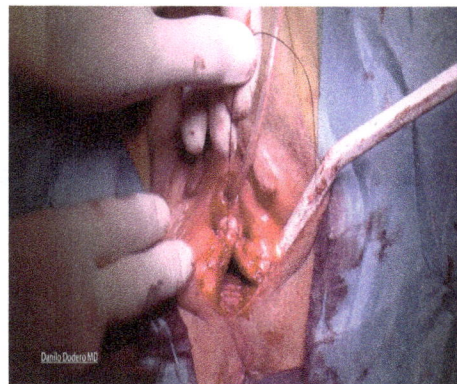

FIGURE 10

which are generally found as thick paracervical remnants or parts of the vaginal chorion on each side. Cardinal ligaments are then held by Allis clamps in view of delayed transfixion with no adsorbable 2-0 sutures to the upper arms of the H shaped Tutomesh (Figures 6 and 7).

As soon as all the surgical landmarks are localized and exposed, the Tutomesh graft, previously adequately molded and cut, is then placed in situ. After suturing the vaginal apex with interrupted stiches of Vicryl 0, the posterior colporrhaphy is started using Vicryl 2-0 in a continuous not crossed fashion. When the colporrhaphy reaches the mid portion of the vagina it is halted. The four Tutomesh arms can be now tied as follows: the inferior right arm is sutured to the sacrospinous ligament, the two upper lateral arms are sutured to the cardinal ligaments, and the inferior left arm is sutured to the perineal body (Figures 8 and 9).

In this last case a barbed suture (Quill 2-0, Surgical Specialties Corporation, USA) in a continuous fashion is generally done. Thereafter the colporrhaphy is completed ending with final cosmetic repair of the perineum (Figure 10). Iodine gauze is left in vagina for 24 hours and urinary catheter kept in place for 72 hours. On the day of surgery, cefazolin 2 g was administered. Prophylactic anticoagulant therapy was given for up to 28 days. All patients are advised to start and prosecute for at least 1 month a local estrogen therapy by vaginal route.

3. Results

Operative parameters and short term complications are reported in Table 2. The median operation time was 90 minutes (range 55–166 minutes) and median blood loss was 120 mL (20–790 mL). No patients required a blood transfusion. Importantly, one case of early total surgical failure due to suboptimal suspension to the sacrospinous ligament in a 60-year-old patient with apical prolapse was observed. In this case the visualization and transfixion of the ligament during the intervention resulting were particularly difficult because of paucity and laxity of ischiorectal tissues. This patient was readmitted later soon and reoperated on by means of abdominal sacrocolpopexy. Additional prolapse recurrence occurred in two cases (cystocele) out of 30 and specifically involved only those 2 cases of apical prolapse where a prophylactic repair of the anterior compartment was inadvertently not done. This was observed at 12-month interval. However, only one patient in this subgroup was

TABLE 2: List of operative parameters and postoperative complications at 1 month.

Variable	With hysterectomy	Without hysterectomy
Number of patients	20	10
Hemoglobin drop	2.0 ± 1 g%	1.5 ± 1 g%
Bladder lesions	0	0
Hematoma	0	1 (drained)
Abscess	2 (spontaneous resolution)	0
Bowel lesions	0	0
Concomitant pelvic surgery	Bilateral oophorectomy in 12 cases	0

TABLE 3: POP-Q findings.

	Before surgery	3-month follow-up	12-month follow-up
Aa	1.5	−2	−2.31
Ba	2	−1.9	−2.13
C	1.5	−5.0	−4.99
Gh	5.2	4.2	3
Pb	4.1	4.5	3.44
Ap	1.1	−2.13	−2.37
Bp	1.2	−2.1	−2.22

TABLE 4: Quality-of-life questionnaires.

Months after surgery	PISQ-12	UIQ	CRAIQ	POPIQ
0	28.9	100.22	36.86	76.70
3	33.2	59.11	15.88	16.15
12	36.7	31.7*	4.61*	10.2*

*p value <0.001 in the score between months 12 and 0. PISQ-12: pelvic organ prolapse urinary incontinence sexual function questionnaire-12, UIQ: Urinary Impact Questionnaire, CRAIQ: Colon Rectoanal Impact Questionnaire, and POPIQ: Pelvic Organs Prolapse Impact Questionnaire.

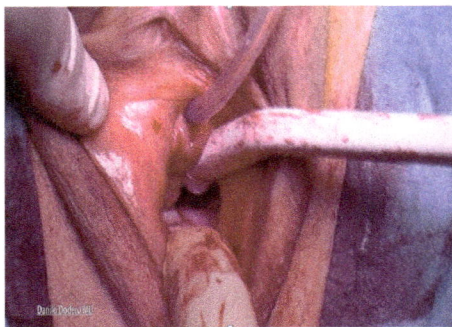

FIGURE 11

symptomatic and required reoperation by anterior colporrhaphy and transobturator mesh urethroplasty (TOT). Finally, in other two patients a de novo urinary stress incontinence at 3 months after hysterectomy was present requiring, again, a TOT operation. Overall in 4 out of 30 cases (13.3%) it was necessary to repeat surgery.

A normalization of the vaginal axis with satisfactory length and width was achieved in all cases with importantly no report of dyspareunia or hyspareunia (male partner complaints due to vaginal axis narrowing as it occurs when one vaginal cuff corner is fixed tightly to the sacrospinous ligament) (Figure 11). Mean total vaginal length was 8.2 cm and the mean point C position as a measure of vaginal apex fixation above the hymen, one year after surgery, was −4.99 (Table 3). A significant improvement in the quality-of-life questionnaires after surgery was found in most cases (Table 4).

4. Discussion

Treatment and prevention of vaginal vault prolapse are challenging as they are shown by the existence of more than 40 different techniques to treat this pathology. Moreover controversy also exists over the choice of vaginal procedure as well as the relative merits of vaginal versus abdominal suspension procedures. In general, for elderly patients whose health status precludes prolonged surgery, an obliterative repair closing vagina and affording symptom relief with minimal morbidity is preferred (colpocleisis) while, for those patients with discrete defects in the endopelvic fascia without ongoing risk factors for recurrence, a restorative procedure accomplished by a vaginal approach is rather favored (sacrospinous ligament suspension or iliococcygeus fascial suspension or uterosacral ligament suspension in variable combination with anterior colporrhaphy or paravaginal repair and posterior colporrhaphy). In other circumstances the native tissue repair however is insufficient and a compensatory operation using grafts materials (meshes) became a more reasonable option (abdominal or laparoscopic sacral colpopexy or anterior and posterior total vaginal wall mesh replacement or infracoccygeal IVS sling colpopexy) [1–3, 5–7]. Nonetheless, graft materials, particularly when used by a vaginal approach, may shrink after placement (mesh erosion) or lead to loss of pelvic floor flexibility (dyspareunia) or be site of late infections [24, 25]. For this reason a novel laparoscopic technique employing only native tissues such as the obliterated umbilical arteries anchored to the vaginal cuff (laparoscopic chordofixation) has more recently been proposed as a safer and faster option [26]. Notwithstanding the above, no technique is as yet fully satisfactory reflecting how poorly the pathophysiology is understood and so its correction [27]. In addition, the choice of procedure is often dependent on the individual surgeon's choice and experience.

Our long time experience of vaginal surgery has allowed addressing an original strategy for the correction of advanced uterine-vaginal prolapse in order to prevent it (at the time of vaginal hysterectomy) and directly cure it as well. We hypothesized that the use of a new biological mesh for a compensatory repair in combination with a restorative one (sacrospinous ligament-mesh fixation) could possibly be of advantage if compared with total wall synthetic mesh repair or sacrospinous ligament suspension as separately considered. Our procedure allows replacing fascial defects with a biological mesh of bovine pericardium properly arranged for being anchored to the sustaining connective structures and ligaments which naturally follow a tridimensional way of disposition and support inside the pelvic floor. Importantly, level I DeLancey apex suspension is obtained indirectly by fixing the mesh to the vaginal chorion and paracervical tissue containing the cardinals and only secondly by suspending the mesh to the right sacrospinous ligament. We believe this point to be a striking feature of our procedure since it reduces a lot the vaginal tension and posterolateral axis deviation as usually reported in case of traditional procedure for sacrospinous ligament fixation. By suturing the mesh also to the perineal body (just over the previously repaired rectovaginal fascia) and completing the operation with an anterior colporrhaphy it is possible at the end to obtain a full restitutio ad integrum of the vaginal support with good urinary continence, vaginal capacity, and coital function. The level I vaginal suspension so executed along with the anterior and posterior fascial and ligamentous repair also would reinforce the pelvic floor thus making unlikely the formation of tears or breaks of the pelvic floor conducing to recurrence. Our results show this to be the case. In fact the only three cases with unsuccessful outcome should be ascribed in one case to an unpredictable severe macroscopic (and probably microscopic) deficiency of the connective tissue of the ischiorectal space (one total failure) and in the other two cases to the missed anterior compartment repair at the time of apical vault surgery (two cystoceles). The cystocele recurrence risk deserves particular and separate consideration whenever a solid apex fixation and efficient posterior reinforcement, such as here done, are provided.

To our knowledge this is the first time that a biological mesh of bovine pericardium (Tutomesh) is used in gynecological surgery even though we took into account the same surgical principles already reported using Tutomesh in case of abdominal wall hernias repair [17]. Tutomesh appears to greatly satisfy many of the requests for a prosthetic graft to be ideal including biocompatibility, inert activity, no allergic or inflammatory reaction, and sterility, no carcinogen, and also handling feasibility. However, despite the significant increase in the use of biological products to overcome the problems of prosthesis erosion and extrusion it is generally still an open question of how long any biological absorbable material has to remain as a scaffold (and not only as bridge) before adequate in-growth of host tissues has occurred to maintain long term support [28]. Up to date whether, among a number of new absorbable and biological meshes proposed, Tutomesh might be more resistant to infections or be particularly suited for avoiding shrinkage and mechanical stress while preserving its intrinsic strength has still to be determined.

In any case, we believe that our procedure is original since we have not been able to find anything similar in the literature.

We refer to the review article of Birch on the use of prosthetics in pelvic reconstructive surgery [28]. In this review two studies using a similar combination of restorative/compensatory surgery (for the cure of separate prolapse compartments) have been reported. Salomon et al. [29] described the use of porcine skin collagen (Pelvicol) introduced through a transobturator approach in combination with a sacrospinous fixation for the anterior compartment repair. Their short term results were encouraging. Dwyer and O'Reilly described the fixation of a Y-shaped polypropylene prosthesis to the sacrospinous ligament bilaterally and an inferior attachment to the perineal body for the posterior compartment repair. In their study of 33 patients, erosions were reported in 4% with no reports of postoperative sexual dysfunction [30].

In conclusion, we have here described a new approach aimed at restoring, in case of severe POP, the first, the third, and only partially the second (posterior half) of DeLancey levels. Despite our encouraging preliminary results here reported using the "Butterfly 3D" Tutomesh (low POP recurrence, no mesh erosions, and no dyspareunia), due to the limited number of cases studied and short follow-up period we cannot, to date, draw firm long term conclusions. At the moment, we are now in the process of extending our studies in a multicenter randomized trial (protocol BioPOP approved by Regional Ethic Committee) involving 15 centers in Italy to enroll at least 300 patients as for adequate statistical power analyses request. At the same time we have initiated a study on fresh cadavers to evaluate the possibility to correct completely also the second DeLancey level by means of a new biological mesh of different size (ASSUT Spa).

Conflict of Interests

The authors declare that there is no conflict of interests regarding the publication of this paper.

Acknowledgments

The authors are historically grateful to Professor Kovac for the surgical hints received and thank Melita for her assistance during data collection.

References

[1] F. Rojas and G. W. Cundiff, "Urogynecology and reconstructive pelvic surgery," in *The John Hopkins Manual of Gynecology and Obstetrics*, pp. 324–342, Walters Kluwer, Lippincott Williams & Wilkins, 3rd edition, 2007.

[2] M. Alperin, M. Weinstein, S. Kivnick, T. H. Duong, and S. Menefee, "A randomized trial of prophylactic uterosacral ligament suspension at the time of hysterectomy for Prevention of Vaginal Vault Prolapse (PULS): design and methods," *Contemporary Clinical Trials*, vol. 35, no. 2, pp. 8–12, 2013.

[3] R. E. Blandon, A. E. Bharucha, L. J. Melton III et al., "Incidence of pelvic floor repair after hysterectomy: a population-based cohort study," *The American Journal of Obstetrics and Gynecology*, vol. 197, no. 6, pp. 664.e1–664.e7, 2007.

[4] J. O. L. DeLancey, "Anatomic aspects of vaginal eversion after hysterectomy," *American Journal of Obstetrics and Gynecology*, vol. 166, no. 6, pp. 1717–1728, 1992.

[5] C. Chaliha and V. Khullar, "Management of vault prolapse," *Reviews in Gynaecological Practice*, vol. 5, no. 2, pp. 89–94, 2005.

[6] R. Afifi and A. T. Sayed, "Post-hysterectomy vaginal vault prolapse," *The Obstetrician & Gynaecologist*, vol. 7, no. 2, pp. 89–97, 2005.

[7] G. R. McCracken and G. Lefebvre, "Mesh-free anterior vaginal wall repair: history or best practice?" *The Obstetrician & Gynaecologist*, vol. 9, no. 4, pp. 233–242, 2007.

[8] A. Uzoma and K. A. Farag, "Vaginal vault prolapse," *Obstetrics and Gynecology International*, vol. 2009, Article ID 275621, 9 pages, 2009.

[9] R. Arbel and Y. Lavy, "Vaginal vault prolapse: choice of operation," *Best Practice and Research: Clinical Obstetrics and Gynaecology*, vol. 19, no. 6, pp. 959–977, 2005.

[10] RCOG and BSUG, "The management of post hysterectomy vaginal vault prolapse," Green-Top Guideline 46, 2007.

[11] A. Khunda, A. Vashisht, and A. Cutner, "New procedures for uterine prolapse," *Best Practice & Research: Clinical Obstetrics & Gynaecology*, vol. 27, no. 3, pp. 363–379, 2013.

[12] P. Petros, *The Female Pelvic Floor: Function, Dysfunction and Management According to the Integral Theory*, Springer, Heidelberg, Germany, 2010.

[13] A. E. Bent, D. R. Ostegard, G. W. Cundiff, and S. Swift, Eds., *Ostergard's Urogynecology and Pelvic Floor Dysfunction*, Lippincott Williams & Wilkins, Philadelphia, Pa, USA, 5th edition, 2003.

[14] M. Halaska, K. Maxova, O. Sottner et al., "A multicenter, randomized, prospective, controlled study comparing sacrospinous fixation and transvaginal mesh in the treatment of posthysterectomy vaginal vault prolapse," *The American Journal of Obstetrics and Gynecology*, vol. 207, no. 4, pp. 301.e1–301.e7, 2012.

[15] B. Shull and M. M. Karram, "Concerns regarding pelvic reconstructive surgery," *International Urogynecology Journal and Pelvic Floor Dysfunction*, vol. 16, no. 4, pp. 251–252, 2005.

[16] L. T. Prodigalidad, Y. Peled, S. L. Stanton, and H. Krissi, "Long-term results of prolapse recurrence and functional outcome after vaginal hysterectomy," *International Journal of Gynecology and Obstetrics*, vol. 120, no. 1, pp. 57–60, 2013.

[17] L. D'Ambra, S. Berti, C. Feleppa, P. Magistrelli, P. Bonfante, and E. Falco, "Use of bovine pericardium graft for abdominal wall reconstruction in contaminated fields," *World Journal of Gastrointestinal Surgery*, vol. 4, no. 7, pp. 171–176, 2012.

[18] S. R. Kovac, "Route of hysterectomy: an evidence-based approach," *Clinical Obstetrics and Gynecology*, vol. 57, no. 1, pp. 58–71, 2014.

[19] S. H. Cruikshank and S. R. Kovac, "Randomized comparison of three surgical methods used at the time of vaginal hysterectomy to prevent posterior enterocele," *American Journal of Obstetrics and Gynecology*, vol. 180, no. 4, pp. 859–865, 1999.

[20] S. H. Cruikshank, "Operations for support of the vaginal vault," *The Global Library of Women's Medicine*, 2009.

[21] D. H. Nichols and C. L. Randall, *Vaginal Surgery*, Williams & Wilkins, Baltimore, Md, USA, 3rd edition, 1989.

[22] C. L. Randall and D. H. Nichols, "Surgical treatment of vaginal inversion," *Obstetrics and Gynecology*, vol. 38, no. 3, pp. 327–332, 1971.

[23] S. H. Cruikshank, "Sacrospinous fixation—should this be performed at the time of vaginal hysterectomy?" *American Journal of Obstetrics and Gynecology*, vol. 164, no. 4, pp. 1072–1076, 1991.

[24] D. Biller and W. G. Davila, "Choosing the best technique for vaginal vault prolapse," *OBG Management Journal*, vol. 16, no. 12, 2004.

[25] C. B. Iglesia, "STOP using synthetic mesh for routine repair of pelvic organ prolapse," *OBG Management Journal*, vol. 25, no. 4, 2013.

[26] M. Koppan, A. Hackethal, I. A. Muller-Funogea et al., "Laparoscopic chordofixation: a new technique for vaginal vault suspension," *Pelviperineology*, vol. 31, pp. 70–73, 2012.

[27] A. Lukanovič and K. Dražič, "Risk factors for vaginal prolapse after hysterectomy," *International Journal of Gynecology and Obstetrics*, vol. 110, no. 1, pp. 27–30, 2010.

[28] C. Birch, "The use of prosthetics in pelvic reconstructive surgery," *Best Practice & Research: Clinical Obstetrics and Gynaecology*, vol. 19, no. 6, pp. 979–991, 2005.

[29] L. J. Salomon, R. Detchev, E. Barranger, A. Cortez, P. Callard, and E. Darai, "Treatment of anterior vaginal wall prolapse with porcine skin collagen implant by the transobturator route: preliminary results," *European Urology*, vol. 45, no. 2, pp. 219–225, 2004.

[30] P. L. Dwyer and B. A. O'Reilly, "Transvaginal repair of anterior and posterior compartment prolapse with Atrium polypropylene mesh," *BJOG: An International Journal of Obstetrics & Gynaecology*, vol. 111, no. 8, pp. 831–836, 2004.

18

To Investigate the Effect of Colchicine in Prevention of Adhesions Caused by Serosal Damage in Rats

İhsan Yıldız and Yavuz Savas Koca

Department of General Surgery, School of Medicine, Suleyman Demirel University, Isparta, Turkey

Correspondence should be addressed to İhsan Yıldız; drihsanyildiz@gmail.com

Academic Editor: Todd Pesavento

Introduction and Aim. Adhesion formation is a process which starts with an inflammation caused by a number of factors and eventually results in fibrosis. Colchicine prevents adhesion formation which is antifibrous process. The effectivity of colchicine in the prevention of adhesions was investigated. *Materials and Methods.* A total of 36 rats were equally divided into three groups: (I) control group 1 ($n = 12$), (II) abrasion group 2 ($n = 12$), and (III) abrasion + colchicine group 3 ($n = 12$). Group 1 underwent laparotomy and was orally given physiological serum 2 cc/day for 10 days. In Group 2, injury was created in the cecum serosa following laparotomy and they were orally given physiological serum 2 cc/day for 10 days. In Group 3, injury was created in the cecum serosa following laparotomy and the rats were orally given colchicine 50 mcg kg/day mixed with physiological serum 2 cc/day for 10 days. Laparotomy was performed and adhesions were examined both macroscopically and microscopically. Both macroscopic and microscopic examinations were performed using Zühlke's score. *Results.* A significant difference was observed among the adhesion scores of the groups both macroscopically and microscopically. Macroscopic score was lower in group 3 than group 2. Microscopic score was lower in group 3 than group 2. *Conclusion.* Oral administration of colchicine is effective in the prevention of adhesions.

1. Introduction

Intraperitoneal adhesions remain a challenging surgical problem. These adhesions often cause a number of clinical problems including intestinal obstruction, chronic abdominal pain, and infertility. During abdominal surgery, serosal adhesions may lead to organ injuries and thus may lead to higher morbidity and mortality. For a long period of time, numerous studies have been conducted to investigate the pathophysiology of adhesion formation and to prevent adhesion formation in light of the results obtained [1–9]. Adhesion formation starts with the accumulation of fibrin matrix, which becomes organized and eventually results in fibrous adhesions within 5–7 days. Postsurgical adhesions occur among the traumatic serosal surfaces induced by the trauma during surgery. Wound healing process starts when the inflammation following tissue injury occurs [3]. During the wound healing process, a gel fibrin structure oozes out and if this structure is not destroyed by the fibrinolytic activity, a fibrin clot is formed, leading to permanent fibrous bands [4, 5].

Colchicine is a natural drug which provides various effects including antifibrotic activity, anti-inflammatory effect, membrane stabilization, and the inhibition of lipid peroxidation. Due to these effects, colchicine is considered to be effective in the diseases closely associated with inflammatory events and cell division [6]. Colchicine inhibits the macrophage release of fibronectin and the release of growth factor from the macrophages and also suppresses the cellular replication by connecting to the tubulin and the release of cytokines from the polymorphonuclear leukocytes. Pharmacodynamic studies have demonstrated that the biological effect of colchicine is associated with the plasma concentration. Colchicine exerts antimitotic effect in a dose-dependent manner. This effect takes 30–120 min to occur. The oral bioavailability of colchicine is 50%. The elimination half-life of colchicine ranges between 20 and 40 h. Most common side effects of colchicine include diarrhea, nausea, and vomiting [4, 5].

Colchicine prevents adhesion formation during the healing process of serosal injury by altering the neutrophil migration and the distribution of adhesion molecules on neutrophils and endothelial cells [5]. The aim of this experimental study was to investigate the effectivity of colchicine in the prevention of adhesions induced by serosal injury.

2. Materials and Methods

The study included 36 young adult Wistar Albino rats weighing 210–280 g. The rats were divided into three groups as follows: (I) control group ($n = 12$), (II) abrasion group ($n = 12$), and (III) abrasion + colchicine group ($n = 12$). Intramuscular anesthesia was performed using 80 mg/kg ketamine hydrochloride (Ketalar, Parke-Davis, Morris Plains) and 10 mg/kg xylazine hydrochloride (Rompun, Bayer). All the surgical procedures were performed in sterile conditions. In all the rats, the abdominal skin was shaved and cleaned with povidone-iodide solution. The surgical site was covered with green sterile drape with a hole. Laparotomy was performed through a 3-cm midline incision. The cecum and the terminal ileum were localized and wet gauze was placed on them. Abrasion was performed on the antimesenteric surface of the cecum using dry gauze. The procedure was continued until petechial bleeding foci were seen on the surfaces (cecal abrasion model).

2.1. Groups. The control group underwent laparotomy only and was orally given physiological serum 2 cc/day for 10 days. In the abrasion group, injury was created in the cecum serosa following laparotomy. This group was also orally given physiological serum 2 cc/day for 10 days. In the abrasion + colchicine group, injury was created in the cecum serosa following laparotomy and the rats were orally given colchicine 50 mcg/kg/day with physiological serum 2 cc/day for 10 days (using gavage).

Laparotomy was performed on postoperative day 10 in order to monitor and score the adhesions. The adhesions were examined both macroscopically (see the Zühlke Macroscopic Classification, Figure 1) and microscopically (see the Zühlke Microscopic Classification) using Zühlke's grading system.

The Zühlke Macroscopic Classification. The classification is as follows:

Grade 1: filmy and easy to separate by blunt dissection.

Grade 2: blunt dissection possible, partly sharp dissection necessary, and beginning vascularization.

Grade 3: lysis possible by sharp dissection only, clear vascularization.

Grade 4: lysis possible by sharp dissection only, organs strongly attached with severe adhesions, and damage of organs hardly preventable.

The Zühlke Microscopic Classification. The classification is as follows:

TABLE 1: The Zülhke macroscopic classification.

Groups	Adhesion scores			
	1	2	3	4
Control ($n = 12$)	2	0	0	0
Abrasion ($n = 12$)	1	3	5	3
Abrasion + colchicine ($n = 12$)	4	5	2	1

TABLE 2: The Zülhke microscopic classification.

Groups	Adhesion scores			
	1	2	3	4
Control ($n = 12$)	2	0	0	0
Abrasion ($n = 12$)	0	3	5	4
Abrasion + colchicine ($n = 12$)	3	4	3	2

Grade 1: loose connective tissue, cell-rich, old and new fibrine, fine reticular fibers.

Grade 2: connective tissue with cells capillaries, few collagen fibers.

Grade 3: connective tissue more firm, fewer cells, more vessels, and few elastic and smooth-muscle fibers.

Grade 4: old firm granulation tissue, cell-poor, serosal layers hardly distinguishable.

The crude drugs were examined under a light microscope and then photographed. The results were evaluated using the microscopic classification system developed by Zühlke (Figure 1).

Statistical analyses were performed using Mann-Whitney U Test. A p value of <0.05 was considered significant.

3. Results

No subjects were lost and no healing problems such as infection and delayed wound closure occurred in any group. No side effects of colchicine such as diarrhea, hair loss, and bone marrow depression were detected. No serious feeding disorder, inappetence, or weight loss was observed in the postoperative period.

The macroscopic adhesion scores were significantly higher in the abrasion and abrasion + colchicine groups compared to the control group ($p < 0.01$ and $p < 0.05$, resp.) (Table 1). Similarly, the microscopic adhesion scores were significantly higher in the abrasion and abrasion + colchicine groups compared to the control group ($p < 0.01$ and $p < 0.05$, resp.) (Table 2).

The macroscopic adhesion scores were significantly higher in the abrasion group compared to the abrasion + colchicine group ($p < 0.01$) (Table 1). Likewise, the microscopic adhesion scores were significantly higher in the abrasion group compared to the abrasion + colchicine group ($p < 0.01$) (Table 2).

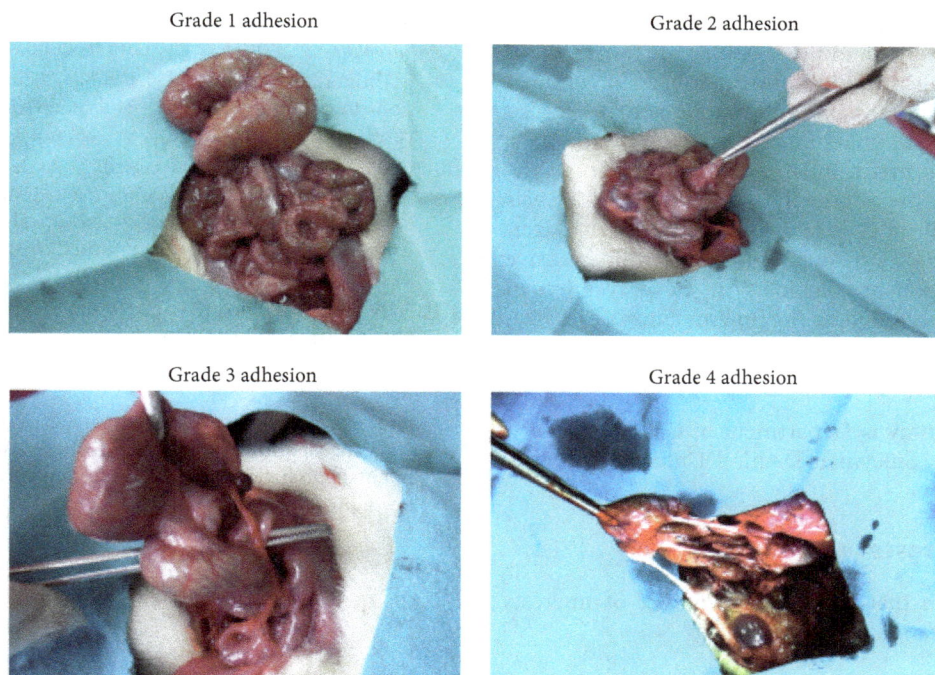

FIGURE 1: Macroscopic scoring of adhesions.

4. Discussion

Adhesions occur in 90% of the patients undergoing intra-abdominal surgery and they lead to intestinal obstruction in 3% of these patients. These adhesions often cause numerous clinical problems including mechanical intestinal obstruction, infertility, and chronic abdominal pain [2–6]. However, it is difficult to predict when adhesions may cause intestinal obstruction. The experimental model used in this study was a cecal abrasion model which mimics the trauma caused by laparotomy. However, the absence of postoperative symptoms such as inappetence, nausea, and vomiting in our rats was attributed to the absence of adhesion-induced obstruction.

Numerous studies have been conducted to prevent intraperitoneal adhesions [2–14]. These studies have utilized various substances including the mechanic effects of solid-liquid and organic barriers, fibrinolytic agents, anticoagulants, and antibiotics [2–14]. In order to prevent adhesions, surgeons have investigated the methods of migrating the fibrin glue from the peritoneum and have tried a number of techniques including peritoneal washing, dilution of the fibrin glue, melting of the fibrin gel with hyaluronidase gel or fibrinolysin, and enzymatic digestion of the fibrin glue; however, limited success has been obtained [4].

Tarhan et al. reported that a fibrinolytic activator was detected on the mesothelial surfaces and the activator exhibited a significant decrease following the creation of serosal trauma with phenol and formaldehyde [10]. As a result of the decrease in the serosal fibrinolytic activation system, intra-abdominal adhesions develop approximately on day 10 after the decrease [3]. Since the fibrin is not destroyed due to the reduction of tissue plasminogen activator (t-PA) release,

fibrinous adhesions occur. These adhesions then become organized and turn into fibrous adhesions [4, 5]. Depending on this process, we performed laparotomy on day 10 in order to monitor adhesion formation.

Dargenio et al. compared the effect of colchicine and dexamethasone in the prevention of adhesions and reported that colchicine yielded better outcomes [12]. The study administered the colchicine intramuscularly or intraperitoneally, whereas we administered it orally. Ince et al. conducted a dose-dependent experiment on rabbits and used various doses of colchicine in the prevention of adhesions caused by intraperitoneal infection [4]. The study reported that the response obtained with a dose of 1 mg/kg was sufficient for the prevention of the adhesions. Rojkind and Kershenobich, demonstrating the colchicine as a collagen synthesis inhibitor, used colchicine in the prevention of fibrosis in liver cirrhosis and obtained successful outcomes in 5- and 10-year follow-ups [13]. Similarly, Ben-Chetrit et al. investigated the anti-inflammatory effects of colchicine in rheumatological patients in 2006 and obtained successful results [5]. On the other hand, Granat et al. reported that the intraserosal administration of colchicine 50 mcg/day provided better results when mixed with dexamethasone [7]. In our study, colchicine was administered orally at a dose of 50 mcg/kg/day.

In our study, the highest adhesion score was in the abrasion group, followed by the colchicine and control groups, respectively. The presence of the lowest score in the control group was attributed to the absence of cecal abrasion in this group. In the abrasion + colchicine group, colchicine was highly effective.

The results suggested that colchicine is an effective agent in the prevention of adhesions. Colchicine is considered to inhibit collagen synthesis by restraining the mitotic activity and fibroblastic response and thus prevent the formation of fibrotic adhesions which lead to obstruction. As mentioned above, since colchicine inhibits the mitotic activity, it also reduces the activity of the macrophages as well as macrophage migration and thus prevents inflammation. In this study, the macroscopic parameters were analyzed but no evaluation was performed for the phagocytic activities of the macrophages. Therefore, further studies are needed to perform an extensive analysis on the effects of colchicine in the prevention of adhesions and an evaluation on the inflammation process.

The Source of Study

The source of the study is Department of General Surgery, School of Medicine, Suleyman Demirel University, Isparta, Turkey.

Conflict of Interests

The authors declare that there is no conflict of interests regarding the publication of this paper.

Authors' Contribution

İhsan Yıldız contributed approximately 60% and Yavuz Savas Koca contributed approximately 40% to this study.

References

[1] H. V. Zühlke, E. M. Lorenz, E. M. Straub, and V. Savvas, "Pathophysiology and classification of adhesions," in *Langenbecks Archiv für Chirurgie. Supplement II, Verhandlungen der Deutschen Gesellschaft für Chirurgie*, pp. 1009–1016, Springer, Berlin, Germany, 1990.

[2] B. Özçelik, I. S. Serin, M. Basburg, S. Uludag, F. Narin, and M. Tayyar, "Effect of melatonin in the prevention of post-operative adhesion formation in a rat uterine horn adhesion model," *Human Reproduction*, vol. 18, no. 8, pp. 1703–1706, 2003.

[3] S. A. Müller, K. H. Treutner, M. Anurov, S. Titkova, A. P. Oettinger, and V. Schumpelick, "Experimental evaluation of phospholipids and icodextrin in re-formation of peritoneal adhesions," *British Journal of Surgery*, vol. 90, no. 12, pp. 1604–1607, 2003.

[4] A. Ince, A. Eroglu, O. Tarhan, and M. Bülbül, "Peritoneal fibrinolytic activity in peritonitis," *The American Journal of Surgery*, vol. 183, no. 1, pp. 67–69, 2002.

[5] E. Ben-Chetrit, S. Bergmann, and R. Sood, "Mechanism of the anti-inflammatory effect of colchicine in rheumatic diseases: a possible new outlook through microarray analysis," *Rheumatology*, vol. 45, no. 3, pp. 274–282, 2006.

[6] I. Marcovici, B. A. Rosenzweig, A. I. Brill, and A. Scommegna, "Colchicine and post-inflammatory adhesions in a rabbit model: a dose-response study," *Obstetrics and Gynecology*, vol. 82, no. 2, pp. 216–218, 1993.

[7] M. Granat, I. T. Kaspa, E. Zylber Katz, and J. G. Schenker, "Reduction of peritoneal adhesion formation by colchicine: a comparative study in the rat," *Fertility and Sterility*, vol. 40, no. 3, pp. 369–372, 1983.

[8] R. C. Dinsmore, W. C. Calton Jr., S. B. Harvey, and M. W. Blaney, "Prevention of adhesions to polypropylene mesh in a traumatized bowel model," *Journal of the American College of Surgeons*, vol. 191, no. 2, pp. 131–136, 2000.

[9] I. Altuntas, O. Tarhan, and N. Delibas, "Seprafilm reduces adhesions to polypropylene mesh and increases peritoneal hydroxyproline," *American Surgeon*, vol. 68, no. 9, pp. 759–761, 2002.

[10] O. R. Tarhan, I. Barut, R. Sutcu, Y. Akdeniz, and O. Akturk, "Pentoxifylline, a methyl xanthine derivative, reduces peritoneal adhesions and increases peritoneal fibrinolysis in rats," *Tohoku Journal of Experimental Medicine*, vol. 209, no. 3, pp. 249–255, 2006.

[11] A. Ar'Rajab, M. Snoj, K. Larsson, and S. Bengmark, "Exogenous phospholipid reduces postoperative peritoneal adhesions in rats," *European Journal of Surgery*, vol. 161, no. 5, pp. 341–344, 1995.

[12] R. Dargenio, C. Cimino, G. Ragusa, N. Garcea, and C. Stella, "Pharmacological prevention of postoperative adhesions experimentally induced in the rat," *Acta Europaea Fertilitatis*, vol. 17, no. 4, pp. 267–272, 1986.

[13] M. Rojkind and D. Kershenobich, "Effect of colchicine on collagen, albumin and transferrin synthesis by cirrhotic rat liver slices," *Biochimica et Biophysica Acta*, vol. 378, no. 3, pp. 415–423, 1975.

[14] O. R. Tarhan, I. Barut, and M. Sezik, "An evaluation of normal saline and taurolidine on intra-abdominal adhesion formation and peritoneal fibrinolysis," *Journal of Surgical Research*, vol. 144, no. 1, pp. 151–157, 2008.

19

Long-Term Outcomes of Sacrococcygeal Germ Cell Tumors in Infancy and Childhood

Rangsan Niramis,[1,2] **Maitree Anuntkosol,**[1,2] **Veera Buranakitjaroen,**[1,2]
Achariya Tongsin,[1,2] **Varaporn Mahatharadol,**[1,2] **Wannisa Poocharoen,**[1,2]
Suranetr La-orwong,[1,2] **and Kulsiri Tiansri**[1,2]

[1]*Department of Surgery, Queen Sirikit National Institute of Child Health, Bangkok 10400, Thailand*
[2]*College of Medicine, Rangsit University, Bangkok 10400, Thailand*

Correspondence should be addressed to Rangsan Niramis; rniramis@hotmail.com

Academic Editor: Hiroo Uchida

Purpose. The aim of this study was to evaluate long-term outcomes of sacrococcygeal germ cell tumors (SC-GCTs) over a 15-year period. *Materials and Methods.* A retrospective review was conducted of all pediatric patients treated for SC-GCTs at our hospital from 1998 to 2012. *Results.* Fifty-seven patients were treated for SC-GCTs with the most common in Altman's classification type I. Age at surgery ranged from one day to 5.6 years. Tumor resection and coccygectomy were primarily performed in about 84% of the cases. Pathology revealed mature, immature, malignant sacrococcygeal teratomas (SCTs), and endodermal sinus tumors (ESTs) in 41 (72%), 4 (77%), 6 (10.5%), and 6 (10.5%), respectively. Recurrence of discase occurred in 3 of 41 patients with mature teratomas (7.3%); 2 recurrences with mature teratomas and one recurrence with EST. Five of 6 malignant SCTs and 3 of 6 ESTs responded well to the treatment. Alpha-fetoprotein (AFP) level was elevated in both malignant teratomas and ESTs. No immediate patient death was noted in any of the 57 cases, but 4 patients with malignant tumors and distant metastasis succumbed at home within 2 years of the initial treatment. *Conclusion.* Benign SCTs have a significant recurrence rate of approximately 7%. Close follow-up with serial AFP level monitoring should be done for 5 years after initial tumor resection and coccygectomy. The survival rate for malignant SC-GCTs with distant metastasis was unfavorable in the present study.

1. Introduction

Pediatric germ cell tumors (GCTs) are neoplasms derived from primodial germ cells and may occur both inside the gonads and in extragonadal organs. The five main histologic categories of GCTs are dysgerminomas (in the ovary), seminomas (in the testes), teratomas, choriocarcinomas, and endodermal sinus tumors (ESTs) or yolk sac tumors [1, 2] (Figure 1). The most common site of extragonadal GCTs in the pediatric population is the sacrococcygeal region followed by the anterior mediastinum, intracranial region, retroperitonium, neck, stomach, and vagina [2]. The most common sacrococcygeal germ cell tumors (SC-GCT) are teratomas which mostly behave as benign tumors and, less commonly, as malignant ones [1–3]. The least common SC-GCT is EST which characteristically presents as a malignant tumor. Sacrococcygeal teratomas (SCTs) are classified as mature, immature, and malignant forms [4–6]. A mature SCT is a benign tumor containing only mature teratomatous components while immature SCTs contain immature tissues which are not frankly malignant, and malignant SCTs are composed of mature or immature teratomatous tissues and any of the other 4 malignant GCTs. The behavior of SCT does not depend entirely on histology appearance, but also on the age of patient at surgery. This paper presents a study of a single tertiary institute for pediatrics in order to evaluate long-term outcomes of SC-GCT over a 15-year period.

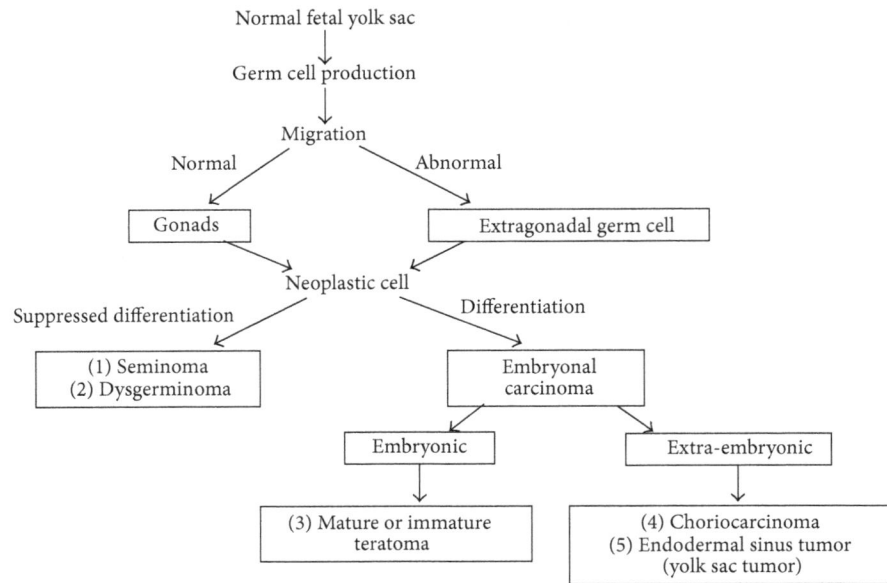

FIGURE 1: Development of germ cell tumors.

2. Materials and Methods

After the study protocol had been approved by the Institutional Reviewer Board (Document number 57-054), medical records were reviewed of all the patients with SC-GCT treated at Queen Sirikit National Institute of Child Health between January 1998 and December 2012. Data were obtained on gestational age (GA), birth weight (BW), age at operation, anatomical types, pathological reports, and results of treatment. The tumors in this region were classified into 4 anatomical types as described by Altman et al. [7]. SCT was categorized into 3 histologic types: mature, immature, and malignant teratomas [4–6]. If a pathologic report revealed one type of malignant GCT without mentioning the presence of teratomatous components, the tumor was diagnosed as a malignant GCT in accordance with the histologic description. The tumor was diagnosed as mixed GCT if it contained more than one type of malignant GCT. The patients were investigated preoperatively by plain film of the pelvis, ultrasonography, computerized tomography (CT) scan, or barium enema in some cases. Preoperative and postoperative alpha-fetoprotein (AFP) levels were determined in all of the patients. An AFP level of 20 ng/mL or lower was considered to be normal in children over 8 months of age [8, 9]. The Pediatric Oncology Group (POG) and Children Cancer Group (CCG) staging of malignant extragonadal GCT was used for analysis of the malignant cases (Table 1). Adjuvant therapy for malignancy was recorded and long-term follow-up of clinical outcomes was evaluated.

3. Results

A total of 57 patients were treated for SC-GCTs during the study period. There were 13 males and 44 females; hence the male to female ratio was approximately 1 : 4. Six patients with

TABLE 1: Pediatric Oncology Group/Children Cancer Group (POG/CCG) staging for malignant extragonadal germ cell tumors.

Stage	Characteristics
I:	Complete resection at any site; coccygectomy for sacrococcygeal site; negative tumor margins; tumor markers positive or negative
II:	Microscopic residual; lymph nodes negative; tumor markers positive or negative
III:	Gross residual or tumor biopsy only; retroperitoneal nodes negative or positive; tumor markers positive or negative
IV:	Distant metastasis, including liver

SC-GTCs were born at Rajavithi Hospital (previously known as the "Women's Hospital") during the period in which there were 131,851 live births. Therefore, the incidence of SC-GCT at Rajavithi Hospital was 1 : 21,975 live births. The tumors were identified prenatally by ultrasonography, at birth and later in infancy and childhood in 13 (22.8%), 26 (45.6%), and 18 (31.6%) cases, respectively. Average BW was 3250.9 ± 410.5 grams (range from 2700 to 4610 grams) and average GA was 39.1 ± 1.7 weeks (range from 35 to 40 weeks). Three cases had tumor ruptures since birth; 2 of these were cases of vaginal delivery and one of cesarean section. Of the 15 patients diagnosed at over one year of age, the presenting symptoms included constipation, dysuria, palpable suprapubic mass, and abdominal pain in 12, 9, 8, and 3 cases, respectively. Two cases with coccygeal pain and one case with weakness of the lower extremities were identified as having lung and vertebral metastasis at diagnosis.

Age at surgery ranged from one day to 5.6 years (median 43 days, mean 281.9 ± 439.6 days). For the initial treatment, total tumor resection with coccygectomy was performed in 47 cases, while tumor biopsy was done in 8 cases and partial

TABLE 2: Anatomical types of sacrococcygeal germ cell tumors and risk of malignancy.

| Altman's type | Sacrococcygeal teratoma | | | Endodermal sinus tumor | Total |
	Mature	Immature	Malignant		
I	25	4	0	0	29 (50.9%)
II	10	0	2	0	12 (21.0%)
III	3	0	0	2	5 (8.8%)
IV	3	0	4	4	11 (19.3%)
Total	41 (72.0%)	4 (7.0%)	6 (10.5%)	6 (10.5%)	57 (100%)

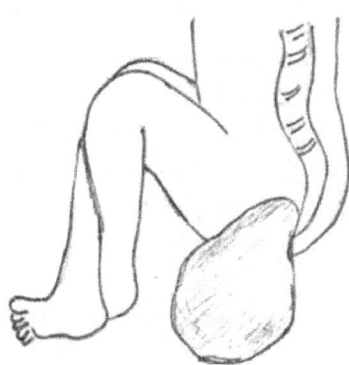

Type I 29 cases (50.9%)

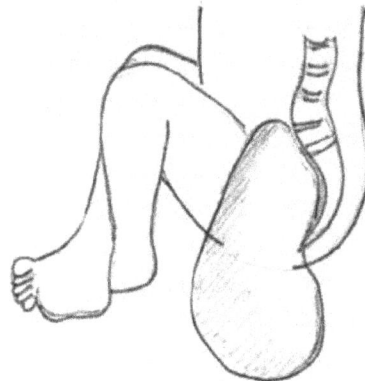

Type II 12 cases (21.0%)

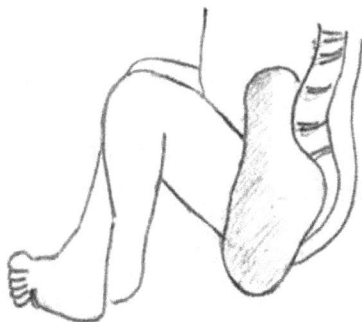

Type III 5 cases (8.8%)

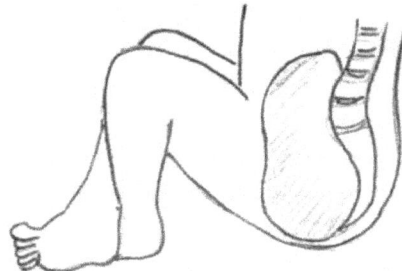

Type IV 11 cases (19.3%)

FIGURE 2: Classification system for 57 sacrococcygeal germ cell tumors based on Altman's American Academy of Pediatrics series [7].

excision in the other 2. The total 57 cases of SC-GCT were customarily grouped into 4 anatomical types according to Altman's classification [7]. Twenty-nine patients (50.9%) were categorized as type I, 12 (21.0%) as type II, 5 (8.8%) as type III, and 11 (19.3%) as type IV (Figure 2). Pathological examination revealed 41 (72.0%) mature teratomas, 4 (7.0%) immature teratomas, 6 (10.5%) malignant teratomas, and 6 (10.5%) pure ESTs. The risk of malignancy varied from zero in type I to approximately 73% in type IV (Table 2). The relation between risk of malignancy and age at surgery is shown in Table 3.

Patients who underwent surgery at or before one year of age had a risk of malignancy of only 2.41% (one in 42 cases) and the risk increased to 73.3% (11 in 15 cases) if the patients underwent surgery at the age of over one year. The youngest malignant case was 1.5 months of age at surgical excision with pathological report of malignant SCTs (including mature teratomas and ESTs).

Of the 41 cases (9 males and 32 females) with mature SCTs, age at surgery ranged from one day to 5.6 years. Thirty-three patients who underwent surgical resection at

TABLE 3: Age distribution and histologic types of sacrococcygeal germ cell tumors.

| Age at operation (years) | Sacrococcygeal teratoma | | | Endodermal sinus tumor | Total |
	Mature	Immature	Malignant		
0-1	37	4	1	0	42 (73.7%)
1-2	1	0	3	4	8 (14.0%)
2-3	1	0	1	1	3 (5.3%)
>3	2	0	1	1	4 (7.0%)
Total	41 (72.0%)	4 (7.0%)	6 (10.5%)	6 (10.5%)	57 (100%)

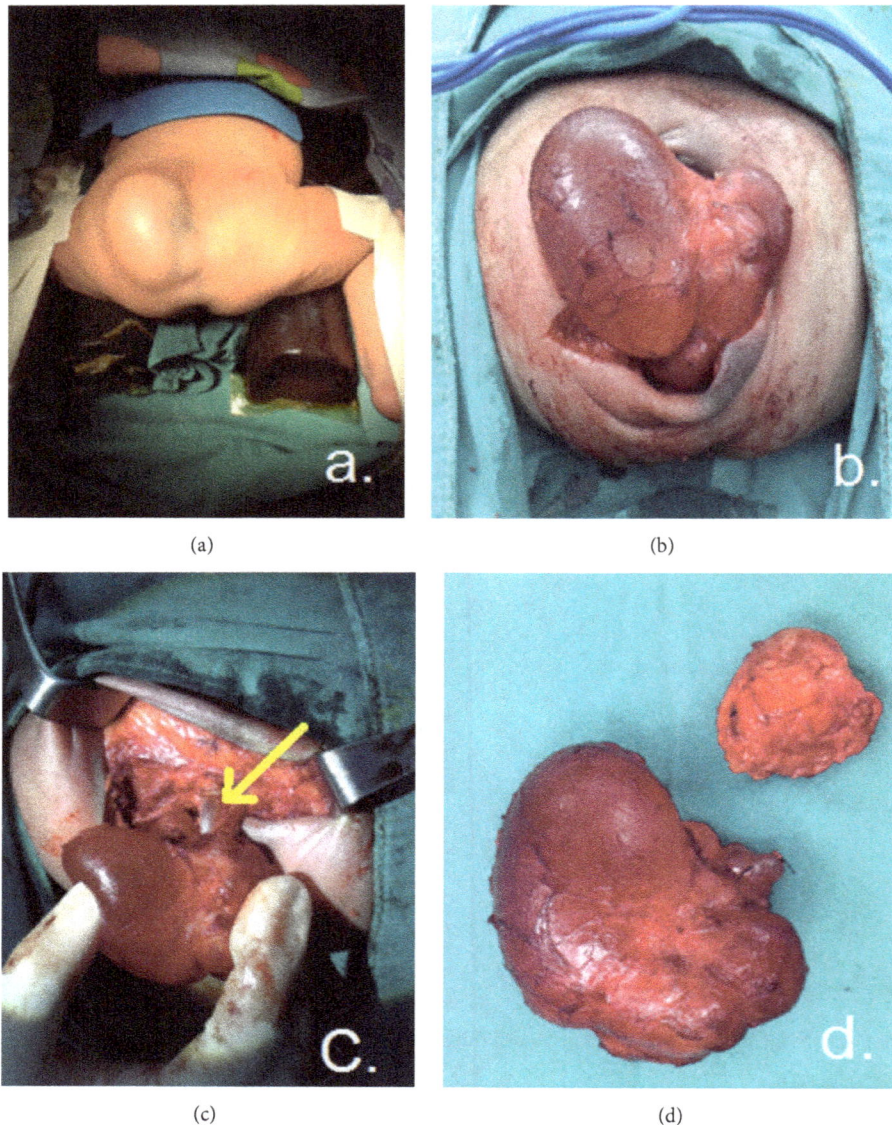

FIGURE 3: Resection of a type I sacrococcygeal teratoma; (a) the patient in frog-legged position (b) mobilization of the tumor, (c) exposure of the coccyx, and (d) removal of the tumor and coccyx.

under 8 months of age had AFP levels ranging from 125.6 to 179,185 ng/mL/. The AFP level declined to normal limits (<20 ng/mL.) at the age of over 8 months after operation. Eight cases aged over 8 months at surgery had normal AFP levels (range from 0.6 to 4.8 ng/mL). All of the 41 patients with mature teratomas underwent tumor resection and coccygectomy (Figure 3). Tumor spillage during surgical excision was noted in 6 cases (14.6%). Three cases with tumor type IV required both a transsacral approach and abdominal laparotomy for removal of the intrapubic mass and coccygectomy. Recurrent disease developed in 3 of the 41 patients (7.3%) with mature teratomas between 3 months and 3.5 years after the initial resection. All of the recurrences were tumors initially categorized into Altman's type I with complete tumor resection and coccygectomy, but there were the evidences of tumor spillage during operation. Two of the recurrences were mature teratomas that were noted on rectal examination at 3 and 8 months after operation and treated with surgery alone. AFP levels at the recurrence period were within normal limits (1.5 and 2.5 ng/mL), and both of these patients are long-term survivors. One of the recurrences was found to be EST in a patient who presented with a presacral mass, a rising AFP level of over 2,000 ng/mL, and lung metastasis proven by a CT scan at 3.5 years after initial operation. The treatment included transsacral tumor biopsy, adjuvant chemotherapy (cisplatin, etoposide and bleomycin-PEB), and pelvic radiation and after 3 months; AFP levels declined to 2.6 ng/mL. At the last 6-year follow-up (9.6 years of age), the patient was doing well, with normal AFP levels and no evidence of lung metastasis from pulmonary CT scan (Table 4).

The tumors of 4 patients (one male and 3 females) with immature teratomas were categorized into type I in 3 cases and type II in the other case. Age at operation ranged from 3 to 45 days with AFP levels ranging from 1,000 to 50,000 ng/mL and declining to normal levels at the age of one year. Histology revealed premature teratomas of both grades I and II in 2 cases. No evidence of recurrence was noted at the follow-up of an average of 18 months.

Of the 6 cases (2 males and 4 females) with malignant SCTs, age at operation ranged from one month to 2.25 years with Altman's types II, III, and IV in 2, 1, and 3 case, respectively. AFP levels at operation ranged from 20,000 to 60,500 ng/mL. The initial surgical procedures included tumor biopsy in 3 cases and tumor resection with coccygectomy in the other 3 cases. Pathological examinations revealed immature teratomas with ESTs in 2 cases and mature teratomas with ESTs in the other 4 (Table 4). After surgery, 4 patients received adjuvant chemotherapy (PEB) and radiotherapy. Two patients, one in stage I and one in stage IV, received only chemotherapy. The patient with lung metastasis at diagnosis did not respond to chemotherapy treatment; his serum AFP level was still high at over 20,000 ng/mL, and he was lost to follow-up approximately one year after surgery and died at home. Five patients followed up for between 3 and 10 years after surgery (average 7 years); and they had a good response to adjuvant therapy, with AFP levels declining to normal levels within 3 months of chemotherapy and radiation. Three of the 5 patients underwent second-look operation for resection of the residual tumors; pathology revealed only mature teratomas in 2 cases and necrotic tissue without tumor cell in the other case.

Of the 6 patients (one male and 5 females) with pure ESTs, age at surgery ranged from 1.1 to 3.2 years with type III (2 cases) and type IV (4 cases). Two patients had evidences of lung metastasis at diagnosis and AFP levels before surgery ranged from 20,000 to 51,260 ng/mL. Their chief complaints included dysuria, constipation, palpable suprapubic mass, abdominal pain, coccygeal pain, and weakness of the lower extremities. Tumor biopsy alone was performed in 5 cases and partial tumor resection with coccygectomy was carried out in the other case. Adjuvant chemotherapy and radiotherapy were added after surgery. One patient developed colonic and bladder neck obstructions within one month of tumor biopsy and she required abdominal laparotomy, right transverse colostomy, and suprapubic cystostomy. Four patients underwent second-look operation with tumor resection and coccygectomy between 4 and 6 months after chemotherapy and radiation; pathology of the second operation showed benign fatty tissue, cartilage, and cell debris in all of 4 cases. Three of the 6 patients with pure ESTs did not respond to treatment and had tumor relapse with lung and brain metastases. They were lost to follow-up within 2 years of the initial treatment and succumbed at home. The remaining 3 cases responded to treatment, and they were doing well at the 3-year follow-up with normal AFP levels and no evidence of relapse or metastasis (Table 4).

4. Discussion

The incidence of sacrococcygeal tumors at Rajavithi Hospital, Bangkok, Thailand, was approximately 1 : 22,000 live births, whereas the incidence of this entity had earlier been reported as 1 : 28,500 to 35,000 live births [10, 11]. As in previous reports, the present study revealed a female predominance with a 1 : 3 to 1 : 4 ratio [2–7, 11, 12]. SC-GCTs usually occur in patients in two clinical patterns: 1, neonates presenting with large benign tumors of mature or immature teratomas, and 2, infants and children presenting with primary malignant SCTs or pure ESTs located in the pelvis, including benign SCTs in some cases. SC-GCTs in neonates frequently present with the characteristic mass protruding from the sacrococcygeal region which can be detected by prenatal ultrasonography. Infants with sacral masses that are prenatally diagnosed as greater than 5 cm in size should be considered for abdominal delivery to avoid dystocia and tumor rupture [13]. Three of our patients were noted to have tumor rupture, even though one case was delivered by cesarean section. SC-GCTs in older infants and children generally have no protruding mass noted at birth. They usually have the clinical presentations related to bladder or rectal compression and a palpable suprapubic mass, and these features were found in 12 of the 15 patients of this study. These tumors presumably arise from normal germ cells deposited in the sacrococcygeal area that undergo malignant transformation or from unrecognized small foci of malignancy present at birth which eventually become the major tissue type in the tumor [14, 15].

The risk of malignancy of sacrococcygeal tumors is related to its anatomical type and age of patient at surgery. Type I tumors have the lowest risk and type IV have the highest risk of malignancy. This was well demonstrated in our series, in keeping with the report of Altman et al. [7]. In the American Academy of Pediatrics survey, the incidence of malignancy was 7–10% in patients operated upon at the age of less than 2 months but 48–67% if they were treated after 2 months of age [7]. In our present study, the incidence of malignancy was only 2.4% in patients who underwent surgery at the age of less than one year and 73.3%

TABLE 4: Malignant sacrococcygeal germ cell tumors and results of the treatment.

Patient/gender/age at operation	Altman's type	Initial operation	AFP level (ng/mL) Histology	Initial staging	Adjuvant therapy	Second operation	Outcomes
Mature teratoma (MT) and recurrence with endodermal sinus tumor (EST)							
1 F 3.5 y (at the recurrence)	IV	Tumor biopsy	2,000 EST	IV (lung metastasis)	Chemotherapy + radiotherapy	None	6-year FU Survival-NED*
Malignant teratoma							
1 F 2.1 y	II	Total resection + coccygectomy	20,000 MT + EST	I	Chemotherapy	None	3-year FU Survival-NED*
2 F 1.2 y	IV	Tumor biopsy	2,000 MT + EST	III	Chemotherapy + radiotherapy	Total resection + coccygectomy	8-year FU Survival-NED*
3 M 9 m	IV	Partial resection + coccygectomy	43,430 MT + EST	III	Chemotherapy + radiotherapy	Total resection	8-year FU Survival- NED*
4 F 1.5 m	II	Partial resection + coccygectomy	6,985 MT + EST	III	Chemotherapy + radiotherapy	None	10-year FU Survival-NED*
5 F 1.2 y	IV	Tumor biopsy	60,500 MT + EST	III	Chemotherapy + radiotherapy	Total resection + coccygectomy	7-year FU Survival-NED*
6 M 3 y	III	Tumor biopsy	60,000 IMT** grade 3 + EST	IV (lung metastasis)	Chemotherapy + radiotherapy	None	Lung metastasis Death at home after one year treatment
Endodermal sinus tumor							
1 F 1.5 y	III	Partial resection + coccygectomy	20,000 EST	III	Chemotherapy + radiotherapy	None	Lung metastasis Death at home after 2-year treatment
2 F 1.1 y	III	Tumor biopsy	58,704 EST	III	Chemotherapy	Total resection + coccygectomy	Lung and brain metastases Death at home after 2-year treatment
3 F 2.3 y	IV	Tumor biopsy	34,144 EST	IV (lung metastasis)	Chemotherapy + radiotherapy	Total resection + coccygectomy	2-year FU Survival-NED*
4 M 1.3 y	IV	Tumor biopsy	2,207 EST	III	Chemotherapy + radiotherapy	Total resection + coccygectomy	3-year FU Survival-NED*
5 F 1.8 y	IV	Tumor biopsy	51,250 EST	IV (lung metastasis)	Chemotherapy + radiotherapy	Laparotomy, colostomy, and cystostomy	Lung, long bone, and vertebral metastases Death at home after 10-month treatment
6 F 3.2 y	IV	Tumor biopsy	30,763 EST	IV (vertebral metastasis)	Chemotherapy + radiotherapy	Laparotomy, partial resection, and coccygectomy	3-year FU Survival-NED*

*NED: no evidence of disease; **IMT: immature teratoma.

in the patients operated upon after one year of age. These findings indicated that SC-GCTs should be surgically treated as soon as possible after birth.

In some cases with a large size tumor of types III and IV, a complete resection requires a combination of abdominal and sacral approach, and the coccyx is removed along with the tumor in every case. Failure to remove the coccyx results in a high recurrence rate [15–17], and Gross et al. [16] reported a recurrence rate as high as 37% when the coccyx was not removed. The other factor associated with recurrence of SC-GCTs is spillage of tumor during surgery [18]. The present study noted a 7.3% recurrence rate with mature SCTs where the coccyx had been completely removed with tumor spillage during surgical resection in all of the patients with tumor recurrence. Many studies have demonstrated a recurrence rate of 10–21% after resection of neonatal sacrococcygeal tumors and incidences of recurrence occurring within 3 years [12, 19]. The longest period to recurrence was reported by Mahour et al. [4] with local recurrence of mature SCT at 4.5 years after initial resection of the previous mature SCT. The recurrent tumor is usually composed of mature teratomatous tissue; however, instances of malignant recurrence after previous resection of a mature SCT have been reported [4–6, 12, 17]. Recurrence with EST in one of our 3 patients occurred as late as 3.5 years after operation of mature SCT; this may possibly be due to the presence of malignant components in the primary tumor which were not recognized during histologic examination as a result of sampling error in a large tumor. Incomplete resection of malignant components may result in tumor recurrence.

Results of treatment of mature and immature SCTs were satisfactory in this study. There was no immediate postoperative death and no long-term sequelae of anorectal function (constipation and soiling) or urinary function (neurogenic bladder and incontinence) as in some reports [10, 20]. In contrast, treatments of malignant SC-GCT obtained unsatisfactory outcomes, especially sacrococcygeal EST or yolk sac tumor. Our patients with malignant SC-GCTs did not respond to adjuvant chemotherapy and radiotherapy; they developed distant metastases to the lung, vertebra, and brain in 53.8% of cases and died at home in 30.8% of cases (Table 4), similar to those in other reports [4, 6, 12, 21]. Several studies have demonstrated markedly improved survival in malignant sacrococcygeal tumors with the use of new regimens of adjuvant chemotherapy such as PVB (cisplatin, vinblastine, and bleomycin), JEB (carboplatin, etoposide, and bleomycin), and PEI (cisplatin, etoposide, and ifosfamide) [18, 22, 23].

Close follow-up after resection of benign SCT should be done, including physical examination of the lower abdomen and buttock region, rectal examination, and serial AFP determinations. AFP levels are proven to be elevated in early infancy before gradually decreasing to normal levels at 8 months of age [8]. The data of the present study and others [16, 24–26] indicate that the presence of EST is associated with elevated serum AFP levels. Serial AFP examinations are useful for diagnosis, determination of the completeness of malignant tumor removal, tumor recurrence during the follow-up period, and formation of the prognosis [8, 22–27]. Based on our present study and other reports, monitoring

of serum AFP level should be carried out every 3–6 months for more than 3 years because malignant recurrence clinically presents within 3.5 years of initial resection of mature SCT.

5. Conclusion

Teratomas are the most common GCTs of the sacrococcygeal region. Benign SCTs have a recurrence rate of approximately 7% after initial tumor resection and coccygectomy. Some cases of recurrence may present with malignant tumors and distant metastasis, and close follow-up with serial AFP monitoring should be done for 5 years. Even though chemotherapeutic regimens are more effective in this era, survival for malignant SC-GCTs with distant metastasis was not satisfactory in the present study.

Conflict of Interests

The authors declare that there is no conflict of interests regarding the publication of this paper.

Acknowledgments

The authors would like to thank Dr. Siraporn Sawasdivorn, Director of Queen Sirikit National Institute of Children Health, for permission to publish this paper and Ms. Nutthaya Pitakwong for her drawings in Figure 2.

References

[1] L. P. Dehner, "Gonadal and extragonadal germ cell neoplasia of childhood," *Human Pathology*, vol. 14, no. 6, pp. 493–511, 1983.

[2] F. J. Rescorla, "Pediatric germ cell tumors," *Seminars in Surgical Oncology*, vol. 16, no. 2, pp. 144–158, 1999.

[3] J. K. McKenney, A. Heerema-Mckenney, and R. V. Rouse, "Extragonadal germ cell tumors: a review with emphasis on pathologic features, clinical prognostic variables, and differential diagnostic considerations," *Advances in Anatomic Pathology*, vol. 14, no. 2, pp. 69–92, 2007.

[4] G. H. Mahour, M. M. Woolley, S. N. Trivedi, and B. H. Landing, "Sacrococcygeal teratoma: a 33-year experience," *Journal of Pediatric Surgery*, vol. 10, no. 2, pp. 183–188, 1975.

[5] M. M. Woolley, "Malignant teratomas in infancy and childhood," *World Journal of Surgery*, vol. 4, no. 1, pp. 39–47, 1980.

[6] W. A. Donnellan and O. Swenson, "Benign and malignant sacrococcygeal teratomas," *Surgery*, vol. 64, no. 4, pp. 834–846, 1968.

[7] R. P. Altman, J. G. Randolph, and J. R. Lilly, "Sacrococcygeal teratoma. American academy of pediatrics surgical section survey-1973," *Journal of Pediatric Surgery*, vol. 9, no. 3, pp. 389–398, 1974.

[8] Y. Tsuchida, Y. Endo, S. Saito, M. Kaneko, K. Shiraki, and K. Ohmi, "Evaluation of alpha-fetoprotein in early infancy," *Journal of Pediatric Surgery*, vol. 13, no. 2, pp. 155–156, 1978.

[9] K. Ohama, H. Nagase, K. Ogino et al., "Alpha-fetoprotein (AFP) levels in normal children," *European Journal of Pediatric Surgery*, vol. 7, no. 5, pp. 267–269, 1997.

[10] J. P. M. Derikx, A. De Backer, L. Van De Schoot et al., "Factors associated with recurrence and metastasis in sacrococcygeal teratoma," *British Journal of Surgery*, vol. 93, no. 12, pp. 1543–1548, 2006.

[11] E. Pantoja, R. Llobet, and B. Gonzalez Flores, "Retroperitoneal teratoma: historical review," *Journal of Urology*, vol. 115, no. 5, pp. 520–523, 1976.

[12] F. J. Rescorla, R. S. Sawin, A. G. Coran, P. W. Dillon, and R. G. Azizkhan, "Long-term outcome for infants and children with sacrococcygeal teratoma: a report from the Childrens Cancer Group," *Journal of Pediatric Surgery*, vol. 33, no. 2, pp. 171–176, 1998.

[13] A. W. Flake, "Fetal sacrococcygeal teratoma," *Seminars in Pediatric Surgery*, vol. 2, no. 2, pp. 113–120, 1993.

[14] K. W. Ashcraft and T. M. Holder, "Congenital anal stenosis with presacral teratoma: case reports," *Annals of Surgery*, vol. 162, no. 6, pp. 1091–1095, 1965.

[15] S. H. Ein, K. Mancer, and S. D. Adeyemi, "Malignant sacro-coccygeal teratoma-endodermal, yolk sac tumor in infants and children: a 32-year review," *Journal of Pediatric Surgery*, vol. 20, no. 5, pp. 473–477, 1985.

[16] R. E. Gross, H. W. Clatworthy, and I. A. Meeker, "Sacrococcygeal teratoma in infants and children," *Surgery, Gynecology, and Obstetrics*, vol. 92, no. 3, pp. 341–354, 1951.

[17] J. L. Grosfeld, T. V. N. Ballantine, D. Lowe, and R. L. Bechner, "Benign and malignant teratomas in children: analysis of 85 patients," *Surgery*, vol. 80, no. 3, pp. 297–305, 1976.

[18] A. De Backer, G. C. Madern, F. G. A. J. Hakvoort-Cammel, P. Haentjens, J. W. Oosterhuis, and F. W. J. Hazebroek, "Study of the factors associated with recurrence in children with sacrococcygeal teratoma," *Journal of Pediatric Surgery*, vol. 41, no. 1, pp. 173–181, 2006.

[19] S. N. Huddart, J. R. Mann, K. Robbinson et al., "Sacrococcygeal teratomas: the UK Children's Cancer Study Group's experience," *Pediatric Surgery International*, vol. 19, no. 1-2, pp. 47–51, 2003.

[20] B. Schmidt, A. Haberlik, E. Uray, M. Ratschek, H. Lackner, and M. E. Höllwarth, "Sacrococcygeal teratoma: clinical course and prognosis with a special view to long-term functional results," *Pediatric Surgery International*, vol. 15, no. 8, pp. 573–576, 1999.

[21] J. Noseworthy, E. E. Lack, H. P. W. Kozakewich, G. F. Vawter, and K. J. Welch, "Sacrococcygeal germ cell tumors in childhood: an updated experience with 118 patients," *Journal of Pediatric Surgery*, vol. 16, no. 3, pp. 358–364, 1981.

[22] D. Misra, J. Pritchard, D. P. Drake, E. M. Kiely, and L. Spitz, "Markedly improved survival in malignant sacro-coccygeal teratomas—16 years' experience," *European Journal of Pediatric Surgery*, vol. 7, no. 3, pp. 152–155, 1997.

[23] F. De Corti, S. Sarnacki, C. Patte et al., "Prognosis of malignant sacrococcygeal germ cell tumours according to their natural history and surgical management," *Surgical Oncology*, vol. 21, no. 2, pp. e31–e37, 2012.

[24] U. Gobel, D. T. Schneider, G. Galaminus et al., "Multimodal treatment of malignant sacrococcygeal germ cell tumors: a prospective analysis of 66 patients of the German cooperative protocols MAKEI 83/86 and 89," *Journal of Clinical Oncology*, vol. 19, no. 7, pp. 1943–1950, 2001.

[25] Y. Tsuchida and H. Hasegawa, "The diagnostic value of alpha-fetoprotein in infants and children with teratomas: a questionnaire survey in Japan," *Journal of Pediatric Surgery*, vol. 18, no. 2, pp. 152–155, 1983.

[26] M. Kawai, T. Kano, F. Kikkawa et al., "Seven tumor markers in benign and malignant germ cell tumors of the ovary," *Gynecologic Oncology*, vol. 45, no. 3, pp. 248–253, 1992.

[27] H. B. Marsden, J. M. Birch, and R. Swindell, "Germ cell tumours of childhood: a review of 137 cases," *Journal of Clinical Pathology*, vol. 34, no. 8, pp. 879–883, 1981.

20

Evaluation of Factor VIII as a Risk Factor in Indian Patients with DVT

Darpanarayan Hazra,[1] **Indrani Sen,**[1] **Edwin Stephen,**[1] **Sunil Agarwal,**[1] **Sukesh Chandran Nair,**[2] **and Joy Mammen**[2]

[1]*Department of Vascular Surgery, The Christian Medical College, Vellore 632004, India*
[2]*Department of Transfusion Medicine and Immunohaematology, The Christian Medical College, Vellore 632004, India*

Correspondence should be addressed to Indrani Sen; dr.indranisen@gmail.com

Academic Editor: Miltiadis I. Matsagkas

Introduction. Elevated factor VIII population in the Indian population has not been studied as a possible risk factor for deep vein thrombosis (DVT). High factor VIII level is considered a predisposing factor for DVT and its recurrence. However it is known to vary between populations and its exact role in the etiopathogenesis of thrombophilia remains unknown. *Material and Methods.* Factor VIII levels of patients with DVT who had undergone a prothrombotic workup as a part of their workup was compared to normal age matched controls in a 1 : 3 ratio. *Results.* There were 75 patients with DVT who had undergone a prothrombotic workup in the course of their treatment for lower limb DVT. In these, 64% had levels of factor VIII more than 150 as compared to 63% of normal controls ($p > 0.05$, not significant). *Conclusion.* Elevated factor VIII in the Indians may not be associated with the same thrombotic risk as seen in the West. We find a variation in the levels of factor VIII with a different "normal" than what is reported in other populations. This needs further study to elucidate the role of factor VIII in the evaluation and treatment of thrombophilia.

1. Introduction

High factor VIII level is considered a predisposing factor for deep vein thrombosis (DVT) and its recurrence. Koster et al. in the Leiden Thrombophilia study reported that elevated levels above 150 IU/dL carried a 5-fold increased risk for DVT [1]. However, factor VIII levels can vary due to a multitude of physiological and disease factors. Normal levels also vary between populations, with higher plasma levels of factor VIII reported from Africa and Japan [2–4]. Many population differences in thrombophilic risk factors are reported in India; however, factor VIII levels have not yet been studied [5–11]. This is the first study to analyze whether a high factor VIII level in Indian patients with DVT was a significant prothrombotic risk factor for venous thromboembolism.

2. Materials and Methods

We designed a retrospective case control study comparing factor VIII levels in a population with DVT to normal controls.

Inclusion criteria were as follows: factor VIII levels from patients who had undergone a thrombophilia workup as a part of management of deep vein thrombosis. Management is in accordance with the ACCP guidelines [12]. A thrombophilia workup is ordered when indicated in patients with an initial episode of unprovoked DVT after the initial treatment phase is over. The patients are not on anticoagulation for at least 6 weeks at the time of testing. Patients with obvious provoking factors or those who are planned for lifelong anticoagulation are not offered thrombophilia testing. Exclusion criteria were as follows: children, pregnant women, and patients with thrombosis of the visceral, cerebral, or pulmonary venous beds were excluded as levels of factor VIII are known to vary in these conditions. Controls were as follows: blood samples from healthy donors were used as controls. There was no history of thrombosis in the control group that was matched for baseline characteristics like age and sex. The design was formulated in discussion with the biostatistics department. As it was mainly a numerical analysis of data, institutional review was not required.

Thrombophilia workup included blood cell counts, coagulation parameters (PT with INR, aPTT), factor levels, d-dimer, thrombin time, fibrinogen levels, proteins C and S, antithrombin, lupus anticoagulant, DDVRT, Ham's test, sucrose lysis, sickle test, homocysteine levels, and Thromboelastogram. Genetic markers of thrombosis were studied when indicated. The "normal" cut-off value used for factor VIII was 150 IU/dL [1]. Data was analysed from a prospectively maintained hospital registry.

2.1. Method of Factor VIII Assessment.

All samples were collected in the laboratory using an evacuated tube system, Vacuette (Greiner) into citrate anticoagulant at the ratio of 1 : 9 following the proper order of draw, and processed with 30 minutes of the collection after double centrifugation. FVIII : C is assayed with 1-2 hrs of the sample collection and for rest of the assays like AT, PC, and PS the citrated samples are frozen in vials and stored at -800°C.

The calibrators have an assigned value traceable to the international standard and the value of the IL calibrator has been verified on the CS2000i after being tested on ACL Top analyser that the laboratory has and this is further validated against 6th World Health Organisation (WHO) International Standard (IS) for factor VIII/VWF plasma (07/316) randomly as we have it in our inventory since our laboratory is enlisted as one of the 22 reference laboratories to assign values to the IS by NIBSC, UK. Any sample which is closest to the samples being tested with no matrix effect is a good reference material and can be used as a precision tool like a control or even as a calibrator (as long as it has an assigned value traceable to a standard), providing that it is stable across days it is being tested. At a temperature of -800°C coagulation factors are stable for at least a period of 6 months. The PNP prepared in our laboratory is stored at -800°C and is prepared once in 4 months as it gets exhausted. It has proven to be a good precision tool like the commercial control that we run along. Only FVIII : C activity assay is done and FVIII : Ag is not performed as part of the thrombophilia screen.

2.2. Statistical Methods.

The sensitivity and specificity were calculated for every cut-off value including the normal. As the design is matched case control design, we have used McNemar's chi-square test to test association between factor VIII in cases and factor VIII in controls. The p value was fixed at 0.05, 5% level of significance. The ROC curve was drawn by taking false positive rate at the x-axis and the sensitivity at the y-axis. R software was used to draw the ROC curve. Data was entered using EPIDATA software and analyzed using SPSS and R software.

3. Results

There were 75 patients with DVT who had undergone a prothrombotic workup in the course of their treatment for unprovoked lower limb DVT. The average age was 40.2 years with a range of 22–64 years. The male : female ratio was 4 : 1. The results of the thrombotic workup were normal in 13% and were positive for lupus anticoagulant in 23% and elevated

TABLE 1: Factor VIII distribution in cases and controls using 150 (IU/dL) as cut-off.

	Factor VIII levels (IU/dL)	
	>150	<150
DVT cases, $n = 75$	48 (64%)	27 (36%)
Controls, $n = 289$	181 (63%)	108 (37%)

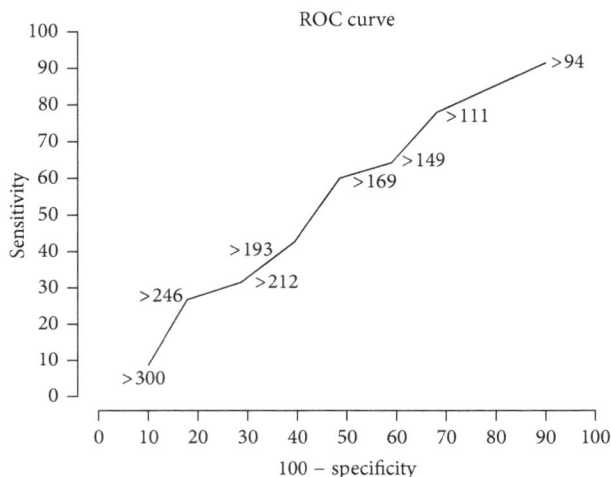

FIGURE 1: ROC curve-Factor VIII, no relevant cutoff.

factor VIII in 56%, with more than one prothrombotic risk factor identified in 8%. Healthy blood donor's samples were analysed for plasma factor VIII as controls ($n = 289$). There was no history of thrombosis, the control group which was matched for baseline characteristics like age and sex.

Amongst cases, 48 patients (64%) had elevated levels of factor VIII (>150); of these, elevated factor VIII was the only abnormality in 42 (56%). In the control population ($n = 289$), 181 patients (63%) had factor VIII levels above the normal cut-off value.

At the cut-off of 150, a 2 × 2 table was generated to determine the association between factor VIII and the presence of DVT (Table 1). This provided a sensitivity of 64% and specificity of 63%, $p < 0.05$ (not significant). As both the sensitivity and specificity at the presently used normal were poor, we calculated these statistics for other proposed (higher and lower) cut-offs (Table 2). The p values at all these proposed cut-offs were calculated; none reached significance.

ROC analysis was plotted to assess whether a higher factor VIII level is necessary as a cut-off in our population (as 63% of controls with no evidence of thrombosis also had elevated plasma levels of factor VIII). This was done to check the diagnostic accuracy of 150 IU/mL as the clinically relevant cut-off (not factor VIII levels as a diagnostic tool for DVT). However, the plot yielded a flat curve without a clinically significant cut-off test result level (Figure 1). This demonstrated that we could not determine a clinically relevant cut-off to determine a "high" factor VIII in our population.

TABLE 2: Sensitivity and specificity value of VIII at different cut-off levels.

Factor VIII cut-off value	Cases (n)	Control (n)	Sensitivity (%)	Specificity (%)	p value
>149	49	169	64.5	40.9	Ns
<149	27	117			
>169	41	139	59.9	51.4	Ns
<169	35	147			
>193	32	112	42.1	60.8	Ns
<193	44	174			
>212	24	82	31.6	71.3	Ns
<212	52	204			
>246	20	51	26.3	82.2	Ns
<246	56	235			
≥300	7	29	9.2	89.9	Ns
<300	69	257			

4. Discussion

The relative risk for venous thrombosis of factor VIII : Ag levels ≥150 IU/dL is 5.3 (95% CI 2.7 to 10.1) compared with levels <100 IU/dL, which is very similar to the risk previously reported for factor VIII activity levels ≥150 IU/dL [1]. Population studies in the African Americans and Japanese have demonstrated that plasma FVIII levels are influenced by ethnicity, with higher levels compared to Caucasians [2–4]. In the studied populations, increased levels above 150 IU/dL have been shown to cause a dose-dependent risk increase in VTE and its recurrence, both when present as an isolated risk factor or in combination with other prothrombotic states [1]. The biological pathway in causation of thrombosis remains unknown [13–16]. In clinical practice we find that our population also has increased plasma FVIII levels but there is no published data on this topic from India. Though most centres include this as a part of screening for thrombophilia, there is considerable variation in interpretation of results with regard to recurrence and further treatment.

The results of the prothrombotic workup for venous thrombosis in our population differ from what is commonly seen in the West [17]. The prevalence of heterozygosity for other prothrombotic risk factors also varies: for example, the factor V Leiden mutation in Indian, Arab, Canadian, and Israeli populations is lower (1 to 8.5%) than European studies (5–8%). Factor II abnormalities are not as common in our patients [5–11]. Regional variations, for example, higher APC mutations from studies done in the Northern and Western parts of the country, are also reported [5–11].

The commonest abnormality seen in our study was elevated factor VIII levels followed by lupus anticoagulant positivity. This is the first study from India which reports this pattern. We believe that the difference in our study is due to population variation in the levels of factor VIII. There is a remote possibility that this difference in the underlying prothrombotic condition is related to the site of occurrence of DVT; this needs further study [1]. Our study found a relatively "high" blood level of factor VIII in normal controls. Again, we attribute this to population variation. This is a relevant finding; such a variation has not been previously reported in India.

Factor VIII or antihaemophilic factor is perhaps better studied in haemophilia. However elevated levels are also known to cause venous and occasionally arterial thrombosis (coronary, cerebrovascular beds). It is considered a prothrombotic risk factor along with factor V Leiden, prothrombin 20210A, elevated fibrinogen, antithrombin/protein C/protein S deficiency, hyperhomocysteinemia, and lupus anticoagulant positivity [1, 18, 19]. Factor VIII circulates bound to von Willebrand factor (vWF). The blood levels are influenced by various patient and disease factors. Patient factors include age (increase of 5 IU/dL with each decade increase in age), sex (higher in females), pregnancy, race, blood group, and genetic factors affecting vWF levels. However, no direct genetic factors affecting factor VIII levels are reported. Obesity, diabetes, insulin, liver disease, increased triglycerides, endothelial stimulation (exercise, V2 receptor analogs, and surgery), fibrinogen, intravascular haemolysis, chronic inflammation, malignancy, hyperthyroidism, and renal disease also cause increase in factor VIII levels [13, 20]. It is considered a risk factor for DVT in women using oral contraceptives; OCPs themselves do not influence factor VIII levels. The estimated population-attributable risk for factor VIII levels ≥150 IU/dL is ≈16% [1, 13]. This makes it an important prothrombotic risk factor. Thus, treatment parallels the other thrombophilias in which a specific genetic mutation is identified [1, 12]. There are no treatment guidelines specific to elevated factor VIII levels especially where the normal population demonstrated increased baseline plasma levels like in our population. Hence identification of a prothrombotic risk factor implies lifelong anticoagulation; this is a major clinical decision and influences all aspects of the patient's life [18, 19]. However, treatment based on assumption of similar "normal" blood levels among populations may be erroneous. The clinical behaviour in the patients with "elevated" levels therefore may not reflect a true prothrombotic tendency and may overtreat this patient group and cause undue anxiety. A cut-off level of 150 IU/dL may not be significant to diagnose elevated factor VIII levels as a prothrombotic risk factor in our population. There is a need for formulation of population specific treatment protocols.

5. Limitations

This study fails to find a suitable cut-off for a "normal" plasma factor VIII level: this is probably due to a small sample size with data from a single centre. The retrospective design and testing factor VIII at a single point are other limitations. The design comparing the levels of FVIII between the patients with unprovoked DVT and healthy people, though not easily justified, is used to highlight the lack of published data in Indian patients. We do not have prospective data to ascertain whether any of the healthy controls with elevated FVIII levels develop an unprovoked DVT during their life. This is also a serious limitation of our study.

6. Conclusion

Elevated factor VIII in the Indians may not be associated with the same thrombotic risk as seen in the West. We find a variation in the levels of factor VIII with a different "normal" than what is reported in other populations. This needs further study to elucidate the role of factor VIII in the evaluation and treatment of thrombophilia.

Conflict of Interests

The authors declare that there is no conflict of interests regarding the publication of this paper.

References

[1] T. Koster, J. P. Vandenbroucke, F. R. Rosendaal, E. Briët, F. R. Rosendaal, and A. D. Blann, "Role of clotting factor VIII in effect of von Willebrand factor on occurrence of deep-vein thrombosis," *The Lancet*, vol. 345, no. 8943, pp. 152–155, 1995.

[2] S. Ota, N. Yamada, Y. Ogihara et al., "High plasma level of factor VIII: an important risk factor for venous thromboembolism," *Circulation Journal*, vol. 75, no. 6, pp. 1472–1475, 2011.

[3] R. K. Patel, E. Ford, J. Thumpston, and R. Arya, "Risk factors for venous thrombosis in the black population," *Thrombosis and Haemostasis*, vol. 90, no. 5, pp. 835–838, 2003.

[4] S. Khan and J. D. Dickerman, "Hereditary thrombophilia," *Thrombosis Journal*, vol. 4, article 15, 2006.

[5] S. G. Anderson, D. C. Hutchings, A. H. Heald, C. D. Anderson, T. A. B. Sanders, and J. K. Cruickshank, "Haemostatic factors, lipoproteins and long-term mortality in a multi-ethnic population of Gujarati, African-Caribbean and European origin," *Atherosclerosis*, vol. 236, no. 1, pp. 62–e72, 2014.

[6] L. V. Baxi, "Hereditary thrombophilia in cerebral venous thrombosis: a study from India," *Blood Coagulation & Fibrinolysis*, vol. 25, no. 1, p. 92, 2014.

[7] P. Amarapurkar, N. Bhatt, N. Patel, and D. Amarapurkar, "Primary extrahepatic portal vein obstruction in adults: a single center experience," *Indian Journal of Gastroenterology*, vol. 33, no. 1, pp. 19–22, 2014.

[8] R. K. Pinjala, L. R. C. Reddy, R. P. Nihar, G. V. A. Praveen, and M. Sandeep, "Thrombophilia—how far and how much to investigate?" *Indian Journal of Surgery*, vol. 74, no. 2, pp. 157–162, 2012.

[9] N. Pai, K. Ghosh, and S. Shetty, "Hereditary protein C deficiency in Indian patients with venous thrombosis," *Annals of Hematology*, vol. 91, no. 9, pp. 1471–1476, 2012.

[10] N. Pai, K. Ghosh, and S. Shetty, "Cause of deep venous thrombosis and pulmonary embolism in young patients from India as compared with other ethnic groups," *Blood Coagulation and Fibrinolysis*, vol. 23, no. 4, pp. 257–261, 2012.

[11] P. Lalita Jyotsna, S. Sharma, and S. S. Trivedi, "Coagulation inhibitors and activated protein C resistance in recurrent pregnancy losses in Indian women," *Indian Journal of Pathology and Microbiology*, vol. 54, no. 4, pp. 752–755, 2011.

[12] S. M. Bates, I. A. Greer, S. Middeldorp, D. L. Veenstra, A. Prabulos, and P. O. Vandvik, "VTE, thrombophilia, antithrombotic therapy, and pregnancy," *Chest*, vol. 141, no. 2, supplement, pp. e691S–e736S, 2012.

[13] P. W. Kamphuisen, J. C. J. Eikenboom, and R. M. Bertina, "Elevated factor VIII levels and the risk of thrombosis," *Arteriosclerosis, Thrombosis, and Vascular Biology*, vol. 21, pp. 731–738, 2001.

[14] P. V. Jenkins, O. Rawley, O. P. Smith, and J. S. O'Donnell, "Elevated factor VIII levels and risk of venous thrombosis," *British Journal of Haematology*, vol. 157, no. 6, pp. 653–663, 2012.

[15] M. G. Conlan, A. R. Folsom, A. Finch et al., "Associations of factor VIII and von Willebrand factor with age, race, sex, and risk factors for atherosclerosis. The Atherosclerosis Risk in Communities (ARIC) study," *Thrombosis and Haemostasis*, vol. 70, no. 3, pp. 380–385, 1993.

[16] I. Martinelli, P. M. Mannucci, V. De Stefano et al., "Different risks of thrombosis in four coagulation defects associated with inherited thrombophilia: a study of 150 families," *Blood*, vol. 92, no. 7, pp. 2353–2358, 1998.

[17] P. M. Ridker, J. P. Miletich, J. E. Buring et al., "Factor V Leiden mutation as a risk factor for recurrent pregnancy loss," *Annals of Internal Medicine*, vol. 128, no. 12, part 1, pp. 1000–1003, 1998.

[18] G. Palareti, C. Legnani, M. Frascaro, G. Guazzaloca, and S. Coccheri, "Factor VIII: C levels during oral anticoagulation and after its withdrawal," *Thrombosis and haemostasis*, vol. 74, no. 6, pp. 1609–1610, 1995.

[19] C. M. Schambeck, K. Hinney, I. Haubitz, B. M. Taleghani, D. Wahler, and F. Keller, "Familial clustering of high factor VIII levels in patients with venous thromboembolism," *Arteriosclerosis, Thrombosis, and Vascular Biology*, vol. 21, no. 2, pp. 289–292, 2001.

[20] W. L. Chandler, C. Ferrell, J. Lee, T. Tun, and H. Kha, "Comparison of three methods for measuring factor VIII levels in plasma," *American Journal of Clinical Pathology*, vol. 120, no. 1, pp. 34–39, 2003.

21

Operative Exposure of a Surgical Trainee at a Tertiary Hospital in Kenya

Daniel Kinyuru Ojuka,[1] Jana Macleod,[2] and Catherine Kwamboka Nyabuto[3]

[1]Department of Surgery, University of Nairobi, P.O. Box 19969-00202, Nairobi, Kenya
[2]Department of Surgery, Kenyatta University, Kenya
[3]Spinal Injury Hospital, Nairobi, Kenya

Correspondence should be addressed to Daniel Kinyuru Ojuka; danielojuka@gmail.com

Academic Editor: Michael J. Brenner

Background. Psychomotor domain training requires repetitive exposure in order to develop proficiency in skills. This depends on many training factors in any training institution. *Objective.* This study sought to look at the operative exposure of surgical trainees in a tertiary hospital in a developing country. *Design and Setting.* This was a six-month retrospective study performed in one surgical firm at Kenyatta National Hospital. *Patients and Methods.* The files of all patients admitted to the unit at that time were retrieved. The demographics, diagnosis at admission, need for surgery, and cadre of operating surgeon among others were recorded. Scientific Package for Social Sciences (SPSS) version 17.0 was used for data entry and analysis. *Results.* The study cohort was 402 patients of the 757 patients admitted in the study period. The average age was 36.7 years, a female to male ratio of 1 : 2.5. The majority (69.7%) of patients required surgery. Trauma was the most common reason for admission (44.5%). Year 2 residents received the most clinical exposure. Consultant was available in only 34.5% of the cases. *Conclusion.* The junior residents performed the vast majority of procedures with an unsatisfactory amount of supervision from the senior residents and faculty.

1. Introduction

Medical educators have in the last decade delineated the domains of competency expected of graduating general surgery residents [1]. The patient care domain in the American model overlaps with the technical skills domain in the Canadian model, both clearly delineating the need for competency to perform certain operative procedures as part of the graduate surgical trainees' skills at the end of their training. Repeated purposeful practice in performing complex psychomotor tasks like surgical operations has been shown to be of paramount importance in achieving this level of competence [2].

In the last 5 years, the surgical education literature has documented a reduced level of operative exposure for skill acquisition for graduating general surgery trainees in England and North America [3–5]. However, the operative exposure and the operative skill development opportunities for Kenyan surgical trainees have not been investigated. The surgical trainee examining board in the United States of America, the American Board of Surgery (ABS), as well as program directors and residents in the American training systems have recorded serious concerns regarding the gap between surgical knowledge and surgical operative experience with a resultant reduced readiness for practice in general surgery [5] Approximately 80% of graduates of general surgical residency programs in an American training system now opt for additional postresidency fellowship training, often citing lack of confidence to start practise immediately as the main reason for the fellowship [6]. This change in surgical trainee operative confidence level at the end of training is often cited to be a result of the reduction in operative exposure for these surgical trainees as well as an increased focus on patient safety and the consultant surgeon's need for accountability. The situation of the graduating surgical trainee in the Kenyan context has not yet been similarly objectively elucidated.

Therefore, we designed a study to analyse the operative exposure and hence skill development opportunities of Kenyan surgical residents in a six month period in a surgical ward within a referral and teaching hospital in Nairobi, Kenya.

2. Patients and Methods

This was a six-month retrospective study between March 2012 and August 2012 in a single general surgical firm of the main referral and teaching hospital in Kenya that trains University of Nairobi surgical trainees (KNH). The trainees have rotations of 3 months each and so during the study time, there were 2 rotations with two different groups of residents. The call system of the hospital is that the resident takes a weekly call of seven days straight in the general surgical wards. This call week will have a maximum of three days of admission. There is no statutory regulation regarding duty hours for doctors in the country because of the inadequate number of doctors. The number of consultants in this unit during the study was 8. The ward has a bed capacity of 45. The residents working in the ward are distributed at random from year 2 to year 5 with the exception of year 3 residents who usually work in the speciality units. The total number of residents working at any one given time depends on the total number of residents available. The surgical patients come to the wards and for surgery in a variety of ways. Some emergencies will have been referred from other institutions as well as those who come to KNH directly for emergency care. Elective patients are chosen by the residents in consultation with the faculty for the purposes of learning. They are chosen most commonly from the surgical outpatient clinic run by the unit. But they can also already be in the ward after an emergency admission and have remained there for an extended period of time for a number of different reasons and they now require elective surgery.

Between March and May 2012, we had 6 residents; 5 were postgraduate year (PGY) 2, and one was PGY 4. Between June and August 2012, we had 6 residents; 3 were PGY 2, one was year 4, and two were year 5. The learning of the resident is expected to take place as they are exposed to patients during the admissions and during the operations. Operating exposure can be as the primary surgeon, meaning the main person operating, or can be as assistant surgeon. During this time, the resident is expected to consult the faculty for input both in decisions regarding the indication for surgery and for nonoperative care of patients. This should be recorded in the patient files. The residents in PGY 3 were operating only on those of head injury and chest injury. This is because acute neurosurgical patients and acute cardiothoracic patients are admitted in general surgical wards but it is the faculty and the residents in those units that will take primary responsibility for those patients. The process of admission and ongoing care of these patients is performed by the residents in the general surgical wards. The calls are taken for a whole week by one resident; it therefore means that, in these 12 weeks, any one resident will have only two call weeks. In any one week, there will be 2-3 days for admitting patients to the unit; given that there are three units, one unit covers the weekend such that weekend calls for each unit are only every three weeks.

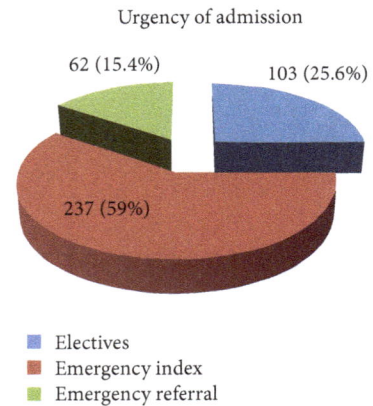

FIGURE 1: Urgency of admission.

Data collection included demographics, diagnosis at admission, admission type, need for surgery, admitting doctor, cancellation of elective surgery, supervision by the faculty, primary surgeon, assistant surgeon, complication, length of stay, and mortality.

These were entered into SPSS version 17 and analysed using frequencies for interval or binary data and means for quantitative data. Differences between frequencies were analysed using the Chi-square statistic or Fisher's exact test as appropriate. Any difference was considered significant if the p value was less than 0.05 as per standard statistical convention.

The study was approved by the Kenyatta National Hospital and University of Nairobi Ethical and Research Committee.

3. Results

The number of patients admitted to the ward during this time was 757, but the number of files we were able to retrieve was 402, the final study cohort. The mean age of the study cohort ($n = 402$) was 36.7 years; males comprised 71.4%. During this study period, 293 of the 402 patients (79.2%) were scheduled for surgery. Most admissions were emergencies (74.9%) (see Figure 1).

The cancellation rate for scheduled surgeries was 7.8%. The majority of the cancellations were because of project-related surgeries preferentially using operating theaters (meaning instead of routine schedule surgery, external expertise in collaboration with administration and local surgeons organize a period where surgeries for particular subspecialty area for a period). Hence, the regularly scheduled surgery is postponed, often without prior arrangement. The final two main reasons were patients who came to the operating room beyond the accepted finishing time of 3:00 pm (2/8) and nonoptimized patients (1/8).

Trauma was the most dominant reason for admission (179/402, 44.5%) (Figure 2). The main body system injured was the head. The largest four diagnoses and their frequency of occurrence are listed in Figure 1 and then each diagnostic category is further detailed in Tables 1–4.

Urological cancers followed by breast cancer were the frequent cancers, while appendicitis was the most frequent infectious surgical pathology seen and hernia was also common (see Tables 1–4).

TABLE 1: Trauma.

Diagnosis	Number ($n = 179$)
Head injury	87
Chest	15
Abdominal	28
Soft tissue injury	28
Snake bite	1
Human bite	2
Multiple	18

TABLE 2: Oncology.

Area	Number ($n = 39$)
Head and neck	4
Gastric	2
Oesophageal	4
Colorectal	3
Urology	21
Gall bladder	1
Cervical	2
Metastasis	2

TABLE 3: Infections.

Area	Number ($n = 52$)
Appendicitis	22
Cholecystitis	3
Cellulitis	9
Necrotizing fasciitis	5
Peritonitis	6
Pyomyositis	1
Urological	6

TABLE 4: Anatomical defect/inflammation.

Diagnosis	Number ($n = 109$)
Hernia	28
Urethral stricture	12
Pancreatitis	2
Hemorrhoids	6
Goitre	10
Undescended testis	3
Urinary calculi	5
Prostatic enlargement	5
Intestinal obstruction	18
Gall stones	7
Benign breast disease	4
Testicular torsion	1
Enterocutaneous fistula	3
Fistula in ano	2
Anal fissure	3

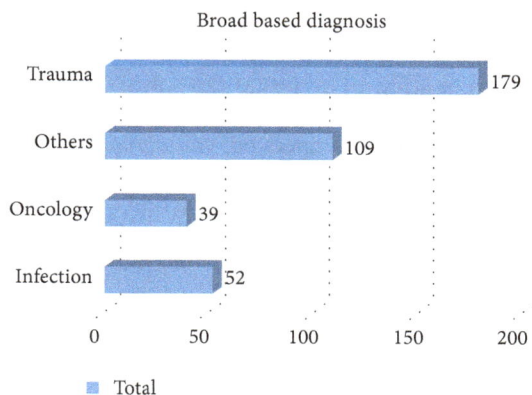

FIGURE 2: Diagnosis by broad categories.

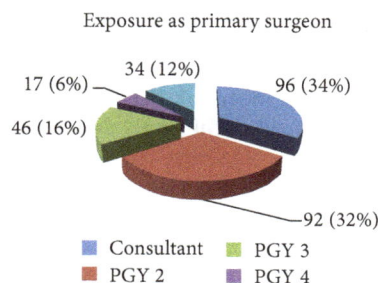

FIGURE 3: Operating doctor.

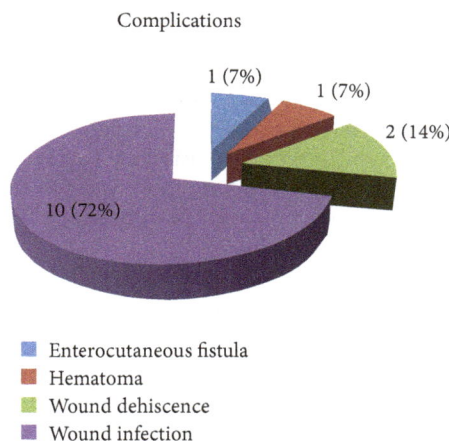

FIGURE 4: Complications.

Exposure by admission shows that the 8 year 2 students shared 392 admissions, which translate to 49 admissions per student, while the two year 4 students shared 6 admissions translating to 1.5 admissions per student; year 5 students shared 2 admissions translating to 1 admission per student.

Exposure as a primary surgeon in this study shows that the eight PGY 2 residents performed 92 operations, which is equivalent to 11.5 operations per PGY 2 resident, while the two PGY 4 residents performed 17 operations, an average of 8.5 operation per PGY 4 resident, and the most operations per resident were completed by the two PGY 5 senior residents who performed 34 operations which is equivalent to an average of 17 operations per PGY 5 resident in the six-month study period (see Figure 3).

Operative exposure gained by operative assisting demonstrated a decreasing exposure as residents became more senior: per resident operation assistance ratio was 16.5 assists per resident for PGY 2, while it reduced to 11.5 and then to 4.5 for PGY 4 and 5 residents, respectively.

Complication rate was 2.8% (14/285) with wound infection being the most common (see Figure 4). The mortality rate for this period was 6.2%.

The consultant was seen, by comments in the file, to supervise and to have been involved in 34.5% of the decisions and assisted in a few cases {8/100 (2.7%)} of all admissions and operations during this period. When the consultants or senior level residents operated, the complications were fewer (p value of 0.001). There was no relationship found between the cadre of resident operating and patient's length of hospital stay (p value of 0.052). Consultants were the primary surgeons in the majority {81/103 (78.6%)} of elective procedures.

4. Discussions

Training as a surgeon is more than just the number of years of training; it involves learning the techniques of operating and the attainment of adequate judgment, overall patient care skills, and professionalism [7].

In Kenya, there has been little system change in the resident training since its inception but the number of trainees in training has increased significantly. In 2009, there was the introduction of a 5-year training curriculum instead of the previous three and half years. Before 2008, the majority of trainees were sponsored by the government for masters of medicine in surgery program (surgery residency training). However, more recently, there has been a dramatic increase in self-sponsored students, who now comprise almost 80% of all the trainees. With these changes, there is a resultant increase in the number of trainees at any particular time in the ward. As a result of this dramatic increase in resident numbers, training experiences such as call have sometimes been reduced to two calls for an entire rotation of 12 weeks. This of course means exposure to fewer patients in terms of both admissions and surgery for residents. This scenario may result in either the resident taking more years in training to meet the required exposure or graduating with less technical experience.

One common approach to learning in residency involves senior residents playing an increasing role in patient care such that the junior students learn and are mentored to a large extent by the seniors as well as consultants. However, in this study it appears that this form of learning for the juniors was unavailable given that we found most senior residents were not present in all or most of the surgeries. In this study, we found that the students in year 2 were actually assisted most often by fellow year 2 students. A solution to this situation may be to introduce a chief residency system.

There were a larger number of PGY 2 residents compared to other years limiting our analysis such that we were unable to compare the exposure between the different years of residency training. This discrepancy in numbers was because of a new curriculum that introduced a large number of trainees in one year, resulting in this larger number of PGY 2 residents. Therefore, our results of increased exposure to admissions and surgeries by postgraduate year 2 residents may in fact be simply a reflection of the absolute numbers of the postgraduate year 2 residents as opposed to a reflection of a type of training system.

Exposure by type of admission demonstrates few elective patients (25.6%). The disadvantage of this in a learning institution is that it means the students have less exposure with the consultant because most of the emergencies are operated without assistance from consultant or at times even without senior residents. In a recent study looking at the changing caseloads for surgical residents, Varley et al. noted that reduced electives exposures should prompt reforms so that the caseloads are taken into account to maintain quality of training [7]. Maddern in an article published about 18 years ago noted that changing times required a requisite change in surgical teaching methods [8]. Our study emphasizes the changes needed are those that will increase the exposure despite the increased number of students with unchanging numbers of patients. One possible solution is to consider introducing the system where chief residents are involved in most of the surgeries both emergency and elective. This way, senior residents take more responsibility in giving service, learning, and teaching. This is the model predominantly followed in surgery resident training systems in North American centers.

We previously reviewed the operative exposure of our residents to emergency surgery but this study is the first to define the elective surgical exposure of our surgery residents [9]. In our previous study, one hundred and forty five patients were admitted. The number of admissions per resident varied between 30 and 41. Operative experience where the resident was the principal surgeon ranged from 11 cases to 23 cases per resident. A second resident assisted in 8 out of the fifty-eight cases operated on and consultant support was infrequent. The previous study was of three-month duration, with a retrieval rate of files at 72%. The duration for the current study is increased but retrieval is less at 53.2%. The admission per student ranges from 1.5 to 49, which demonstrates reduction somewhat, while that of exposure to primary surgery averages at 8.5 to 11.5 per student, and assistance at 4.5 to 16.5 per student. In all areas, this shows reduction, although this probably can be explained more by the lower retrieval rate and increased number of students than by a valid change in exposure per student.

The reduction in numbers in this study is likely reflective of the combination of both elective and emergency surgery together. The PGY 2 resident is meant to perform 15 appendectomies as primary surgeon (The Log Book of department of surgery requirement) in two general surgical rotations that total six months. But in this study of the same duration there were only 20 appendicitis cases in total. The PGY 4-5 residents require 10. In total, one training as a general surgeon requires 25 appendectomies. If the trend above continues, it means that any one PGY 2 resident may not be able to meet the competency requirements to graduate.

This study and our previous study [9] reveal an insignificant level of supervision by the consultant. Though the consultants are involved in elective cases (100%), the same does not hold true during emergency surgery cases. The most critical patient, the emergency surgery patient, is left in the hands of the resident while the least critical patient, elective patients, are operated on by the faculty. The involvement of faculty should improve resident clinical skills and knowledge and, therefore, would be expected to reduce the higher complication rates taking in to account patient acuity.

The limitation of the study is its retrospective nature which results in a reduced retrieval of medical records and the inherent bias of nonrandom record loss as is reflected in a retrieval rate of only 53.2%.

5. Conclusion

In conclusion, this study reveals a reduced clinical exposure rate for surgery residents in both elective and emergency surgery volumes. In particular, in the more senior years of training, there is a reduction in surgeries performed with successive years of training. There is a skew toward emergency surgery exposure with a paucity of elective procedures. To add to this finding, the supervision is the highest during elective surgeries (as reflective in consultant involvement) while exposure by residents at all levels is lowest in these same elective procedures. Concurrently, emergency surgeries are the commonest surgeries for all residents but in particular for the junior residents (PGY 2) and are most often assisted by only similar level residents (PGY 2). This study highlights the need for changes that will enable the resident to acquire necessary technical skills for their work as surgeons when they graduate. There is a need for greater involvement by the faculty in the management of surgical emergency patients, especially as they have the greatest morbidity and mortality.

Conflict of Interests

The authors declare no conflict of interests.

Authors' Contribution

Daniel Kinyuru Ojuka was responsible for study design, questionnaire, collection of data, data entry and cleaning, data analysis, and initial write-up. Jana Macleod was responsible for further analysis, paper preparation, and editing. Catherine Kwamboka Nyabuto was responsible for data collection and initial entry.

Acknowledgments

The authors acknowledge the contribution of Dr. Catherine Kwamboka Nyabuto in the collection of the data, Dr. Daniel Kinyuru Ojuka for the design of the study, and Kenyatta National Hospital department of medical records for assisting in accessing the necessary medical records for data collection. The authors are grateful to Dr. Daniel Kinyuru Ojuka for availing funds for the papers and printing as part of his research work in the department of surgery in surgical education.

References

[1] S. J. Lurie, C. J. Mooney, and J. M. Lyness, "Measurement of the general competencies of the accreditation council for graduate medical education: a systematic review," *Academic Medicine*, vol. 84, no. 3, pp. 301–309, 2009.

[2] K. A. Ericsson, "An expert-performance perspective of research on medical expertise: the study of clinical performance," *Medical Education*, vol. 41, no. 12, pp. 1124–1130, 2007.

[3] G. Morris-Stiff, E. Ball, J. Torkington, M. E. Foster, M. H. Lewis, and T. J. Havard, "Registrar operating experience over a 15-year period: more, less or more or less the same?" *Surgeon*, vol. 2, no. 3, pp. 161–164, 2004.

[4] S. V. Gurjar and A. J. McIrvine, "Working time changes: a raw deal for emergency operative training," *Annals of The Royal College of Surgeons of England*, vol. 87, supplement, pp. 140–141, 2005.

[5] R. H. Bell Jr., T. W. Biester, A. Tabuenca et al., "Operative experience of residents in US general surgery programs: a gap between expectation and experience," *Annals of Surgery*, vol. 249, no. 5, pp. 719–724, 2009.

[6] K. R. Borman, L. R. Vick, T. W. Biester, and M. E. Mitchell, "Changing demographics of residents choosing fellowships: longterm data from the American board of surgery," *Journal of the American College of Surgeons*, vol. 206, no. 5, pp. 782–788, 2008.

[7] I. Varley, J. Keir, and P. Fagg, "Changes in caseload and the potential impact on surgical training: a retrospective review of one hospital's experience," *BMC Medical Education*, vol. 6, article 6, 2006.

[8] G. J. Maddern, "The changing pattern of surgery," *British Journal of Surgery*, vol. 83, no. 2, pp. 145–146, 1996.

[9] K. Ojuka and H. Saidi, "Exposure in emergency general surgery in a time-based residency program: a call for review," *Annals of African Surgery*, vol. 2, pp. 15–18, 2009.

22

Hiatus Hernia Repair with Bilateral Oesophageal Fixation

Rajith Mendis,[1] Caran Cheung,[2] and David Martin[3,4,5]

[1]Westmead Hospital, Sydney, NSW 2145, Australia
[2]University of Sydney, Sydney, NSW 2006, Australia
[3]Department of Upper GI Surgery, Concord Hospital, Sydney, NSW 2139, Australia
[4]Department of Upper GI Surgery, Royal Prince Alfred Hospital, Sydney, NSW 2050, Australia
[5]Department of Upper GI Surgery, Strathfield Private Hospital, Sydney, NSW 2135, Australia

Correspondence should be addressed to Rajith Mendis; rajithmendis@gmail.com

Academic Editor: Michael Hünerbein

Background. Despite advances in surgical repair of hiatus hernias, there remains a high radiological recurrence rate. We performed a novel technique incorporating bilateral oesophageal fixation and evaluated outcomes, principally symptom improvement and hernia recurrence. *Methods.* A retrospective study was performed on a prospective database of patients undergoing hiatus hernia repair with bilateral oesophageal fixation. Retrospective and prospective quality of life (QOL), PPI usage, and patient satisfaction data were obtained. Hernia recurrence was assessed by either barium swallow or gastroscopy. *Results.* 87 patients were identified in the database with a minimum of 3 months followup. There were significant improvements in QOL scores including GERD HRQL (29.13 to 4.38, $P < 0.01$), Visick (3 to 1), and RSI (17.45 to 5, $P < 0.01$). PPI usage decreased from a median of daily to none, and there was high patient satisfaction (94%). 57 patients were assessed for recurrence with either gastroscopy or barium swallow, and one patient had evidence of recurrence on barium swallow at 45 months postoperatively. There was an 8% complication rate and no mortality or oesophageal perforation. *Conclusions.* This study demonstrates that our technique is both safe and effective in symptom control, and our recurrence investigations demonstrate at least short term durability.

1. Introduction

Achieving durable hernia repair and symptom outcomes whilst minimising untoward sequelae are key challenges in hiatus hernia surgery. The technique for repair of the hiatus hernia has evolved significantly from the original approach described in 1919 by Soresi detailing reduction of the hernia with closure of the crus [1]. Current methods favour complete mobilisation with division of adhesions, fundoplication (often around an oesophageal bougie), and crural closure [2]. There remain, however, many variations on this technique and there is no one standardised method which has been proven to be superior.

One of the major issues related to hiatus hernia repair is hernia recurrence, with rates of recurrence varying from 4 to 42% at intermediate followup [3–5]. This rate may deteriorate in the longer term with a more recent study reporting a high radiological recurrence rate of 66% in 35 patients undergoing barium studies at a median followup of 99 months [6], suggesting concerns about the longevity of current repairs. However, despite this higher rate, quality of life (QOL) assessments were not significantly affected and only one patient required reoperation.

Techniques to decrease recurrence and maximise outcomes have been investigated in the literature and include the use of meshes and gastropexy and the degree and type of fundoplication.

Use of nonabsorbable mesh has been associated with improved rates of recurrence [7] but can be associated with local mesh related complications including erosion, hiatal stenosis, and fibrosis [8]. Biologic meshes have been associated with decreased rates of complications with respect to nonabsorbable meshes [9] and short term efficacy [10, 11] but long term studies are awaited.

Partial and full (360°) fundoplication have been shown in meta-analyses to have similar control of reflux symptoms,

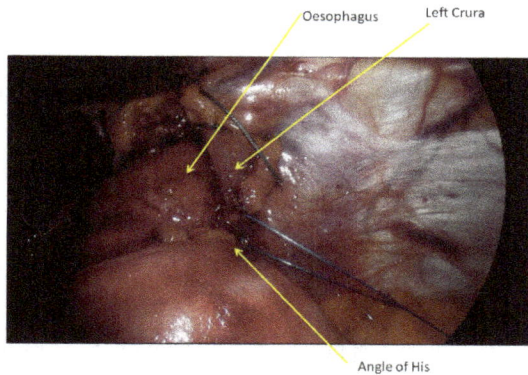

FIGURE 1: Left sided fixation suture with oesophagus and angle of His anchored to left crura.

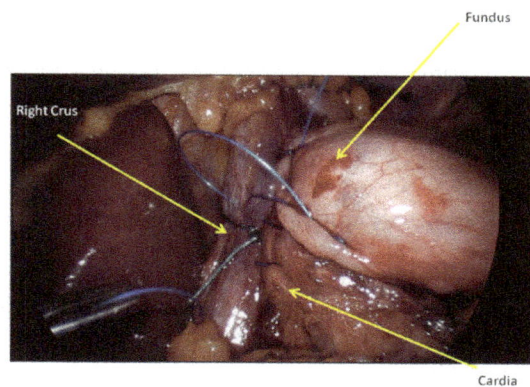

FIGURE 2: Right sided fixation suture involving running bites along entire length of wrap.

with similar satisfaction and reoperative rates. The partial fundoplication group generally has less dysphagia and bloating but a slightly higher attrition rate for reflux with longer followup [12]. One meta-analysis has shown a higher reoperation rate in the total fundoplication group, predominately due to dysphagia [13].

Gastropexy may have some role in reducing postoperative recurrence [14], but bilateral oesophageal fixation as performed in our series has not previously been in any of the randomised control trials evaluating fundoplication techniques.

We performed a novel technique involving bilateral oesophageal fixation to the oesophageal crura coupled with a fixed anterior fundoplication in an effort to reduce the risk of recurrence. Our study evaluates the outcomes using this technique, principally symptom improvement and hernia recurrence.

2. Materials and Methods

2.1. Technique. Our technique involves laparoscopic optical entry, with standard circumferential mobilisation of the phrenooesophageal ligament, followed by dissection and reduction of the peritoneal sac from the mediastinum. The oesophagus is then mobilised high into the mediastinum and the crura is closed with deep interrupted anterior and posterior sutures to maintain the oesophagus in the mid-crura, using a nonabsorbable braided suture (0 Ethibond, Ethicon). A 56 French bougie is used to calibrate the closure.

Left sided fixation of the oesophagus to the crura is then performed, centred at the 3 o'clock position with a figure of 8 suture, with the same suture used to then incorporate the "angle of His" prior to tying (Figure 1). The anterior wrap with right sided oesophageal fixation is then performed with a running suture encompassing the fundus, right oesophagus, and crura, from the 11 o'clock position anteriorly to the 7 o'clock position posteriorly over 3-4 bites (Figure 2). The anterior wrap is then further sutured to the hiatus apex with a figure of 8 suture, including the anterior oesophagus (12 o'clock position) only if the anterior vagus nerve can be identified and excluded from the suture. A nonabsorbable

nonbraided monofilament suture (Novafil, Covidien) is used for all fixation sutures.

Absorbable biological mesh (Surgisis, Cook Medical) is infrequently used on the posterior crus and only if there is marked tension at closure.

This technique has evolved from the phrenooesophageal ligament repair (described by Nathanson) though instead of repairing the damaged structure, we decided to directly fix the two organs being held by it.

By performing an anterior wrap, we were able to fix the fundus to the oesophagus along almost the entire length of the wrap, thereby theoretically decreasing the risk of migration of the wrap into the chest. This form of fixation, essentially across the anterior 180 degrees of the hiatus, involving oesophagus, fundus, and crura, has not been explicitly described previously. Certainly, the incorporation of the left sided fixation of oesophagus and angle of His to the left crura does not seem to be a feature of anterior wraps used in the randomised controlled trials.

All operations were performed under the auspices of the senior author (David Martin) with the senior author scrubbed and either performing the surgery or assisting senior surgical Upper GI fellows.

2.2. Study Design. A retrospective study was performed on a prospectively collected electronic database of patients who had hiatus hernia repair with the abovementioned oesophageal fixation technique, performed by the same surgeon. All patients underwent routine gastroscopy and manometry. 24 hour pH studies were usually performed, if tolerated and nuclear medicine isotope scans were also often performed. The 24-hour pH studies were considered positive if the patients had a pH < 4 for greater than 5% of the time. Many patients also had fluoroscopic swallow studies. Some patients with large symptomatic hiatus hernias did not undergo assessment with nuclear medicine isotope scans or 24-hour pH monitoring.

Retrospective and prospective QOL, Proton Pump Inhibitor (PPI) usage, and patient satisfaction (3-point scale) data were obtained with phone interviews. QOL was assessed using the validated gastrooesophageal reflux disease health related quality of life (GERD HRQL, 10-question, 5-point scale) [15], Visick score (4-point symptom scale) and the Reflux Symptom Index (RSI, 9-question, 5-point scale assessing laryngopharyngeal reflux) [16]. PPI usage was assessed according to frequency.

All patients were contacted postoperatively for preoperative and postoperative data. Some patients had prospectively completed the preoperative assessment.

Hernia recurrence was assessed by either barium swallow or gastroscopy. As part of routine postoperative followup most patients underwent a 6-month gastroscopy. All patients, not having undergone a postoperative gastroscopy within 5 months of their phone interview were also invited to have a barium swallow exam assessing for hiatus hernia recurrence using an established protocol encompassing views of the lower oesophagus, supine fundus, right lateral decubitus fundus, and erect lateral. The reports of any recent gastroscopy were also reviewed for any sign of recurrence. Recurrence was assessed at 6 months or greater postoperatively.

2.3. Statistical Analysis. Data was analysed using SPSS for statistical analysis, with the Wilcoxon Signed-Ranks test used to compare non-normally distributed results, confirmed with the Shapiro-Wilk test.

2.4. Ethical Statement. The project and data collection was approved by Sydney Local Health District Human Research Ethics Committee covering the associated hospitals and as accredited by the NSW Ministry of Health (File Ref: LNR/13/CRGH/194).

3. Results

93 consecutive patients underwent laparoscopic hiatus hernia repair between 2008 and 2012 of which 87 had a minimum of 3 months followup. There were 36 (39%) male and 57 (61%) female patients, with a mean age of 61 (range 24–89). 7 were with recurrent hiatus hernias following previous fundoplication. 46 patients had preoperative 24-hour pH studies and 50 patients had preoperative isotope studies, 31 patients having both. There were no conversions to open surgery, no oesophageal perforations, and no mortality. Absorbable mesh (Surgisis, Cook Medical) was used in 10 patients (11%). There were 6 complications (8%): 1 small volume bile leak in drain following liver laceration from a liver retractor which settled with conservative management, 2 patients with postoperative chest pain, 1 patient with a food bolus obstruction on day 2 postoperatively after inadvertently being started on a full diet, and 2 patients with diarrhoea immediately postoperatively.

Quality of life (QOL) data was obtained from 56 patients, with 36 (66%) of the preoperative assessments being completed retrospectively. The postoperative QOL data was obtained at a mean of 24 months postoperatively (range 3–48 months). Mean HRQL scores improved from 29.13/50 preoperatively to 4.38/50 postoperatively (P < 0.001) (Figure 3). RSI scores improved from a mean of 17.45/45 preoperatively to 5.04 postoperatively (P < 0.001) (Figure 4) and the number of RSI scores above 13 (considered positive for LPR) decreased from 32 preoperatively to 9 postoperatively.

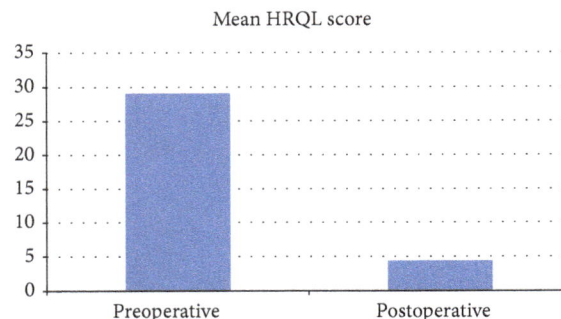

FIGURE 3: Comparison of preoperative and postoperative gastrooesophageal reflux QOL scores.

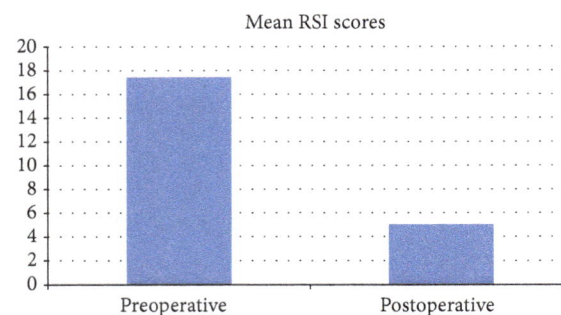

FIGURE 4: Comparison of preoperative and postoperative laryngopharyngeal reflux QOL scores.

TABLE 1: Comparison of preoperative and postoperative PPI usage.

	Preoperative	Postoperative
None	8	33
Less than 1/week	1	6
1–3x/week	1	1
4–6x/week	1	0
Daily	44	15

There was also a significant improvement in Visick scores from a median of 3 preoperatively to 1 postoperatively (P < 0.001).

PPI usage decreased from a median of daily to none postoperatively (P < 0.001), however 15 patients (27.3%) were still using a PPI daily postoperatively (Table 1).

Satisfaction scores were obtained from 53 patients with 50 (94%) being satisfied, 1 (2%) neutral, and 2 (4%) dissatisfied.

Dysphagia scores were analysed pre- and postoperatively and only 3 patients (5%) had increases in dysphagia scores postoperatively. Two patients increased from 0 to 1/5, pre- and postoperatively, and the other from 0 to 3/5 in severity. 28 patients had no difference in dysphagia and 25 patients experienced improvement in dysphagia (Figure 5).

57 patients had either follow-up gastroscopy or fluoroscopy for investigation of recurrence at least 6 months postoperatively, with a mean followup of 17.8 months (range 6–49 months). Gastroscopy was the most recent investigation

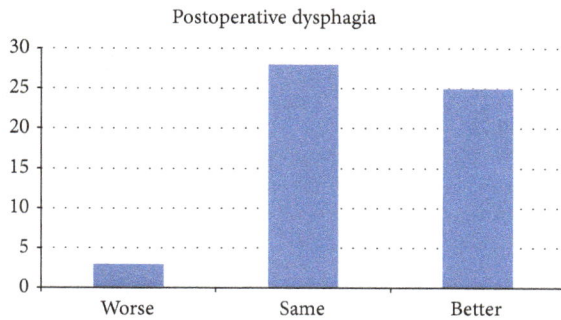

FIGURE 5: Postoperative dysphagia.

in 33 patients (58%) and barium swallow study in 24 (42%). Of these patients, 1 patient (1.8%) had a recurrence on a followup barium swallow study performed at 45 months postoperatively. This patient had undergone repair of a massive hernia containing 100% of the stomach and had some recurrent reflux symptoms which were controlled with a regular PPI. When looking at patients with more than 18 months followup, there were 21 patients, with a mean followup of 33.2 months, with the single recurrence (5%).

4. Discussion

Laparoscopic hiatus hernia repair has been proven to be safe and effective, but the recurrence rate remains not insignificant. The method of bilateral oesophageal fixation utilised with our repair has been performed in attempt to prevent recurrence, specifically from wrap migration and telescoping phenomenon. The incorporation of the angle of His into this fixation was hoped to add further effect to the anterior wrap, plus gastric fixation, thereby hopefully decreasing the attrition of reflux improvement seen in some partial fundoplication studies whilst attempting to maintain the benefits of decreased side effects of dysphagia and bloating seen with the 360-degree wrap. In our series, absorbable mesh was used in 11% of repairs, and only when there was marked tension. We used absorbable mesh to reduce the risk of complications associated with nonabsorbable mesh. The mesh used at the time of the study was an accepted standard though we have since changed to more robust Biomesh. We have analysed data from our database of patients undergoing this novel technique to assess safety, efficacy, and durability.

With 87 patients included in the study and no mortality or oesophageal perforations, it appears that this technique is safe, though we would advise close adherence to correct techniques as described in the following, particularly in suturing the oesophagus and wrap to avoid enteric injury. The complication rate of 8% is comparable to other studies [6, 7].

Surgical Techniques to Avoid Enteric Tears with Oesophageal Fixation Sutures

(1) No tension;

(2) monofilament suture;

(3) single smooth passage of suture through oesophagus with each bite;

(4) minimal traction on the oesophagus by the assistant once fixation is underway.

Initial quality of life data demonstrates that this hernia repair provides very good symptom improvement for both classical heartburn and laryngopharyngeal symptoms, with minimal dysphagia, and resultant high levels of patient satisfaction.

Despite the QOL score improvement, however, a moderate percentage of patients (27.3%) were still using a PPI postoperatively and this remains an area of concern. This is not uncommon, though, with long term studies showing continued use of PPIs in up to 62% of patients having antireflux operations [17]. This may be attributed to previous positive experiences with a PPI preoperatively, resulting in a predilection towards restarting PPI therapy following onset of mild or atypical symptoms. The rate of true reflux as measured by pH monitoring in patients requiring postoperative PPIs has been reported as 26% [18]. The high number of negative studies highlights the need for objective followup and investigation prior to considering any revisional surgery in these patients.

Our study identified one recurrence although the patient's symptoms were controlled with medical therapy. Recurrence was assessed with either a barium swallow study or a gastroscopy. The barium swallow study utilised a defined protocol to maintain the reliability of the study, although a potential for error exists as the films were reviewed and reported by a variety of radiologists. However these radiologists were not aware of the novel technique utlitised in the repair of the hiatus hernia. A potential bias exists in the patients assessed for recurrence with a gastroscopy as most were conducted by the surgical teams at the Upper GI departments at the participating campuses of the senior author and primary surgeon.

5. Conclusion

At intermediate followup, with only one hiatus hernia recurrence in our study population at 45 months, there is potential that this technique may provide improved durability of the hernia repair. With further followup of this growing cohort it will be interesting to further investigate the mode of recurrence and the role of wrap migration or telescoping phenomenon, which we have attempted to prevent by both the oesophageal and anterior wrap fixation.

We believe this technique of hiatus hernia repair offers safe and potentially durable outcomes, with a low likelihood of untoward side effects, and high patient satisfaction.

Conflict of Interests

The authors declare that there is no conflict of interests regarding the publication of this paper.

Acknowledgment

This paper is based on research which has been presented at the ANZGOSA Conference, 2012.

References

[1] N. Stylopoulos and D. W. Rattner, "The history of hiatal hernia surgery: from Bowditch to laparoscopy," *Annals of Surgery*, vol. 241, pp. 185–193, 2005.

[2] B. Dallemagne and S. Perretta, "Twenty years of laparoscopic fundoplication for GERD," *World Journal of Surgery*, vol. 35, no. 7, pp. 1428–1435, 2011.

[3] M. B. Edye, J. Canin-Endres, F. Gattorno, and B. A. Salky, "Durability of laparoscopic repair of paraesophageal hernia," *Annals of Surgery*, vol. 228, no. 4, pp. 528–535, 1998.

[4] R. J. Wiechmann, M. K. Ferguson, K. S. Naunheim et al., "Laparoscopic management of giant paraesophageal herniation," *The Annals of Thoracic Surgery*, vol. 71, no. 4, pp. 1080–1087, 2001.

[5] M. Hashemi, J. H. Peters, T. R. DeMeester et al., "Laparoscopic repair of large type III hiatal hernia: objective followup reveals high recurrence rate," *Journal of the American College of Surgeons*, vol. 190, no. 5, pp. 553–560, 2000.

[6] B. Dallemagne, L. Kohnen, S. Perretta, J. Weerts, S. Markiewicz, and C. Jehaes, "Laparoscopic repair of paraesophageal hernia: long-term follow-up reveals good clinical outcome despite high radiological recurrence rate," *Annals of Surgery*, vol. 253, no. 2, pp. 291–296, 2011.

[7] F. A. Granderath, M. A. Carlson, J. K. Champion et al., "Prosthetic closure of the esophageal hiatus in large hiatal hernia repair and laparoscopic antireflux surgery," *Surgical Endoscopy and Other Interventional Techniques*, vol. 20, no. 3, pp. 367–379, 2006.

[8] R. J. Stadlhuber, A. El Sherif, S. K. Mittal et al., "Mesh complications after prosthetic reinforcement of hiatal closure: a 28-case series," *Surgical Endoscopy*, vol. 23, no. 6, pp. 1219–1226, 2009.

[9] S. A. Antoniou, R. Pointner, and F. A. Granderath, "Hiatal hernia repair with the use of biologic meshes: a literature review," *Surgical Laparoscopy, Endoscopy & Percutaneous Techniques*, vol. 21, no. 1, pp. 1–9, 2011.

[10] B. K. Oelschlager, C. A. Pellegrini, J. Hunter et al., "Biologic prosthesis reduces recurrence after laparoscopic paraesophageal hernia repair: a multicenter, prospective, randomized trial," *Annals of Surgery*, vol. 244, no. 4, pp. 481–490, 2006.

[11] M. Jacobs, E. Gomez, G. Plasencia et al., "Use of surgisis mesh in laparoscopic repair of hiatal hernias," *Surgical Laparoscopy, Endoscopy & Percutaneous Techniques*, vol. 17, no. 5, pp. 365–368, 2007.

[12] J. A. Broeders, D. J. Roks, G. G. Jamieson, P. G. Devitt, R. J. Baigrie, and D. I. Watson, "Five-year outcome after laparoscopic anterior partial versus Nissen fundoplication: four randomized trials," *Annals of Surgery*, vol. 255, no. 4, pp. 637–642, 2012.

[13] M. Catarci, P. Gentileschi, C. Papi et al., "Evidence-based appraisal of antireflux fundoplication," *Annals of Surgery*, vol. 239, no. 3, pp. 325–337, 2004.

[14] J. Ponsky, M. Rosen, A. Fanning, and J. Malm, "Anterior gastropexy may reduce the recurrence rate after laparoscopic paraesophageal hernia repair," *Surgical Endoscopy and Other Interventional Techniques*, vol. 17, no. 7, pp. 1036–1041, 2003.

[15] V. Velanovich, S. R. Vallance, J. R. Gusz, F. V. Tapia, and M. A. Harkabus, "Quality of life scale for gastroesophageal reflux disease," *Journal of the American College of Surgeons*, vol. 183, no. 3, pp. 217–224, 1996.

[16] P. C. Belafsky, G. N. Postma, and J. A. Koufman, "Validity and reliability of the reflux symptom index (RSI)," *Journal of Voice*, vol. 16, no. 2, pp. 274–277, 2002.

[17] S. J. Spechler, E. Lee, D. Ahnen et al., "Long-term outcome of medical and surgical therapies for gastroesophageal reflux disease: follow-up of a randomized controlled trial," *The Journal of the American Medical Association*, vol. 285, no. 18, pp. 2331–2338, 2001.

[18] S. K. Thompson, G. G. Jamieson, J. C. Myers, K.-F. Chin, D. I. Watson, and P. G. Devitt, "Recurrent heartburn after laparoscopic fundoplication is not always recurrent reflux," *Journal of Gastrointestinal Surgery*, vol. 11, no. 5, pp. 642–647, 2007.

23

Teamwork Assessment Tools in Modern Surgical Practice: A Systematic Review

George Whittaker,[1] Hamid Abboudi,[2,3] Muhammed Shamim Khan,[2,3] Prokar Dasgupta,[2,3] and Kamran Ahmed[2,3]

[1]*School of Medical Education, King's College London, London SE1 1UL, UK*
[2]*Department of Urology, Guy's and St. Thomas' NHS Foundation Trust, London SE1 9RT, UK*
[3]*MRC Centre for Transplantation, King's College London, London SE1 9RT, UK*

Correspondence should be addressed to Kamran Ahmed; kamran.ahmed@kcl.ac.uk

Academic Editor: Eelco de Bree

Introduction. Deficiencies in teamwork skills have been shown to contribute to the occurrence of adverse events during surgery. Consequently, several teamwork assessment tools have been developed to evaluate trainee nontechnical performance. This paper aims to provide an overview of these instruments and review the validity of each tool. Furthermore, the present paper aims to review the deficiencies surrounding training and propose several recommendations to address these issues. *Methods.* A systematic literature search was conducted to identify teamwork assessment tools using MEDLINE (1946 to August 2015), EMBASE (1974 to August 2015), and PsycINFO (1806 to August 2015) databases. *Results.* Eight assessment tools which encompass aspects of teamwork were identified. The Nontechnical Skills for Surgeons (NOTSS) assessment was found to possess the highest level of validity from a variety of sources; reliability and acceptability have also been established for this tool. *Conclusions.* Deficits in current surgical training pathways have prompted several recommendations to meet the evolving requirements of surgeons. Recommendations from the current paper include integration of teamwork training and assessment into medical school curricula, standardised formal training of assessors to ensure accurate evaluation of nontechnical skill acquisition, and integration of concurrent technical and nontechnical skills training throughout training.

1. Introduction

Due to the sporadic and potentially catastrophic consequences of errors in surgery, the operating theatre environment has been described as a high-reliability organisation (HRO) [1]. Effective teamwork is a vital component of minimising human error and maintaining high reliability, hence the importance of enhancing nontechnical performance of surgical teams. Analysis of adverse events in surgery reveals deficiencies in nontechnical skills (NTS), the cognitive and interpersonal skills required for effective cooperation, as a major contributing factor to surgical errors [2]. These skills also have a direct impact on the technical performance of surgeons [3]. Furthermore, inadequate teamwork has been linked to a higher incidence of adverse events [4], whilst improvement of team-working ability with training correlates

with reduced technical errors [5] and perioperative mortality [6]. This body of evidence highlights the importance of effective teamwork in surgery and, due to the inability of surgeons to accurately self-assess their level of this essential skill [7], the need for NTS assessment.

Surgical trainee performance is continually evaluated with a variety of validated tools. Technical skills assessments such as Procedure-Based Assessment (PBA) and Objective Structured Assessment of Technical Skills (OSATS) are used to measure procedural competence. NTS assessment tools are also used to scrutinise the generic interpersonal (teamwork, leadership, and communication) and cognitive (decision-making, situation awareness, and task management) qualities which complement technical skills [8]. Specific teamwork assessment tools aim to evaluate team-working ability by assessing observable behaviours using a skills taxonomy and behavioural marker system within several areas identified for successful teamwork such as communication and cooperation.

Developing tools for evaluating teamwork can be problematic due to the difficulty in quantifying inherently complex behaviours [9]. Like many other constructs, nontechnical surgical skills have no unique or specific criterion to predict outcomes, and the domain of content to sample is very broad and inclusive (e.g., respect, integrity, accountability, and communications). Before introduction, it must therefore be established as psychometrically robust with numerous sources of evidence confirming validity and reliability [10].

Validity represents the extent to which a test or assessment tool accurately measures the domains it has been designed to measure, whereas reliability refers to the ability of a test to produce consistent results. There are three main types of internal test validity (construct, content, and criterion), each of which can be subdivided. Legitimate proof for each of these attributes is required for a tool to be fully validated.

Construct validity is the extent to which a test measures the intended construct, demonstrated by linkages between expected and acquired measurements (e.g., participants with more experience achieving higher test scores). The linkages may be correlation-based (Pearson's r, regression, factor analysis, etc.) or experimentally based hypothesis testing specifying between group differences (analyses of variance, etc.). Convergent validity, the degree of relation between two similar constructs, and discriminant (divergent) validity, which concerns the degree of dissimilarity between two unrelated concepts, are the two subtypes construct validity.

Content validity concerns the extent to which a test represents all possible items in the domain being assessed and is subjectively determined by a group of experts with the appropriate background. Face validity is the participant's subjective estimate of whether the test appears to be effective at what it purports to be measuring.

Criterion validity relates to the accuracy of a test at predicting outcomes from other variables and is demonstrated by correlation of test scores with a criterion measure. There are two subtypes of criterion validity: concurrent and predictive. Concurrent validity is illustrated by correlation of test scores with simultaneous results from a previously validated tool that measures the same construct. Predictive validity is demonstrated when future test scores are accurately predicted following an initial assessment with a time period between the tests, although accurate prognostication of behaviours also constitutes evidence for predictive validity.

This paper aims to provide an overview of the teamwork assessment tools available for surgery and review the internal validation evidence supporting each instrument. Deficiencies of the current surgical training pathway will also be highlighted with subsequent formation of recommendations for training.

2. Methods

The Preferred Reporting Items for Systematic Reviews and Meta-Analyses (PRISMA) method was used as a guideline for the systematic review. A comprehensive literature search

was conducted to identify teamwork assessment tools and supportive literature using MEDLINE (1946 to August 2015), EMBASE (1974 to August 2015), and PsycINFO (1806 to August 2015) databases. The following keywords were used in combination using the Boolean operators "OR" and "AND": "teamwork," "team work," "team-working," "nontechnical skills," "nontechnical skills," "assessment," "assessing," "surgery," "surgical," and "surgeons." The title of each study was screened for relevance, with retrieval of the abstract and full article if any doubt was present, followed by a selective process in which articles that failed to meet the criteria were excluded.

A wide variety of studies concerning teamwork assessment instruments were included. Original articles regarding the development process of specific instruments were used to identify the assessment tools. Validation studies were also included in addition to those which evaluated reliability and feasibility. Other articles which offered valuable information on teamwork assessment tools were included, encompassing studies which utilised the instruments for other development processes. Conference abstracts were also included.

Teamwork assessment tools developed for a specific surgical subspecialty were excluded because the authors' aim was to provide a broad overview of the general instruments available. Studies regarding assessment tools for technical skills were also excluded. Reviews, case reports, letters, and editorials were excluded in addition to articles in other languages. Duplicates were also removed.

3. Results

The literature search retrieved 994 publications and conference abstracts of potential relevance. Of these, 960 were determined as irrelevant and were subsequently excluded. Of the 34 articles remaining, further nine were excluded as they either failed to meet the inclusion criteria or fell under the exclusion criteria. After reference checking a final total of 25 articles were included in this review (Figure 1).

Eight teamwork assessment tools were identified from the search results generated (Table 1). These tools were developed for a range of healthcare professionals including surgeons, anaesthetists, and operating department practitioners. A total of 13 validation studies were included, some examples of which are presented in (Table 2). The amount and variety of validation evidence differed greatly between each tool.

4. Discussion

4.1. Observational Teamwork Assessment for Surgery (OTAS). The OTAS tool, created from a generalised model of teamwork [24], assesses the NTS of the entire surgical team. Procedures are divided into three phases (preoperative, intraoperative, and postoperative), each of which incorporates three stages. In each stage, a psychologist rates behaviours observed in each theatre subteam (surgeons, anaesthetists, and nurses) against a list of exemplary conducts using a 7-point scale ranging from 0 (severely hindering team function) to 6 (greatly enhancing team function). Analysis of behaviours is implemented in five domains: communication, cooperation,

TABLE 1: Teamwork assessment tools and the types of validity established in the surgical environment.

Assessment tool name	Domains assessed	Scoring system	Types of validity established
OTAS	Communication, cooperation, coordination, shared leadership, and team monitoring & situation awareness	7-point Likert scale and generic checklist	Construct [11] and content [12]
NOTSS	Situation awareness, decision-making, communication & teamwork, and leadership	4-point numeric scale	Face [13], content [13, 14], concurrent [15], and construct [13, 14]
NOTECHS	Leadership & management, teamwork & cooperation, problem-solving & decision-making, and situation awareness	4-point numeric scale	Concurrent [16], convergent [16], face [16], content [16], and construct [16]
ANTS	Task management, team-working, situation awareness, and decision-making	5-point numeric scale	Content [17]
MSF	Clinical care, good medical practice, learning & teaching, and teamwork & communication	3-point Likert scale and 3-point GSS	Content [18], face [18], and concurrent [19]
CbD	Medical record keeping, clinical assessment, diagnostic skills, patient management, leadership, clinical judgement, communication & team-working skills, and reflection	3-point Likert scale and 5-point GSS	None[†]
EBSTAF	Communication, knowledge, clinical skills, teamwork, and technical skills	3-point Likert scale	Construct [20] and concurrent [21]
SPLINTS	Communication & teamwork, situation awareness, and task management	4-point Likert scale	Content [22]

OTAS, Observational Teamwork Assessment for Surgery; NOTSS, Nontechnical Skills for Surgeons; NOTECHS, Oxford Nontechnical Skills; ANTS, Anaesthetists' Nontechnical Skills; MSF, Multisource Feedback; EBSTAF, Edinburgh Basic Surgical Training Assessment Form; SPLINTS, Scrub Practitioners' List of Nontechnical Skills; GSS, Global Summary Score.
[†]Construct and face validities established in other medical specialties.

TABLE 2: Sources of validation evidence for teamwork assessment tools in surgery.

Study	Assessment tool name	Method of validation	Participants	Types of validity established
Sevdalis et al. [11]	OTAS	Assessment of teamwork during surgical procedures	Surgical trainees, human factors experts, and psychologists	Construct
Hull et al. [12]	OTAS	Content validity metric scoring by expert panel performing surgical procedures	Expert surgeons, nurses, anaesthetists supervisors, anaesthetists, and scrub nurses	Content
Yule et al. [13]	NOTSS	Structured interviews regarding difficult nonroutine cases	Consultant surgeons	Face
Crossley et al. [15]	NOTSS	Assessment of NTS during surgical procedures	Surgical trainees, surgical care practitioners, scrub nurses, and anaesthetists	Concurrent
Beard et al. [14]	NOTSS	Assessment of trainees performing surgical procedures	Surgical trainees, clinical supervisors, anaesthetists, and scrub nurses	Construct and content
Mishra et al. [16]	NOTECHS	Assessment of NTS during laparoscopic cholecystectomies	Surgical trainees, nurses, and anaesthetists	Concurrent, convergent, face, content, and construct
Fletcher et al. [17]	ANTS	Assessment of NTS observed in 8 clinical scenario videos	Consultant anaesthetists	Content
Violato et al. [18]	MSF	Assessment of surgeons using MSF	Surgeons from various specialties and their nominated colleagues	Content and face
Paisley et al. [20]	EBSTAF	Assessment of trainees before and after 1 year of training	Surgical trainees (SHO)	Construct
Mitchell et al. [22]	SPLINTS	Assessment of scrub practitioners in 7 scenarios	Scrub practitioners	Content

OTAS, Observational Teamwork Assessment for Surgery; NOTSS, Nontechnical Skills for Surgeons; NOTECHS, Oxford Nontechnical Skills; ANTS, Anaesthetists' Nontechnical Skills; MSF, Multisource Feedback; EBSTAF, Edinburgh Basic Surgical Training Assessment Form; SPLINTS, Scrub Practitioners' List of Intraoperative Nontechnical Skills.

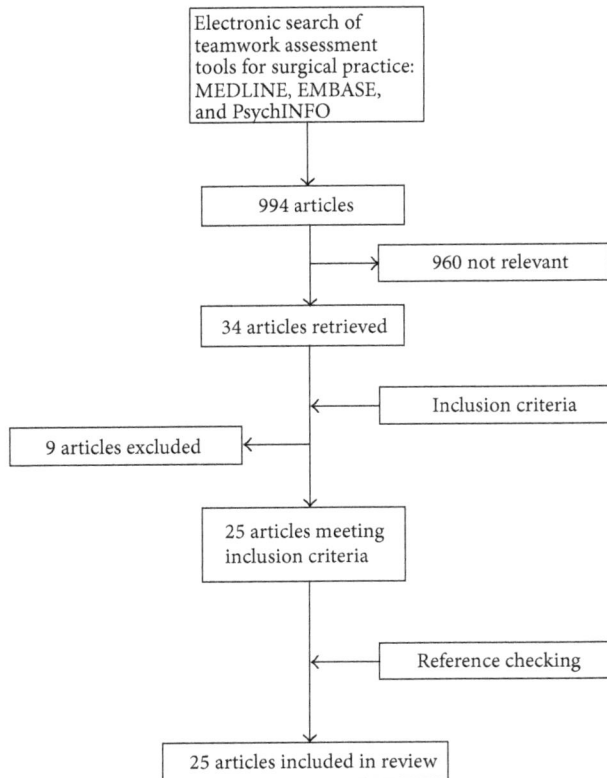

FIGURE 1: Flowchart depicting literature search strategy and results.

coordination, shared leadership, and team monitoring and situation awareness. A generic checklist is employed simultaneously, with individual marks being awarded for each task completed in three categories (patient-related, equipment-related, and communication-related).

Construct validity was illustrated in an article which compared behavioural ratings given by an expert/expert pair and expert/novice pair of assessors for 12 surgical procedures [11]. Significant consistency was observed in the expert/expert pair for 12 of the 15 behaviours (r_s = 0.51–0.94, p < 0.05), whilst significant consistency was observed in the expert/novice pair for only 3 of the 15 behaviours (r_s = 0.52–0.60, p < 0.05). Exemplary behavioural markers were analysed in another article, wherein a panel of 15 experienced theatre practitioners (5 surgeons, 5 anaesthetists, and 5 scrub nurses) rated a substantial amount of markers as key factors of teamwork, indicating a high level of content validity [12]. Furthermore, two blinded assessors observed 30 operations to evaluate the observability of the exemplary behaviours provided, with high agreement (Cohen's κ ≥ 0.41) found for 84% of markers. In the second phase of this study, a group of three experts in nontechnical skills and patient safety reviewed each individual exemplar, resulting in the removal of 21 exemplars and the modification of further 23 markers.

OTAS is a robust tool for precisely assessing NTS due to inclusion of exemplar behaviours for reference, variety of nontechnical domains, and subdivision of procedure and staff. There is good evidence of construct and content validity. The instrument has also demonstrated high reliability [25]

and feasibility [26] in other studies. However, intensive training of assessors is required [11] and determination of criterion validity (concurrent or predictive) is necessary.

4.2. Nontechnical Skills for Surgeons (NOTSS). NOTSS is a behavioural rating system which aims to evaluate the intraoperative NTS of individual trainees. The tool was created by devising an appropriate skills taxonomy using a variation of the Delphi method in which consultant surgeons were interviewed about challenging emergency procedures they had performed, ensuring face validity [13]. An accompanying behavioural marker system was then developed to rate the identified skills within four constructs: situation awareness, decision-making, communication and teamwork, and leadership. Each domain is comprised of three elements which are numerically scored from 1 (poor) to 4 (good) (Table 3). A successive feedback session allows the trainees to reflect and develop their NTS for future procedures.

Multiple validities have been established for NOTSS. Concurrent validity was illustrated in a prospective observational study involving assessment of 85 surgical trainees throughout 404 procedures using NOTSS, PBA, and OSATS tools [15]. A total of 715 assessments were made by 100 staff members including anaesthetists, scrub nurses, surgical care practitioners, and independent assessors. Results showed significant positive correlations between NOTSS, PBA (r = 0.43–0.55, p < 0.001), and OSATS (r = 0.40–0.58, p < 0.001) in all four domains. In a similar experiment, 85 surgical trainees were rated by 148 assessors (including consultants, anaesthetists, nurses, surgical care practitioners, and independent assessors) across 437 cases [14]. NOTSS, PBA, and OSATS tools were employed simultaneously to produce 1635 completed assessments. Associations were observed between training grade and NOTSS scores (r = 0.40–0.57, p < 0.001), and within the four behavioural categories (r = 0.74–0.76, p < 0.001), demonstrating construct and content validities, respectively.

NOTSS has shown high levels of validity and acceptability in practice and has the potential to become a fundamental tool in surgical curricula due to its comprehensive coverage of NTS. Furthermore, interobserver reliability has been established [27], though assessors need a high level of training to obtain accurate results [28]. NOTSS therefore appears to be a valuable tool for the assessment of teamwork in surgery.

4.3. Oxford Nontechnical Skills System (NOTECHS). NOTECHS is an evaluation tool which has been translated from the aviation industry to surgical practice via expert consultation and task analysis [16]. It is used to assess the nontechnical performance of surgical teams in four areas: leadership and management, teamwork and cooperation, problem-solving and decision-making, and situation awareness. An assessor observes the entire team during a procedure and scores individuals in each domain using a 4-point scale ranging from 1 (below standard) to 4 (excellent), with summation of the scores being used to examine the performance of subteams or the team overall (Table 4). A list of behaviours, known as subteam modifiers, rewards positive

TABLE 3: Nontechnical Skills for Surgeons (NOTSS) scoring form Yule et al. (2008) [23].

Hospital				
Trainer name				
Date				
Trainee name				
Operation				
Category	Category rating*	Element	Element rating*	Feedback on performance and debriefing notes
Situation awareness		Gathering information		
		Understanding information		
		Projecting and anticipating future state		
Decision-making		Considering options		
		Selecting and communicating option		
		Implementing and reviewing decisions		
Communication and teamwork		Exchanging information		
		Establishing a shared understanding		
		Coordinating team activities		
Leadership		Setting and maintaining standards		
		Supporting others		
		Coping with pressure		

*1 poor; 2 marginal; 3 acceptable; 4 good; NA not applicable.
1 poor: performance endangered or potentially endangered patient safety; serious remediation is required.
2 marginal: performance indicated cause for concern; considerable improvement is needed.
3 acceptable: performance was of a satisfactory standard but could be improved.
4 good: performance was of a consistently high standard, enhancing patient safety; it could be used as a positive example for others.
NA: not applicable.

actions and penalises negative actions, thus influencing scores.

Validity was investigated in the original article by the use of NOTECHS to evaluate surgical teams performing 65 laparoscopic cholecystectomies before ($n = 26$) and after ($n = 39$) teamwork training [16]. Cases were observed by one ($n = 30$), two ($n = 24$), or three ($n = 11$) assessors. Face and content validity could be assumed as the scale had been adapted for surgery in conjunction with expert theatre practitioners. Concurrent validity was established via positive correlation of scores between NOTECHS and the previously validated Safety Attitudes Questionnaire (SAQ). Construct validity was supported by significant improvement of scores after training ($t = -3.019$, $p = 0.005$). OTAS was also used in parallel with NOTECHS to examine convergent validity, which was successfully demonstrated by the excellent agreement between scores ($r = 0.886$, $p = 0.046$).

NOTECHS is a potentially valuable tool due to its detailed analysis of teamwork and subteam modifiers, with recent utilisation to guide the development of a robotic training curriculum [29]. However, aside from the aforementioned study, very little validation evidence of this tool in the surgical setting exists. Further evidence studies from a variety of sources are therefore desired to reinforce validity.

4.4. Anaesthetists' Nontechnical Skills (ANTS). Anaesthetists' Nontechnical Skills (ANTS) is an anaesthetist-specific teamwork assessment tool that was devised from psychological research which identified requisite teamwork skills and structured them into a hierarchal taxonomy based on NOTECHS [30]. Behaviours are examined in 15 elements within four categories: task management, team-working, situation awareness, and decision-making. Exemplar markers are included to guide the assessor in grading the anaesthetist in each element using a 4-point numeric scale ranging from 1 (poor) to 4 (good), with a summary score given for each behavioural category. There is also an option to mark behaviours as "not observed" and each element possesses a comment box for qualitative feedback.

To explore the content validity of the tool, the original designers recruited 50 consultant anaesthetists of varying experience onto a validity study [17]. The practitioners received training in using ANTS and were then asked to rate eight experimental video scenarios with the tool, scoring every element for each scenario. An evaluation questionnaire was also completed. Results showed a high level of content validity as 100% of consultant anaesthetists stated the tool addressed the key behaviours in question, and 84% agreed that no elements appeared to be absent from the tool.

A comprehensive tool encompassing several behavioural aspects, ANTS, has potential value in assessing the NTS of anaesthetists. Analogous to NOTECHS, no other validation evidence exists apart from this study. Construct and criterion validity therefore need to be ascertained before the true value of the assessment can be realised.

TABLE 4: Oxford Nontechnical Skills (NOTECHS) scoring system, Mishra et al. (2009) [16].

(a)

Leadership and management	
Leadership	Involves/reflects on suggestions/visible/accessible/inspires/motivates/coaches
Maintenance of standards	Subscribes to standards/monitors compliance to standards/intervenes if deviation occurs/deviates with team approval/demonstrates desire to achieve high standards
Planning and preparation	Team participation in planning/plan shared/understanding confirmed/projects/changes in consultation
Workload management	Distributes tasks/monitors/reviews/tasks prioritised/allots adequate time/responds to stress
Authority and assertiveness	Advocates position/values team input/takes control/persistent/appropriate assertiveness
Teamwork and cooperation	
Team building/maintaining	Relaxed/supportive/open/inclusive/polite/friendly/use of humour/does not compete
Support of others	Helps others/offers assistance/gives feedback
Understanding team needs	Listens to others/recognises ability of team/condition of others considered/gives personal feedback
Conflict solving	Keeps calm in conflicts/suggests conflict solutions/concentrates on what is right
Problem-solving and decision-making	
Definition and diagnosis	Uses all resources/analytical decision-making/reviews factors with team
Option generation	Suggests alternative options/asks for options/reviews outcomes/confirms options
Risk assessment	Estimates risks/considers risk in terms of team capabilities/estimates patient outcome
Outcome review	Reviews outcomes/reviews new options/objective, constructive, and timely reviews/makes time for review/seeks feedback from others/conducts posttreatment review
Situation awareness	
Notice	Considers all team elements/asks for or shares information/aware of available resources/encourages vigilance/checks and reports changes in team/requests reports/updates
Understand	Knows capabilities/cross-checks above/shares mental models/speaks up when unsure/updates other team members/discusses team constraints
Think ahead	Identifies future problems/discusses contingencies/anticipates requirements
Below standard = 1	Behaviour directly compromises patient safety and effective teamwork
Basic standard = 2	Behaviour in other conditions could directly compromise patient safety and effective teamwork
Standard = 3	Behaviour maintains an effective level of patient safety and teamwork
Excellent = 4	Behaviour enhances patient safety and teamwork, a model for all other teams

(b) Nontechnical Skills (NOTECHS) subteam modifiers

	Surgical subteam	Anaesthetic subteam	Nursing subteam
	Leadership and management		
Positive modifiers	(i) Raises team morale	(i) Takes control when required	(i) Scrub provides clear instructions to circulating nurse(s)
	(ii) Intervenes if deviation occurs	(ii) Demonstrates desire for high standard	(ii) Senior nurse makes sure protocols are followed
	(iii) Prioritises tasks	(iii) Appropriately distributes tasks between rest of team	(iii) Speaks up when unhappy
Negative modifiers	(i) Deflates or fails to motivate team	(i) Does not take control when required	Senior nurse does not support juniors

(b) Continued.

	Surgical subteam	Anaesthetic subteam	Nursing subteam
	(ii) Does not attempt to build cohesion	(ii) Does not set standards	
		(iii) Inappropriate task distribution	
Teamwork and cooperation			
Positive modifiers	(i) Open	(i) Supportive of other subteams	(i) Nurses cooperate and support each other well
	(ii) Appropriate use of abilities within team	(ii) Appreciates functions of other subteams	(ii) Senior nurse covers for junior scrub
	(iii) Supportive of other subteams when necessary		
Negative modifiers	(i) Aggressive in conflicts	(i) Remains idle when problems arise	Poor coordination between equipment needs and those provided
	(ii) Does not appreciate others' abilities	(ii) Functions separately from other subteams	
Problem-solving and decision-making			
Positive modifiers	(i) Demonstrates generation of options	(i) Participates in solving problems	(i) Takes an active part in decision-making
	(ii) Open discussion and agreement over anatomy	(ii) Raises suggestions	(ii) Suggests solutions to problems, for example, alternative equipment
	(iii) Incorporates other subteam issues		
Negative modifiers	(i) Decisions made unsystematically	Does not consider anaesthetic options when faced with problem	Blames the surgeons when faced with problems
	(ii) Does not utilise team where it may benefit		
Situation awareness			
Specific to subteams			
Positive modifiers	Periodically gathers awareness of surroundings	Anticipates surgical and process needs	Anticipates equipment needs
Negative modifiers	Is fixated on operative field	Is not present at important stages of the operation or for long periods of time	Absent at stages when needed to provide service
For all subteams			
Positive modifiers	(i) Patient: has awareness of patient condition/comorbidity		
	(ii) Procedure: appreciates stage of operation		
	(iii) People: who is present in theatre, what skills they have, and what they are doing		

4.5. Multisource Feedback (MSF). MSF, or 360° feedback, is a peer assessment tool currently used to review the overall performance of every clinician in the National Health Service (NHS), with results serving as evidence for revalidation. The assessment entails a structured questionnaire designed to relay feedback regarding performance and professional behaviour, which is completed by self-nominated colleagues and patients. Surgical trainees are categorically rated using a 3-point qualitative scale for 16 competencies specified on the form provided by the ISCP, including procedural skills and teamwork.

Face and content validity of MSF in the surgical setting was investigated in a study which recruited 201 surgeons from various specialties who asked 25 consecutive patients to complete the survey, with subsequent analysis of response rates [18]. Face validity was confirmed via endorsement of the included assessment items by the College of Physicians and Surgeons of Alberta, and content validity was established as tool development was based on a list of core nontechnical competencies provided by the surgical committee. The tool has also demonstrated concurrent validity in this field through a study which examined the correlation of scores between MSF and a small-scale combination of an Objective Structural Clinical Examination (OSCE), Direct Observation of Procedural Skills (DOPS), and Internal Medicine In-Training Examination (IM-ITE) [19]. The 209 participants were in their first year of postgraduate residency and a strong positive correlation was observed between the MSF scores and the OSCE + DOPS + IM-ITE scores ($r = 0.85$, $p < 0.016$). However, there is currently no evidence of validity for the ISCP MSF form. There is, however, a lack of evidence supporting construct validity in the surgical setting. Exploration of this area is necessary to provide complete validation, though the MSF tool does appear to be useful due to the variety of feedback sources engaged.

4.6. Case-Based Discussion (CbD).

CbD, an adaptation of the valid Chart-Stimulated Recall (CSR) tool [31], is another current instrument which principally evaluates clinical judgement and decision-making. The appraisal involves detailed discussion of a clinical case in the form of a structured interview between the trainee and assessor. Eight domains (including team-working skills) are assessed, with factors such as case complexity accounted for. The trainee is given a 3-point qualitative rating in each domain, a 5-point GSS, and verbal feedback after the discussion.

Surprisingly, very little validation evidence for CbD has been published despite its widespread use in clinical practice, including the ISCP curriculum. Moreover, studies appear to have conflicting conclusions depending on clinical setting. For instance, Foundation Year 1 trainees were found to have increased CbD scores following training progression, demonstrating construct validity [32], whilst CbD assessment of surgical trainees revealed no correlation between scores and training grade, providing evidence against construct validity [33]. This paper also raised concerns about assessor bias, further questioning the validation evidence for this tool.

The value of CbD is questionable due to the insufficient and contradictory validation evidence presented, highlighting the need to conduct further studies and ascertain the validity of this tool in the surgical environment.

4.7. Edinburgh Basic Surgical Training Assessment Form (EBSTAF).

The EBSTAF tool was created from a previous list of 70 skills deemed necessary for surgical competence by consultant surgeons using a modified Delphi method [34]. The test encompasses rating of behaviours observed in five domains (communication, knowledge, teamwork, clinical skills, and technical skills) using a 3-point qualitative scale. The assessment forms are completed by various healthcare professionals in multiple departments to provide a comprehensive overview of the trainee's performance.

Validation evidence for EBSTAF is scarce despite having existed for several years. The tool designers presented evidence of construct validity via assessment of 36 surgical trainees using EBSTAF at the beginning and end of the training year [20]. A total of 101 assessments were conducted after a year of training, with results showing a significant improvement in EBSTAF scores across all domains except clinical skills (time 0 to time 1 year median: 81 to 100,

$p = 0.008$; 17 to 72, $p = 0.015$; 85 to 100, $p = 0.018$; 82 to 92, $p = 0.211$; 27 to 76, $p = 0.004$). Concurrent validity has also been established in a recent analysis [21].

Although there is great potential in the EBSTAF tool, limited supportive evidence indicates further investigation into the validity of the tool, particularly content validity.

4.8. Scrub Practitioners' List of Intraoperative Nontechnical Skills (SPLINTS).

The SPLINTS system is a new teamwork assessment tool for scrub practitioners such as nurses and operating department practitioners [35]. The SPLINTS taxonomy is organised into three skillset categories, each containing three elements against which subjects are marked using a 4-point rating scale. The "situation awareness" category assesses information gathering, information recognition and understanding, and anticipation; "communication and teamwork" contains acting assertively, exchanging information, and coordinating with others; "task management" involves planning and preparation, providing and maintaining standards, and coping with pressure.

As this tool is a recent development, an insufficient amount of time has elapsed to allow for full review of its validity, with only content validity currently established [22]. In the study 34 experienced scrub practitioners completed an evaluation questionnaire following SPLINTS assessment training and practice. Results from the questionnaire showed that 100% of participants agreed that the tool addressed key nontechnical behaviours observed and that no elements listed were unnecessary. 62% and 50% of participants found the tool to be easy to associate observed behaviours with SPLINTS categories and elements, respectively, with 0% and 3% finding it difficult to use the tool. Reliability and internal consistency were also established in this study.

The SPLINTS system shows promise as valuable tool for assessing the teamwork skills of scrub practitioners. However, other forms of validity must be evaluated in order to fully appraise the tool.

4.9. Deficiencies in Current Training.

As surgery is traditionally viewed as a practical profession, current surgical curricula focus has been towards the development of clinical knowledge and surgical skill, with a distinct absence of formal NTS training [8]. In response to this concern and others regarding current surgical training, an independent inquiry into the Modernising Medical Careers (MMC) training pathway was conducted by Sir John Tooke, who proposed several changes to meet evolving healthcare needs [36]. Recommendations included alteration of the postgraduate training structure from two years of foundation training followed by two years of core specialty training to one year of foundation training followed by three years of core specialty training, with complete abolition of run-through specialist training. The document also comments on the lack of cognitive (NTS) assessment in junior doctor posts.

The final report of another independent review of MMC was authored by Greenaway in 2013 detailing further recommendations to resolve the continual failings of the training pathway, including the necessity to implement NTS training into surgical curricula [37]. Propositions include bringing full GMC registration forward to medical school graduation and the introduction of a formal framework for training teamwork skills outlined in the GMC's *Good Medical Practice* document including communication and leadership training. The former recommendation necessitates that medical students possess some nontechnical competence prior to graduation, indicating the introduction of NTS training into the medical school curriculum. Meier et al. investigated the integration of a simulation-based NTS module adapted from the TeamSTEPPS teamwork training programme into the elective period of the medical school curriculum, with positive results showing a substantial increase in teamwork skills ($p < 0.001$), reinforcing the potential advantage of medical student NTS training [38].

Despite evidence that surgical trainees are safe to operate under direct supervision [39], the increasing patient expectation of surgeons to be technically competent before live operating has instigated significant research into the area of simulation. The benefits of a simulated environment are evident: acquisition of surgical skill without risk of causing harm to the patient, assessment of competence in a controlled reproducible environment, and preparation for crisis scenarios [40]. However, training opportunities with simulation are usually limited and do not form part of the current curriculum. Simulation is an integral part of robotic training curricula, particularly in the field of urology with the modular robotic urology fellowship curriculum devised by the European Robotic Urology Section (ERUS). To date no standardised curriculum exists for such training [41], resulting in varied knowledge and skills between institutions.

There is an increasing awareness of the value of simulation in NTS training and assessment. The feasibility of using a moderate-fidelity simulated operating theatre environment to train surgeons in technical and nontechnical skills simultaneously was explored, with participants confirming the positive immersive experience of realistic simulation environments alongside increased technical skill performance [40]. Similarly, a centralised urological simulation-based program incorporating both technical and nontechnical skills training has been trialled in London, utilising several simulator training materials including laparoscopic and robotic virtual reality simulators and bench top models for technical skills and a high-fidelity simulated operating theatre for NTS [42]. Possessing acceptable face and content validity with a high level of construct validity ($p < 0.001$), realism, acceptability, and feasibility, this dichotomous simulation-based approach may be at the forefront of future surgical training.

4.10. Recommendations for Future Training. Based on the current training deficiencies and validation evidence of teamwork assessment tools, the authors suggest the following recommendations to the current UK surgical training curricula:

(1) Formal training of the essential NTS that underpin effective teamwork should be assimilated into the medical school curriculum so that graduates possess a basic level of NTS before entering the clinical setting.

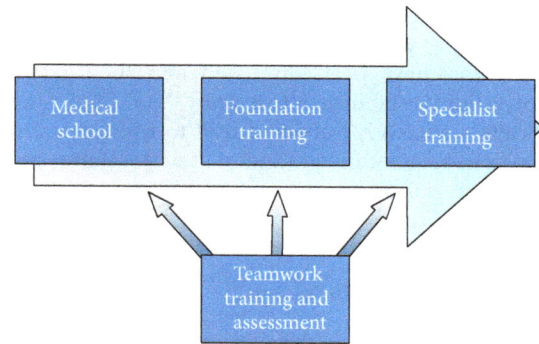

FIGURE 2: Recommended implementation of teamwork training and assessment.

This training should continue throughout foundation and specialty training (Figure 2).

(2) In the current economic climate, high-fidelity simulation should be reserved for senior surgical training as low-fidelity bench models are more cost-effective for training junior trainees [43].

(3) Training should also be supplemented with distributed simulation, an inflatable low-fidelity simulator, which may serve as a useful adjunct for junior trainees in encouraging operative confidence between bench model and live operations [44].

(4) Concurrent training of technical and nontechnical skills should be a central theme of the surgical curricula.

(5) Assessors should receive formal tool training in accordance with national guidelines developed by an expert consensus panel [45].

(6) Progression of NTS acquisition should be monitored using the NOTSS teamwork assessment tool.

(7) A standardised multistep curriculum should be developed and validated for robotic surgical training with inclusion of NTS assessment.

5. Conclusions

Teamwork is a fundamental component of a successful surgical procedure with minimal compromise of patient safety. Current surgical training does not formally encompass development and assessment of the NTS necessary for enhancing team performance. Implementation of NTS training into surgical (or medical school) curricula therefore needs prioritisation to meet the evolving requirements of surgeons and further reduce the occurrence of perioperative adverse events. Training of these skills should ideally be delivered through simulation models to increase skill without risking patient safety, and formal assessment of teamwork must become an integral part of surgical training.

Teamwork assessments are complex tools which focus on evaluating behavioural aspects of each team member. These can be challenging to develop as the tool must possess complex qualities such as the ability to accurately quantify behaviours in a way that is acceptable in practice. A wide range of tools have been discussed and their respective levels of validity established. Currently, NOTSS is the most appropriate sufficiently validated tool to use for teamwork assessment in surgery. Integration of these tools into surgical training is crucial to ensure competent surgeons and safe surgery.

Conflict of Interests

The authors declare that there is no conflict of interests regarding the publication of this paper.

Acknowledgments

Prokar Dasgupta and Kamran Ahmed acknowledge support from the Department of Health via the National Institute for Health Research (NIHR) comprehensive Biomedical Research Centre award to Guy's and St. Thomas' NHS Foundation Trust in partnership with King's College London and King's College Hospital NHS Foundation Trust. Prokar Dasgupta also acknowledges the support of the MRC Centre for Transplantation, London Deanery, London School of Surgery. Kamran Ahmed, Prokar Dasgupta, and Muhammed Shamim Khan acknowledge funding from The Urology Foundation (TUF).

References

[1] D. P. Baker, R. Day, and E. Salas, "Teamwork as an essential component of high-reliability organizations," *Health Services Research*, vol. 41, no. 4, part 2, pp. 1576–1598, 2006.

[2] A. A. Gawande, M. J. Zinner, D. M. Studdert, and T. A. Brennan, "Analysis of errors reported by surgeons at three teaching hospitals," *Surgery*, vol. 133, no. 6, pp. 614–621, 2003.

[3] L. Hull, S. Arora, R. Aggarwal, A. Darzi, C. Vincent, and N. Sevdalis, "The impact of nontechnical skills on technical performance in surgery: a systematic review," *Journal of the American College of Surgeons*, vol. 214, no. 2, pp. 214–230, 2012.

[4] K. Mazzocco, D. B. Petitti, K. T. Fong et al., "Surgical team behaviors and patient outcomes," *American Journal of Surgery*, vol. 197, no. 5, pp. 678–685, 2009.

[5] P. McCulloch, A. Mishra, A. Handa, T. Dale, G. Hirst, and K. Catchpole, "The effects of aviation-style non-technical skills training on technical performance and outcome in the operating theatre," *Quality & Safety in Health Care*, vol. 18, no. 2, pp. 109–115, 2009.

[6] J. Neily, P. D. Mills, Y. Young-Xu et al., "Association between implementation of a medical team training program and surgical mortality," *Journal of the American Medical Association*, vol. 304, no. 15, pp. 1693–1700, 2010.

[7] S. Arora, D. Miskovic, L. Hull et al., "Self vs expert assessment of technical and non-technical skills in high fidelity simulation," *The American Journal of Surgery*, vol. 202, no. 4, pp. 500–506, 2011.

[8] S. Yule, R. Flin, S. Paterson-Brown, and N. Maran, "Non-technical skills for surgeons in the operating room: a review of the literature," *Surgery*, vol. 139, no. 2, pp. 140–149, 2006.

[9] E. Boyle, A. M. Kennedy, E. Doherty, D. O'Keeffe, and O. Traynor, "Coping with stress in surgery: the difficulty of measuring non-technical skills," *Irish Journal of Medical Science*, vol. 180, no. 1, pp. 215–220, 2011.

[10] M. Tavakol, M. A. Mohagheghi, and R. Dennick, "Assessing the skills of surgical residents using simulation," *Journal of Surgical Education*, vol. 65, no. 2, pp. 77–83, 2008.

[11] N. Sevdalis, M. Lyons, A. N. Healey, S. Undre, A. Darzi, and C. A. Vincent, "Observational teamwork assessment for surgery: construct validation with expert versus novice raters," *Annals of Surgery*, vol. 249, no. 6, pp. 1047–1051, 2009.

[12] L. Hull, S. Arora, E. Kassab, R. Kneebone, and N. Sevdalis, "Observational teamwork assessment for surgery: content validation and tool refinement," *Journal of the American College of Surgeons*, vol. 212, no. 2, pp. 234.e5–243.e5, 2011.

[13] S. Yule, R. Flin, S. Paterson-Brown, N. Maran, and D. Rowley, "Development of a rating system for surgeons' non-technical skills," *Medical Education*, vol. 40, no. 11, pp. 1098–1104, 2006.

[14] J. D. Beard, J. Marriott, H. Purdie, and J. Crossley, "Assessing the surgical skills of trainees in the operating theatre: a prospective observational study of the methodology," *Health Technology Assessment*, vol. 15, no. 1, 2011.

[15] J. Crossley, J. Marriott, H. Purdie, and J. D. Beard, "Prospective observational study to evaluate NOTSS (Non-Technical Skills for Surgeons) for assessing trainees' non-technical performance in the operating theatre," *The British Journal of Surgery*, vol. 98, no. 7, pp. 1010–1020, 2011.

[16] A. Mishra, K. Catchpole, and P. McCulloch, "The Oxford NOTECHS system: reliability and validity of a tool for measuring teamwork behaviour in the operating theatre," *Quality and Safety in Health Care*, vol. 18, no. 2, pp. 104–108, 2009.

[17] G. Fletcher, R. Flin, M. McGeorge, R. Glavin, N. Maran, and R. Patey, "Anaesthetists' non-technical skills (ANTS): evaluation of a behavioural marker system," *British Journal of Anaesthesia*, vol. 90, no. 5, pp. 580–588, 2003.

[18] C. Violato, J. Lockyer, and H. Fidler, "Multisource feedback: a method of assessing surgical practice," *British Medical Journal*, vol. 326, no. 7388, pp. 546–548, 2003.

[19] Y.-Y. Yang, F.-Y. Lee, H.-C. Hsu et al., "Assessment of first-year post-graduate residents: usefulness of multiple tools," *Journal of the Chinese Medical Association*, vol. 74, no. 12, pp. 531–538, 2011.

[20] A. M. Paisley, P. Baldwin, and S. Paterson-Brown, "Feasibility, reliability and validity of a new assessment form for use with basic surgical trainees," *American Journal of Surgery*, vol. 182, no. 1, pp. 24–29, 2001.

[21] P. J. Driscoll, N. Maran, and S. Paterson-Brown, "The high fidelity patient simulator and surgical critical care," in *Proceedings of the Annual Scientific Meeting of the Association for the Study of Medical Education*, Edinburgh, UK, 2003.

[22] L. Mitchell, R. Flin, S. Yule, J. Mitchell, K. Coutts, and G. Youngson, "Evaluation of the scrub practitioners' list of intraoperative non-technical skills (SPLINTS) system," *International Journal of Nursing Studies*, vol. 49, no. 2, pp. 201–211, 2012.

[23] S. Yule, R. Flin, N. Maran, D. Rowley, G. Youngson, and S. Paterson-Brown, "Surgeons' non-technical skills in the operating room: reliability testing of the NOTSS behavior rating system," *World Journal of Surgery*, vol. 32, no. 4, pp. 548–556, 2008.

[24] A. N. Healey, S. Undre, and C. A. Vincent, "Developing observational measures of performance in surgical teams," *Quality & Safety in Health Care*, vol. 13, supplement 1, pp. i33–i40, 2004.

[25] S. Undre, N. Sevdalis, A. N. Healey, A. Darzi, and C. A. Vincent, "Observational teamwork assessment for surgery (OTAS): refinement and application in urological surgery," *World Journal of Surgery*, vol. 31, no. 7, pp. 1373–1381, 2007.

[26] S. Undre, A. N. Healey, A. Darzi, and C. A. Vincent, "Observational assessment of surgical teamwork: a feasibility study," *World Journal of Surgery*, vol. 30, no. 10, pp. 1774–1783, 2006.

[27] S. Yule, D. Rowley, R. Flin et al., "Experience matters: comparing novice and expert ratings of non-technical skills using the NOTSS system," *ANZ Journal of Surgery*, vol. 79, no. 3, pp. 154–160, 2009.

[28] J. M. Schraagen, T. Schouten, M. Smit et al., "Assessing and improving teamwork in cardiac surgery," *Quality & Safety in Health Care*, vol. 19, no. 6, article e29, 2010.

[29] P. Patki, S. Undre, N. Sevdalis, L. Hull, N. Wilson, and B. Maddison, "67 Crisis simulations for robotic procedures: development of a training module and initial results," *European Urology Supplements*, vol. 10, no. 8, pp. 565–566, 2011.

[30] G. Fletcher, R. Flin, P. McGeorge, R. Glavin, N. Maran, and R. Patey, "Rating non-technical skills: developing a behavioural marker system for use in anaesthesia," *Cognition, Technology & Work*, vol. 6, no. 3, pp. 165–171, 2004.

[31] Z. Setna, V. Jha, K. A. M. Boursicot, and T. E. Roberts, "Evaluating the utility of workplace-based assessment tools for speciality training," *Best Practice and Research: Clinical Obstetrics and Gynaecology*, vol. 24, no. 6, pp. 767–782, 2010.

[32] H. Davies, J. Archer, L. Southgate, and J. Norcini, "Initial evaluation of the first year of the foundation assessment programme," *Medical Education*, vol. 43, no. 1, pp. 74–81, 2009.

[33] I. Eardley, M. Bussey, A. Woodthorpe, C. Munsch, and J. Beard, "Workplace-based assessment in surgical training: experiences from the Intercollegiate Surgical Curriculum Programme," *ANZ Journal of Surgery*, vol. 83, no. 6, pp. 448–453, 2013.

[34] P. J. Baldwin and S. P. Brown, "Consultant surgeons' opinion of the skills required of basic surgical trainees," *British Journal of Surgery*, vol. 86, no. 8, pp. 1078–1082, 1999.

[35] L. Mitchell, R. Flin, S. Yule, J. Mitchell, K. Coutts, and G. Youngson, "Development of a behavioural marker system for scrub practitioners' non-technical skills (SPLINTS system)," *Journal of Evaluation in Clinical Practice*, vol. 19, no. 2, pp. 317–323, 2013.

[36] T. Delamothe, "Modernising medical careers: final report," *BMJ*, vol. 336, article 54, 2008.

[37] D. Greenaway, *Shape of Training: Securing the Future of Excellent Patient Care. Final Report of the Independent Review Led by Professor David Greenaway*, General Medical Council, 2013.

[38] A. H. Meier, M. L. Boehler, C. M. McDowell et al., "A surgical simulation curriculum for senior medical students based on TeamSTEPPS," *Archives of Surgery*, vol. 147, no. 8, pp. 761–766, 2012.

[39] K. Ahmed, H. Ashrafian, L. Harling et al., "Safety of training and assessment in operating theatres—a systematic review and meta-analysis," *Perfusion*, vol. 28, no. 1, pp. 76–87, 2013.

[40] R. Aggarwal, S. Undre, K. Moorthy, C. Vincent, and A. Darzi, "The simulated operating theatre: comprehensive training for surgical teams," *Quality & Safety in Health Care*, vol. 13, no. 1, pp. i27–i32, 2004.

[41] R. Khan, K. Ahmed, and A. Mottrie, "Towards a standardised training curriculum for robotic surgery: a consensus of an international multidisciplinary group of experts," in *Proceedings of the EAU Robotic Urology Section Congress*, London, UK, 2013.

[42] M. Shamim Khan, K. Ahmed, A. Gavazzi et al., "Development and implementation of centralized simulation training: evaluation of feasibility, acceptability and construct validity," *BJU International*, vol. 111, no. 3, pp. 518–523, 2013.

[43] K. Ahmed, M. Jawad, M. Abboudi et al., "Effectiveness of procedural simulation in urology: a systematic review," *The Journal of Urology*, vol. 186, no. 1, pp. 26–34, 2011.

[44] A. Harris, E. Kassab, J. K. Tun, and R. Kneebone, "Distributed simulation in surgical training: an off-site feasibility study," *Medical Teacher*, vol. 35, no. 4, pp. e1078–e1081, 2013.

[45] L. Hull, S. Arora, N. R. Symons et al., "Training faculty in nontechnical skill assessment: national guidelines on program requirements," *Annals of Surgery*, vol. 258, no. 2, pp. 370–375, 2013.

24

Patient Satisfaction and Quality of Life in DIEAP Flap versus Implant Breast Reconstruction

Rossella Sgarzani,[1] **Luca Negosanti,**[1] **Paolo Giovanni Morselli,**[1] **Veronica Vietti Michelina,**[1] **Luigi Maria Lapalorcia,**[2] **and Riccardo Cipriani**[1]

[1]*Plastic Surgery Department, Sant'Orsola-Malpighi Hospital, University of Bologna, Via Massarenti 9, 40138 Bologna, Italy*
[2]*Plastic Surgery Department, Asl 1 of Umbria, Citta di Castello, Località Chioccolo, 06012 Perugia, Italy*

Correspondence should be addressed to Luca Negosanti; luca.negosanti81@gmail.com

Academic Editor: Jose Maria Serra-Renom

The psychological impact of breast reconstruction has widely been described, and multiple studies show that reconstruction improves the well-being and quality of life of patients. In breast reconstruction, the goal is not only the morphological result, but mainly the patient's perception of it. The objective of our study is to compare the physical and psychosocial well-being and satisfaction concerning the body image of patients who had reconstruction with breast implants to those of patients who had reconstruction with deep inferior epigastric artery perforator flaps. Our results demonstrated a similar quality of life between the two groups, but the satisfaction level was significantly higher in patients who had reconstruction with autologous tissue. Feedback from patients who have already received breast reconstruction may be useful in the decision-making process for future patients and plastic surgeons, enabling both to choose the reconstructive technique with the best long-term satisfaction.

1. Introduction

Many studies evaluate the outcomes of breast reconstruction, but only a few examine the satisfaction of patients who received breast reconstruction with autologous tissues [1].

Despite the continuous increase of early diagnosis and conservative treatments for breast cancer, in 25% of patients, a mastectomy remains the gold standard [2, 3]. This mutilating procedure is a traumatizing event, and many psychological disorders have been linked to this surgery in the literature [4–9].

The role of breast reconstruction after a mastectomy has been widely demonstrated [10], and multiple studies have shown that breast reconstruction improves patients' well-being and quality of life [11, 12].

Several reports show that women who undergo breast reconstruction after mastectomy have less psychological distress and have an improved quality of life compared to women who refuse any reconstructive option [13, 14].

The aim of the present study is to evaluate the physical and psychosocial well-being of patients who underwent breast reconstruction as well as compare the long-term satisfaction of patients who underwent reconstruction with implants with patients who underwent reconstruction with a Deep Inferior Epigastric Artery Perforator (DIEAP) flap.

These two techniques represent the gold standards in breast reconstruction.

The present study is based on a self-evaluating questionnaire to acquire new data concerning the personal satisfaction of patients who have already undergone breast reconstruction and analyze the feelings of patients concerning different reconstruction phases.

2. Materials and Methods

Retrospective observational single center study (S. Orsola-Malpighi Hospital, Bologna, Italy) was performed.

The inclusion criteria of the study were as follows:

(i) adult patients;

(ii) unilateral mastectomy for breast cancer or prophylaxis;

(iii) immediate or delayed breast reconstruction with expander/implant or DIEAP flap;

(iv) reconstruction performed between 2007 and 2011 (in order to have a minimum follow-up time of 36 months).

Patients who met these criteria were identified through our hospital database and were contacted by telephone. They were presented with the opportunity to take part in the study and were offered an appointment at the Plastic Surgery Outpatient Clinic to independently complete the questionnaire; the aim of the study and the average time to complete the questionnaire were explained.

We followed the Dillman method to maximize the percentage of responders including subsequent calls to nonresponders [15].

We contacted 129 patients by telephone, and 87 of them answered.

Sixty-three patients agreed to participate in the study; 4 patients deceased and 20 refused.

Each of the 63 patients participating in the study was welcomed in the Plastic Surgery Outpatient Clinic by a staff member. The purpose of the study was reemphasized, they were informed that all data would remain anonymous, and they signed an informed consent and a sensitive data consent. The questionnaire was delivered to the patient alone, so it could be completed independently.

2.1. Self-Evaluation Questionnaire.
The Breast-Q questionnaire (Memorial Sloan-Kettering Cancer Center and The University of British Columbia, 2006, all rights reserved), designed for patients undergoing breast surgery and specifically for patients undergoing breast reconstruction, was used [16, 17].

The conceptual framework of the questionnaire is formed by two main domains: one related to the quality of life (investigating physical, psychosocial, and sexual well-being) and the other regarding satisfaction (satisfaction with the breast, overall outcome, and the care process).

The average time to administer the questionnaire was 15–20 minutes.

2.2. Data Analysis.
The population was divided into two groups. Group A included 33 patients (52.4%) who had reconstruction with autologous tissue (all of these procedures were DIEAP flaps performed by the same senior surgeon). Group B included 30 patients (47.6%) who had reconstruction using expanders and implants (these surgeries were performed by four senior consultants).

The obtained data were reported in Excel (Microsoft Corp., Redmond, WA, USA) and were analyzed using SPSS statistical software package version 17.0 (SPSS Inc., Chicago, IL, USA).

The average, median, and mode were assessed as position indexes considering the inherent characteristics of our group of responders that did not show a Gaussian distribution for most of the parameters. The evaluation of the median and quartiles was considered more appropriate as the values of skewness and kurtosis were far from 0.

TABLE 1: Demographical data of the two groups, showing no statistically significant differences between them.

	DIEAP	Expander/implant	P
Number of patients	33 (52.4%)	30 (47.6%)	
Age	52.45	53.7	0.432
(Range)	(from 32 to 74)	(from 31 to 71)	
Marital status			
Married	22	20	
Unmarried	7	4	
Separated	0	4	0.087
Divorced	1	2	
Widowed	3	0	
Follow-up time	3.39	3.17	0.922
(Range)	(from 1 to 6 years)	(from 1 to 5 years)	

Mann-Whitney and Student's t-tests for parametric variables were used to compare the two groups, that is, DIEAP flap and expander/implant; the Wilcoxon test was also used for the same assessments.

Correlation studies were performed using nonparametric Spearman's rho.

Pearson Chi-Square and Fisher's exact tests were used to determine the association between a dependent variable and an independent one (a P value < 0.05 was considered to be statistically significant).

3. Results

A total of 129 patients were contacted by telephone, and 87 of them answered (67%).

Of these, 63 patients agreed to take part in the study. The percentage of responders was 72.4%; this is comparable to other studies [18].

The patients were divided into two groups. Group A included 33 patients (52.4%) who underwent reconstruction with DIEAP flaps, and group B included 30 patients (47.6%) who underwent reconstruction with expanders/implants.

The mean age was 53.03 years (ranging between 31 and 74 years); 17.5% were unmarried, 66.7% were married, 11.1% were divorced, and 4.8% were widowed.

We evaluated the differences between the two groups; no statistically significant differences in age ($P < 0.432$), marital status ($P < 0.087$), or follow-up time ($P < 0.922$) were found (Table 1).

The evaluation of the collected data demonstrated a good level of satisfaction with the reconstructed breast (3.1038 out of 4) and a high satisfaction with the overall result (2.714 out of 3). These results emphasize the positive value of breast reconstruction after mastectomy.

In all subscales, patients undergoing breast reconstruction with a DIEAP flap reported higher scores, but the score reached statistical significance only in satisfaction with the reconstructed breast (Figure 1) (implants 2.8393 out of 4; DIEAP 3.3427 out of 4) ($P < 0.002$), overall result (implants 2.6667 out of 3; DIEAP 2.7576 out of 3) ($P < 0.041$),

TABLE 2: The statistical significance of differences between the two groups. The Mann-Whitney and Wilcoxon nonparametric tests allow comparing samples without a normal distribution.

	Reconstructed breast	Overall outcome	Psychosocial well-being	Sexual well-being	Physical well-being	NAC	Information	Surgeon	Medical team	Administrative team
U Mann-Whitney	225,500	350,000	383,000	368,000	390,500	112,000	284,000	419,500	358,000	412,000
W Wilcoxon	631,500	815,000	848,000	746,000	951,500	265,000	635,000	884,500	823,000	847,000
Z	−3,169	−2,004	−1,549	−0,386	−1,244	−2,721	−1,744	−1,143	−2,219	−1,194
P	0,002	0,041	0,121	0,699	0,214	0,007	0,081	0,253	0,027	0,232

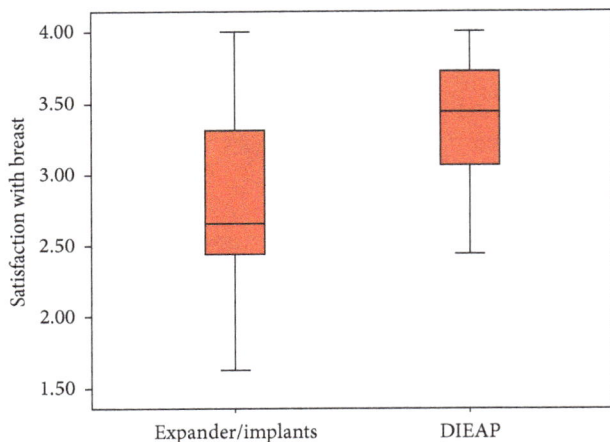

FIGURE 1: Box plot showing satisfaction with the reconstructed breast.

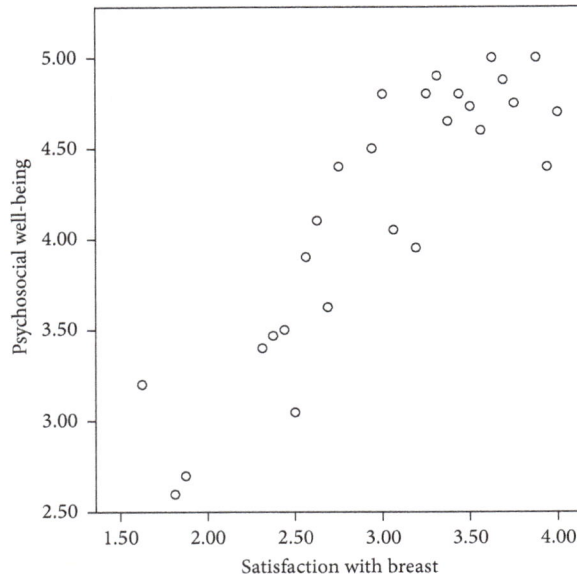

FIGURE 2: Correlation between reconstructed breast satisfaction and psychosocial well-being.

and nipple areola complex (NAC) reconstruction (implants 2.6471 out of 4; DIEAP 3.2208 out of 4) ($P < 0.007$) (Table 2).

Concerning the sexual well-being scale, DIEAP flap patients were more satisfied than the expander/implant patients, 3.2644 versus 3.1358, respectively, but this difference did not reach statistical significance ($P < 0.699$). Patients undergoing DIEAP flap reconstruction reported higher scores in psychosocial and physical well-being, which did not reach statistical significance ($P < 0.121$ and $P < 0.214$, resp.).

Patients undergoing DIEAP flap breast reconstruction reported greater satisfaction with the medical team ($P < 0.027$), which was statistically significant, in addition to greater satisfaction with the surgeon ($P < 0.253$) and the administrative team ($P < 0.232$).

Satisfaction with the reconstructed breast correlates with overall satisfaction and with psychosocial and sexual well-being, reaching statistical significance in both groups (all $P < 0.000$) (Figure 2).

Another finding was that satisfaction about the information given preoperatively was linked to satisfaction with the surgeon ($P < 0.002$ in both groups) and the medical team ($P < 0.002$ for group B; $P < 0.035$ for group A).

We assessed how the follow-up time affected patient satisfaction, but no statistically significant differences were found. The average follow-up time was 3.1587 years (ranging from 3 to 6 years). We compared the two groups using the Mann-Whitney test, which did not show a statistically significant difference ($P < 0.922$).

Regarding NAC reconstruction among the 63 patients who participated in the study, only 47 had undergone NAC reconstruction (74.6%). Three of the patients had not yet received the tattoo to match the color of the contralateral areola at the time of this study.

All patients received a nipple reconstruction using the same technique (star-flap), avoiding bias resulting from different techniques.

With NAC, we found greater satisfaction in patients undergoing autologous tissue reconstruction ($P < 0.007$) (Figure 3). We assessed the satisfaction related to shape, general appearance, naturalness, color, and NAC projection in the two groups. We dichotomized responses into "satisfied" for patients who provided values of 3 (somewhat satisfied) or 4 (very satisfied) and "dissatisfied" for values of 1 (somewhat dissatisfied) or 2 (very dissatisfied).

In the expander/implant group, 68.4% were satisfied with the shape and appearance; in the DIEAP flap group, 85.7% were satisfied with those metrics. This difference did not reach statistical significance ($P < 0.155$).

A significant difference between the two groups was found regarding the NAC naturalness. Of the patients reconstructed with a DIEAP flap, 78.7% declared themselves satisfied, compared with 31.6% in the expander/implant group.

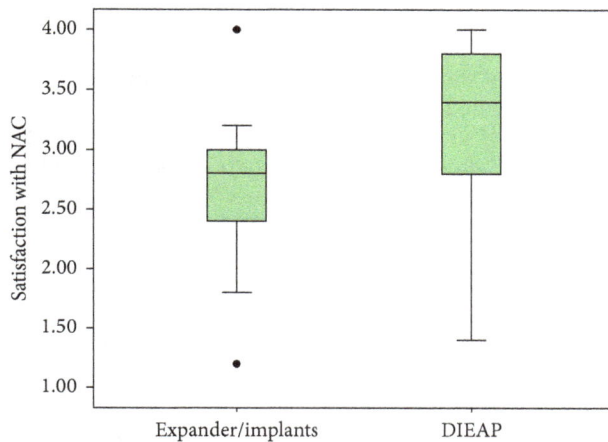

FIGURE 3: Box plot showing satisfaction with the reconstructed NAC.

The significance was assessed using Pearson's Chi-Square ($P < 0.001$) and Fisher's exact tests ($P < 0.002$). Patients whose breasts were reconstructed using a DIEAP flap were also more satisfied with the NAC projection (85.7% versus 78.9% in second group).

We also found a statistically significant correlation between satisfaction with the nipple naturalness and the marital status of the patient; single women showed a greater significance than the married patients ($P < 0.005$ for single and $P < 0.033$ for married women).

Correcting the natural satisfaction of the nipple in relation to marital status, women reconstructed using a DIEAP flap were 2 to 33 times more satisfied than the others; the odds ratio was corrected according to a Mantel-Haenszel value of 8.438 (confidence limits 95%) (2.138–33.303) ($P < 0.002$).

4. Discussion

The decision-making process of a patient undergoing breast cancer surgery is very complex. Many initiatives have been developed recently to provide patients with correct and complete information on reconstructive and nonreconstructive options, such as Breast Reconstruction Awareness Day [19].

Identifying the best source of information for the patient is one question that remains. Medical and paramedical staff in hospitals can provide objective details on surgical options, surgical time needed for each procedure, risks, complication rates, postoperatory recovery times, and hospitalizations [20].

The Internet is a very useful tool for patients to seek information, but not all the information on the Internet is reliable and not all of it meets the expectations of the patients [21]. Many surgical centers currently provide their patients with booklets [22] or website references where they can find correct information [23, 24].

Other patient experiences can be another important source of information. The possibility to provide objective information about other patients' satisfaction levels following different procedures is very useful [25].

Perceived outcome information can be collected through self-evaluating questionnaires assessing the quality of life and patient satisfaction regarding several aspects, including appearance, psychological well-being, and sexual well-being.

Breast-Q, the questionnaire administered in the present study, is designed for patients undergoing breast surgery and reconstruction. It was developed following qualitative and quantitative psychometric methods and meets the international criteria for the outcome assessment [26, 27].

In our study, we decided to include only unilateral breast reconstruction because we believe that the most important aspect of a reconstruction is symmetry. Symmetry influences the posture of the patient and her confidence in her appearance. A bilateral reconstruction with an implant or autologous tissue is more often symmetrical both in the immediate postoperation period and in the long term. The real challenge is reaching and maintaining symmetry in unilateral reconstructions, and our study aims to investigate this aspect.

Through statistical analysis, our results showed that patients who underwent autologous tissue reconstruction were more satisfied than those who received an expander/implant reconstruction, reaching statistical significance in satisfaction with the breast, overall outcome, and NAC reconstruction.

These data confirm previous reports in the literature, with a general consensus suggesting that patients whose breasts are reconstructed using autologous tissue are more satisfied [18, 28, 29].

In this study, only DIEAP flap breast reconstruction was considered in the autologous tissue reconstructive method because the Transverse Rectus Abdominis Muscle flap or the Latissimus Dorsi flap are not performed in our Plastic Surgery Division because of donor site morbidity.

Yueh et al. [18] showed that patients who underwent reconstruction using perforator flaps are more likely to have a higher overall satisfaction compared to those who underwent reconstruction using nonperforator flaps (82.7% versus 65.8%; $P < 0.002$).

The same authors showed that patients undergoing autologous tissue reconstruction were more satisfied with the reconstructed breast than patients receiving implants. Among women who had reconstruction with autologous tissue, those who received a flap taken from the abdominal region were more satisfied than patients who underwent reconstruction with a Latissimus Dorsi flap. When comparing patients who received either TRAM or DIEAP flaps, the difference was no longer statistically significant, although the difference between those two methods in terms of donor site morbidity is well described [30].

Other authors reported satisfaction with breast reconstruction using an abdominal flap but also dissatisfaction with the donor site [31].

We did not include any Superficial Inferior Epigastric Artery (SIEA) flap reconstruction in the study in order to have a uniform group of autologous reconstructed patients and avoid bias linked to the "easier" postoperative period and donor site recovery of the SIEA flap compared to DIEAP flap reconstruction.

In our study, 91% of the DIEAP patients perceived their reconstructed breast as a natural part of their own body, while only 40% of patients who underwent prosthetic reconstruction stated the same.

In our study, we did not demonstrate a significant difference in satisfaction with increasing follow-up time. This evaluation had been made in relation to a previous work published by Hu et al. [32] in which the authors stressed that both breast implants and autologous tissue reconstruction would experience an "aging" process, resulting in different long-term complications that can variably influence the aesthetic result.

The authors noted that patients who underwent TRAM, compared to patients who underwent expander/implant reconstruction, showed greater long-term aesthetic satisfaction. The satisfaction reduction in patients who underwent breast reconstruction using an expander/implant could be related to the high incidence of complications and reoperations that this technique requires [33–35]. Women who undergo reconstruction using silicone gel implants have a 20% risk of developing grade III or IV Baker capsular contracture [36] and a 30% risk of having to remove or replace the prosthesis, resulting in an overall reoperation rate of 45–50% [37].

Interestingly, our result showed no significant reduction in satisfaction over time in both groups, and this allows us to comment that patient perception of the reconstruction is a very complex process in the elaboration of a new body image that is not only correlated to actual symmetry.

It is important to note that our minimal follow-up time of 36 months might be considered insufficient to show the long-term differences between implants and autologous tissues. However, with this timing, we were able to demonstrate that, already at 3 years, autologous breast reconstruction is more satisfactory than implant reconstruction in most of the parameters.

In the quality of life evaluation, we found that DIEAP flap patients reported higher scores in all aspects, but these scores did not reach statistical significance for psychosocial well-being ($P < 0.121$), sexual well-being ($P < 0.699$), or physical well-being ($P < 0.214$).

Patients undergoing a DIEAP flap for breast reconstruction reported statistically significantly greater satisfaction with the medical team ($P < 0.027$) and greater satisfaction with the surgeon ($P < 0.253$) and the administrative team ($P < 0.232$).

Another aspect specifically investigated in our study is the NAC reconstruction.

Although not all patients decide to proceed with NAC reconstruction, several psychological benefits for this reconstruction have been demonstrated in the literature [32]. In our study, 47 of the 63 women (74.6%) underwent nipple reconstruction; three had not yet completed the process of reconstruction or had avoided the intradermal tattoo of the areola.

We showed a statistically significant difference regarding satisfaction with the NAC between the two groups that were studied. Women who underwent breast reconstruction using autologous tissue are, according to our data, more satisfied with their nipple areola complex than those in the implant group.

Our study showed that satisfaction with the NAC projection depended on marital status. Single women were significantly ($P < 0.005$ versus $P < 0.033$) more satisfied with the NAC projection as opposed to women who did not undergo NAC reconstruction, a figure which may correlate with the need for these patients to relate to new partners.

In general, by correcting the satisfaction as a function of marital status, women whose breasts were reconstructed using DIEAP flaps were 2 to 33 times more satisfied with the NAC projection, compared with patients receiving implants, with an odds ratio of 8.438, corrected using Mantel-Haenszel (95%) (2.138–33.303) ($P < 0.002$).

As evidenced by Handel [33], a predictable outcome in the long term is the loss of projection, although this phenomenon is difficult to quantify. A reduction of the average nipple projection of at least 50% must be considered in the reconstruction; this flattening occurs especially in the first months after surgery.

The total and partial loss of nipple sensitivity, investigated in previous research [38], was mentioned by many women as a limiting factor that superseded the result of the reconstruction itself.

Satisfaction concerning the information given preoperatively was linked to satisfaction with the surgeon ($P < 0.002$ in both groups) and the medical team ($P < 0.002$ for the group expander prostheses; $P < 0.035$ for the DIEAP group). This result emphasizes the central role of the information process, which makes a more accurate and aware choice possible and allows for greater satisfaction in the postoperative phases.

Limitations are present in our study. A selection bias is unavoidable because patients cannot be randomized to the types of surgery or reconstruction they received. It appears impossible to control different personal characteristics of patients, such as adversity to risks or personality traits. Patients choosing reconstruction with implants may be systematically different from patients choosing reconstruction using autologous tissue (DIEAP flap), which could affect the results.

Another bias can be linked to responders. It is more likely that only patients who were very satisfied or very dissatisfied with the result decided to participate in the study.

This is a retrospective study, and it has a recall bias; patients were asked to remember different details of their reconstruction process, which may have taken place up to 6 years earlier.

All surgeries in group A were performed by the same surgeon, while patients in group B underwent surgery performed by 4 different consultants in our department who used the same technique. The use of different surgeons could have also affected the results concerning satisfaction related to the surgeon and the information process.

To improve the reliability of the study, a prospective study in which patients are subjected to self-evaluation both preoperatively and postoperatively may be undertaken.

We believe that the high response rate made our data reliable.

Further studies must be developed to understand the different components that work together and affect the overall satisfaction of patients undergoing reconstructive breast surgery.

5. Conclusion

Our results demonstrated an overall higher satisfaction in patients who underwent unilateral breast reconstruction using autologous tissue even 3 years after reconstruction, with a comparable quality of life between the autologous tissue and expander/implant groups.

Feedback from patients who have already gone through the difficult choices related to mastectomy and breast reconstruction may be useful in guiding future patients.

Conflict of Interests

The authors declare that there is no conflict of interests regarding the publication of this paper.

References

[1] J. H. Yueh, S. A. Slavin, E. D. Bar-Meir et al., "Impact of regional referral center for microsurgical breast recontrusctions: the New England perforator flap program experience," *Journal of the American College of Surgeons*, vol. 208, no. 2, pp. 246–254, 2009.

[2] L. C. Hartmann, D. J. Schaid, J. E. Woods et al., "Efficacy of bilateral prophylactic mastectomy in women with a family history of breast cancer," *The New England Journal of Medicine*, vol. 340, no. 2, pp. 77–84, 1999.

[3] S. A. Deppen, M. C. Aldrich, P. Hartge et al., "Cancer screening: the journey from epidemiology to policy," *Annals of Epidemiology*, vol. 22, no. 6, pp. 439–445, 2012.

[4] P. Foibar, S. L. Steward, S. Chang, C. D'Onofrio, P. J. Banks, and J. R. Bloom, "Body image and sexual problema in young women with breast cancer," *Psycho-Oncology*, vol. 15, no. 7, pp. 579–594, 2006.

[5] R. Renneker and M. Cutler, "Psychological problems of adjustment to cancer of the breast," *The Journal of the American Medical Association*, vol. 148, no. 10, pp. 833–838, 1952.

[6] M. H. Frost, D. J. Schaid, T. A. Sellers et al., "Long-term satisfaction and psychological and social function following bilateral prophylactic mastectomy," *The Journal of the American Medical Association*, vol. 284, no. 3, pp. 319–324, 2000.

[7] M. J. Asken, "Psychoemotional aspects of mastectomy: a review of recent literature," *The American Journal of Psychiatry*, vol. 132, no. 1, pp. 56–59, 1975.

[8] M. M. Roberts, I. G. Furnival, and A. P. Forrest, "The morbidity of mastectomy," *British Journal of Surgery*, vol. 59, no. 4, pp. 301–302, 1972.

[9] P. Maguire, "The psychological and social sequelae of mastectomy," in *Modern Perspectives in the Psychiatric Aspects of Surgery*, J. G. Howells, Ed., pp. 390–421, Brunner/Mazel, New York, NY, USA, 1976.

[10] C. K. Christian, J. Niland, S. B. Edge et al., "A multi-institutional analysis of the socioeconomic determinants of breast reconstruction: a study of the National Comprehensive Cancer Network," *Annals of Surgery*, vol. 243, no. 2, pp. 241–249, 2006.

[11] E. E. Elder, Y. Brandberg, T. Björklund et al., "Quality of life and patient satisfaction in breast cancer patients after immediate breast reconstruction: a prospective study," *Breast*, vol. 14, no. 3, pp. 201–208, 2005.

[12] D. M. Harcourt, N. J. Rumsey, N. R. Ambler et al., "The psychological effect of mastectomy with or without breast reconstruction: a prospective, multicenter study," *Plastic and Reconstructive Surgery*, vol. 111, no. 3, pp. 1060–1068, 2003.

[13] C. Dean, U. Chetty, and A. P. M. Forrest, "Effects of immediate breast reconstruction on psychosocial morbidity after mastectomy," *The Lancet*, vol. 321, no. 8322, pp. 459–462, 1983.

[14] S. Franchelli, M. S. Leone, P. Berrino et al., "Psychological evaluation of patients undergoing breast reconstruction using two different methods: autologous tissues versus prostheses," *Plastic and Reconstructive Surgery*, vol. 95, no. 7, pp. 1213–1220, 1995.

[15] D. Dillman, *Mail and Telephone Surveys: The Total Design Method*, John Wiley & Sons, New York, NY, USA, 1978.

[16] A. L. Pusic, C. M. Chen, S. Cano et al., "Measuring quality of life in cosmetic and reconstructive breast surgery: a systematic review of patient-reported outcomes instruments," *Plastic and Reconstructive Surgery*, vol. 120, no. 4, pp. 823–837, 2007.

[17] A. L. Pusic, S. Cano, and A. F. Klassen, "Measuring quality of life in breast surgery: content development of a new modular system to capture patient-reported outcomes (The MSKCC Breast-Q)," in *Proceedings of the IOQOL Annual Meeting*, Lisbon, Portugal, October 2006.

[18] J. H. Yueh, S. A. Slavin, T. Adesiyun et al., "Patient satisfaction in postmastectomy breast reconstruction: a comparative evaluation of DIEP, TRAM, latissimus flap, and implant techniques," *Plastic and Reconstructive Surgery*, vol. 125, no. 6, pp. 1585–1595, 2010.

[19] http://www.bra-day.com/.

[20] N. Causarano, J. Platt, N. N. Baxter et al., "Pre-consultation educational group intervention to improve shared decision-making for postmastectomy breast reconstruction: a pilot randomized controlled trial," *Supportive Care in Cancer*, vol. 23, no. 5, pp. 1365–1375, 2015.

[21] C. W. Joyce, C. M. Morrison, R. Sgarzani, and P. N. Blondeel, "Patient preferences in an online breast reconstruction resource," *Journal of Plastic, Reconstructive and Aesthetic Surgery*, vol. 66, no. 12, pp. e380–e381, 2013.

[22] https://www.breastcancercare.org.uk/.

[23] http://www.beautifulabc.com/.

[24] http://www.myreconstruction.ca/.

[25] R. L. Kane, *Understanding Health Care Outcomes Research*, Jones and Barlett Publisher, Sudbury, Mass, USA, 2005.

[26] K. N. Lohr, "Assessing health status and quality-of-life instruments: attributes and review criteria," *Quality of Life Research*, vol. 11, no. 3, pp. 193–205, 2002.

[27] U.S. Food and Drug Administration, *Patient Reported Outcome Misures: Use in Medical Product Development to Support Labeling Claims*, 2006.

[28] A. K. Alderman, E. G. Wilkins, J. C. Lowery, M. Kim, and J. A. Davis, "Determinants of patient satisfaction in postmastectomy breast reconstruction," *Plastic and Reconstructive Surgery*, vol. 106, no. 4, pp. 769–776, 2000.

[29] A. S. Saulis, T. A. Mustoe, and N. A. Fine, "A retrospective analysis of patient satisfaction with immediate postmastectomy breast reconstruction: comparison of three common procedures," *Plastic and Reconstructive Surgery*, vol. 119, no. 6, pp. 1669–1678, 2007.

[30] P. N. Blondeel, G. G. Vanderstraeten, S. J. Monstrey et al., "The donor site morbidity of free DIEP flaps and free TRAM flaps for breast reconstruction," *British Journal of Plastic Surgery*, vol. 50, no. 5, pp. 322–330, 1997.

[31] T. Zhong, C. McCarthy, S. Min et al., "Patient satisfaction and health-related quality of life after autologous tissue breast reconstruction: a prospective analysis of early postoperative outcomes," *Cancer*, vol. 118, no. 6, pp. 1701–1709, 2012.

[32] E. S. Hu, A. L. Pusic, J. F. Waljee et al., "Patient-reported aesthetic satisfaction with breast reconstruction during the long-term survivorship period," *Plastic and Reconstructive Surgery*, vol. 124, no. 1, pp. 1–8, 2009.

[33] N. Handel, "Managing local implant-related problems," in *Surgery of the Breast: Principles Ans Art*, S. L. Spear, Ed., Linppincott-Raven, Philadelphia, Pa, USA, 1998.

[34] D. T. Netscher, S. Sharma, J. Thornby et al., "Aesthetic outcome of breast implant removal in 85 consecutive patients," *Plastic and Reconstructive Surgery*, vol. 100, no. 1, pp. 206–219, 1997.

[35] E. P. Melmed, "A review of explantation in 240 symptomatic women: a description of explantation and capsulectomy with reconstruction using a periareolar technique," *Plastic and Reconstructive Surgery*, vol. 101, no. 5, pp. 1364–1373, 1998.

[36] G. Little and J. L. Baker Jr., "Results of closed compression capsulotomy for treatment of contracted breast implant capsules," *Plastic and Reconstructive Surgery*, vol. 65, no. 1, pp. 30–33, 1980.

[37] Inamed Corporation, "Summary of safetyand effectiveness data: McGhan silicone filled breast implants," Tech. Rep. PMA P020056, Inamed Corporation, Santa Barbara, Calif, USA, 2004.

[38] L. Negosanti, M. Santoli, R. Sgarzani, S. Palo, and R. Cipriani, "Return of sensitivity and outcome evaluation of breast reconstruction with the DIEP free flap," *Plastic and Reconstructive Surgery*, vol. 126, no. 1, pp. 36e–38e, 2010.

A EWTD Compliant Rotation Schedule Which Protects Elective Training Opportunities Is Safe and Provides Sufficient Exposure to Emergency General Surgery: A Prospective Study

Andrew Emmanuel, Ezzat Chohda, Carolyn Sands, Joseph Ellul, and Hamid Khawaja

Department of General Surgery, Princess Royal University Hospital, Kings College NHS Foundation Trust, Farnborough Common, Orpington, Kent BR6 8ND, UK

Correspondence should be addressed to Andrew Emmanuel; arhemmanuel@gmail.com

Academic Editor: Ahmed H. Al-Salem

Introduction. Training opportunities have decreased dramatically since the introduction of the European Working Time Directive (EWTD). In order to maximise training we introduced a rotation schedule in which registrars do not work night shifts and elective training opportunities are protected. We aimed to determine the safety and effectiveness of this EWTD compliant rotation schedule in achieving exposure of trainees to acute general surgical admissions and operations. *Methods.* A prospective study of consecutive emergency surgical admissions over a 6-month period. Exposure to acute admissions and operative procedures and patient outcomes during day and night shifts was compared. *Results.* There were 1156 emergency admissions covering a broad range of acute conditions. Significantly more patients were admitted during the day shift and almost all emergency procedures were performed during the day shift (2.1 versus 0.3, $p < 0.001$). A registrar was the primary operating surgeon in 49% of cases and was directly involved in over 65%. There were no significant differences between patients admitted during the day and night shifts in mortality rate, length of stay, admission to ICU, requirement for surgery, or readmission rates. *Conclusion.* A EWTD compliant rotation schedule that protects elective training opportunities is safe for patients and provides adequate exposure to training opportunities in emergency surgery.

1. Introduction

There continues to be heated debate around the effects of the European Working Time Directive (EWTD) on surgical training. The Royal College of Surgeons of England (RCSEng) and surgical trainee organisations strongly advocate opting out of the EWTD and extending working hours [1–3]. Although some studies have not found significant reductions in exposure to operative procedures after the introduction of working time restrictions [4], the majority of published studies conclude that training opportunities and operative exposure for trainees have decreased dramatically since the introduction of the EWTD [5–14]. However, many of these studies are based only on trainee questionnaires and surveys or retrospective logbook reviews. As a result, most studies tend to be based on the views of trainees rather than actual data on trainees' exposure. Furthermore, most studies do

not take into account many other factors that have had an important impact on operative training volume such as increases in the number of trainees and changes in surgical management and practice. They also tend to concentrate only on operative experience, which is merely one of several skills required of a surgeon. Exposure to other training opportunities such as assessment of acute surgical patients is generally not assessed by these studies. Furthermore, most studies have not compared this perceived reduced exposure to any standard indicative number of procedures that should be achieved.

The RCSEng has previously recommended that, in order to maximise training opportunities, senior trainees should not work full shifts at night unless a significant opportunity for training exists [15]. Night shifts in surgical specialities such as trauma and orthopaedics clearly provide minimal opportunities for training, but it is less clear what opportunities exist during the night shift in general surgery which has acutely unwell patients, some requiring urgent surgery, presenting unpredictably at any time. As a result of the RCSEng recommendations, our institution introduced a EWTD compliant rotation schedule in which senior trainees do not work full night shifts and therefore do not require compensatory rest periods and are available to attend their normal elective theatre and endoscopy lists and clinics. As no elective opportunities are missed with this system, the only potential problem is lack of exposure to emergency general surgery.

The aim of our study was to determine the safety and effectiveness of a EWTD compliant rotation schedule, which retains full exposure to elective opportunities, in achieving exposure of trainees to acute general surgical admissions and operations.

2. Methods

Our institution has adopted an emergency rotation schedule for registrars which is EWTD compliant but avoids a full shift pattern in order to protect day-time exposure to training opportunities. Registrars work an emergency day-time shift from 08:00 to 21:00. The night shift (21:00–08:00) is covered by two senior house officers with a senior nontraining middle grade surgeon and consultant surgeon on call but off-site.

A prospective study was undertaken of all consecutive emergency general surgical admissions over a 6-month period from 27 January 2012 to 26 July 2012. Data on significant events during the hospital stay such as the need for surgery or admission to the intensive care unit (ICU) was obtained from patients' records and data on the timing of emergency procedures and operating surgeon were obtained from electronic and written theatre logs. Data collected included time of admission, diagnosis, length of stay (LOS), admission to ICU, readmission within 30 days of discharge, in-hospital mortality, emergency procedures and the time they were performed, the grade of the primary surgeon performing the procedures, and the grade of assistant. Admissions, outcomes, and operative procedures were compared between day shifts (08:00–21:00) and night shifts (21:00–08:00). Means were compared using one-way analysis of variance (ANOVA) or Mann-Whitney U test for nonnormally distributed data and proportions compared using the chi-squared test.

3. Results

There were 1156 emergency general surgery admissions over the study period. The mean age of the patients was 55 years and 58% were female. The diagnoses on admission covered a broad range of emergency general surgical conditions (Table 1). The majority of patients were admitted during the day shift with few admitted during the night shift (mean 4.9 versus 1.6, $p < 0.001$).

Almost all patients requiring an emergency procedure had this performed during the day shift with very few operations carried out during the night shift (mean 2.1 versus 0.3 procedures, $p < 0.001$). Table 2 shows there were

TABLE 1: Emergency general surgical admissions.

Diagnosis	Frequency
Biliary disease	137
Appendicitis	103
Abscess/soft tissue infection	98
GI bleed	145
Bowel obstruction	73
Pancreatitis	45
Diverticulitis	44
Constipation/pseudoobstruction	39
Hernias	37
Abdominal pain	238
Trauma	19
Malignancy	27
Perforated viscus	13
Intra-abdominal sepsis	10
Postoperative complication	63
IBD	16
Other surgical diagnosis	29
Gynaecology problem	9
Medical problem	11
Total	1156

TABLE 2: Emergency procedures performed overall and during the day shift.

Procedure	Total	Day shift
Appendicectomy	120	101
Endoscopy (CEPOD)	117	98
I&D	76	66
Laparotomy	63	51
Hernia repair	26	23
Laparoscopy	23	22
Hartmann's procedure	9	6
Small bowel resection	22	19
Large bowel resection	10	9
Adhesiolysis	15	10
Stoma	9	8
Cholecystectomy	8	8
Other	25	23

a broad range of emergency procedures performed which included most emergency procedures to which general surgical trainees would be expected to gain exposure. Very few operative training opportunities were lost by not working night shifts.

There were no significant differences in a variety of outcomes between patients admitted during the day and night shifts, including mortality rate, length of hospital stay, 30-day readmission rate, the need for intensive care admission, or the need for an emergency surgical procedure (Table 3).

For the emergency procedures performed during the day shift, a registrar was the primary operating surgeon in 49% of cases and there was a consultant or associate specialist

TABLE 3: Comparison of outcomes between patients admitted during day and night shifts.

	Shift admitted		p value
	Day	Night	
Mortality (%)	3.5	4.3	0.57
ICU admission (%)	2.2	3.2	0.32
Mean length of stay (days)	5.1	5.7	0.18*
Readmission, 30 days (%)	8.1	7.1	0.60
Need for surgery (%)	43.5	39.6	0.26

*Mann-Whitney U test.

assisting the registrar in 24% of these cases. A registrar was directly involved in over 65% of cases.

4. Discussion

Although there has been debate about the effect of the EWTD on surgical training, the bulk of published opinion is that the EWTD has led to substantial decreases in the quantity and quality of surgical training. These studies largely cite significantly reduced numbers of procedures being performed by trainees following the introduction of the EWTD compared to traditional work patterns and conclude therefore that there is a deficit in training.

However, there are a number of problems with many of the published studies to date and the reasoning that has led to a broad acceptance of the idea that surgical training in the EWTD era is inadequate. For example, many studies that show reduced operative experience for trainees are based on retrospective analysis of surgeons logbooks and operative logs or questionnaires applied to trainees and conclusions about training extrapolated from these [5, 14]. Logbooks do not give a full picture of training and clearly questionnaires merely gauge the prevailing opinion amongst trainees without being based on reliable data. Also, these studies do not take into account the totality of emergency surgery training which in large part involves the assessment of acute surgical patients in the emergency department, making diagnostic decisions and initiating appropriate management. There are few if any prospective studies which assess exposure to the emergency general surgical take as a whole, including exposure to the range of acute general surgical conditions as well as to emergency procedures, with a EWTD compliant rotation schedule.

Another problem with the conclusions drawn from many of the studies critical of the EWTD is that they can be seen as overly simplistic. A finding of reduced operative numbers amongst trainees has many potential explanations other than simply poor training in a EWTD era. There is no doubt that surgical practice is changing. The type and number of operative procedures are changing, with trends in many areas toward conservative management of conditions which in the past were thought to mandate surgery and minimally invasive techniques in other areas. For example, one US study showed a trend toward major increases in percutaneous techniques and sharp declines in traditional open surgical techniques [16]. One result of the increased use of minimally invasive

techniques is that consultant surgeons are likely to perform more procedures that would traditionally have been carried out by a trainee when doing an open operation [17]. The duties and competencies expected of a modern surgeon have also changed. Surgeons qualifying in the current era take on a more subspecialised role than surgeons in the past who may have required greater operative volume of a broader range of procedures to fulfil their role. There is also a trend toward greater consultant lead and delivered care with less reliance on trainees to deliver patient care than in the past [18]. Rather than all effects on procedure volume for trainees being attributable to EWTD changes, these factors may also impact on the numbers of procedures being performed by trainees but could have significant positive effects on the quality of training and the skill set that modern surgeons require. For example, very few studies concluding that the EWTD has had a negative impact on training consider changes to the levels of consultant supervision of trainees performing procedures. There is evidence that consultant supervision of registrars performing procedures has increased dramatically after the introduction of the EWTD [19]. This will clearly have an impact on the quality of training and it is feasible that significantly fewer procedures are required to gain competence if there is quality training with adequate supervision, an issue which most studies do not address.

The Royal College of Surgeons of England recommends that, in order to protect training in the EWTD era, full shift working should be avoided wherever possible for senior trainees (ST3 and above) and that senior trainees should only work as part of a full shift system if it is required for training purposes [15]. This view is supported by other professional surgical bodies [20]. It therefore seems reasonable that for craft specialties such as surgery there is little to be gained from a training perspective by working night shifts. However, whilst this may more definitively be the case for disciplines such as orthopaedic surgery, a general surgical emergency take involves the assessment and management of acute patients who can present at any time of day or night and potentially require emergency surgery as well. Hence, it is necessary to evaluate the level of exposure and therefore potential training, to the broad range of emergency general surgical conditions and procedures during day and night shifts.

Our institution has been using a rotation schedule that is EWTD compliant but ensures that trainees do not work night shifts and are therefore not subject to the mandatory periods of rest which follow night shifts. As a result, they are available to attend all of the firm's elective commitments such as elective surgery, endoscopy, and clinics. Elective training opportunities are therefore unaffected by this rotation schedule, and the only issue is whether there is adequate exposure to emergency general surgical patients and procedures and furthermore whether such a system represents safe practice. Following the NCEPOD report [17] and in common with many other UK hospitals, our institution runs a separate, dedicated emergency theatre which is staffed by dedicated on call anaesthesiology, theatre nurse, and on call general surgery teams. This allows cases requiring surgery presenting at night that are not limb- or life-threatening to be deferred until the day shift while eliminating the struggle to find theatre time and staff to accommodate such cases on a daily basis.

Our study shows that this rotation schedule is safe with no difference between patients admitted during the night shift and those admitted during the day shift in in-hospital mortality, admission to ICU, length of hospital stay, or 30-day readmission rates. It shows that patients with a broad range of emergency general surgical conditions present during the day shift and, in comparison, very few present during the night shift. Similarly, the vast majority of operative exposure is to be gained during the day shift with very few operations performed during the night shift. Very few training opportunities are missed as a result of not working a night shift. In addition, if the exposure to emergency procedures in this study is indicative of the type of exposure a trainee can expect during the course of their training, this rotation schedule should provide sufficient exposure to emergency surgery.

Although several surgical bodies advocate against the EWTD, it is likely to remain in force for the foreseeable future and most trainees will complete their training under this system. It is therefore imperative that innovative solutions are sought to protect training. Such solutions include improved training and supervision with a focus on quality rather than quantity [21], the use of surgical simulation [22, 23], improvements in surgical curricula [24], and, perhaps most importantly, innovations in emergency rotation schedules for trainees to protect exposure to elective training opportunities whilst allowing adequate training in the emergency take and procedures in comparison to trainees at the end of their training applying for a certificate of completion of training [25, 26]. Our study supports the notion that innovative rotation schedules can protect all training opportunities [27].

We recognise some limitations of our study. It is difficult to accurately predict the mortality and morbidity risk of this patient population who presented with a variety of acute surgical conditions and underwent different management strategies. Many were treated nonoperatively. As a result, we did not perform any risk adjustment calculations for patients admitted during the day and night shifts. However, we would not expect this to significantly affect our conclusions as intuitively we would expect patients presenting at night to be more acutely unwell than those presenting during the day, but we did not find that these patients experienced worse outcomes using our rotation schedule. Another limitation is the paucity of trauma cases at our institution. However, trauma cases in the UK are now transferred directly to a limited number of nominated major trauma centres and so our experience is typical of an acute district hospital general surgery service. Departments such as ours provide the bulk of emergency general surgery care in the UK and general surgery trainees who do not elect to have an interest in major trauma would spend most of their training time in a similar setting.

We conclude that a EWTD compliant rotation schedule that protects elective opportunities is safe for patients and provides adequate exposure to training opportunities in emergency surgery.

Conflict of Interests

The authors declare that there is no conflict of interests regarding the publication of this paper.

References

[1] Royal College of Surgeons of England, *Surgery and the European Working Time Directive—Background Briefing*, Royal College of Surgeons of England, 2013, http://www.rcseng.ac.uk/policy/documents/EWTDBackgroundBriefingJune2013Final.pdf.

[2] J. E. Fitzgerald and B. C. Caesar, "The European Working Time Directive: a practical review for surgical trainees," *International Journal of Surgery*, vol. 10, no. 8, pp. 399–403, 2012.

[3] Association of Surgeons in Training, *Optimising Working Hours to Provide Quality in Training and Patient Safety: A Position Statement by the Association of Surgeons in Training*, Association of Surgeons in Training, 2009, http://www.asit.org/assets/documents/ASiT_EWTD_Position_Statement.pdf.

[4] E. Lim and S. Tsui, "Impact of the European Working Time Directive on exposure to operative cardiac surgical training," *European Journal of Cardio-Thoracic Surgery*, vol. 30, no. 4, pp. 574–577, 2006.

[5] N. Kara, P. V. Patil, and S. M. Shimi, "Changes in working patterns hit emergency general surgery training," *Annals of The Royal College of Surgeons of England, Supplement*, vol. 90, no. 2, pp. 60–63, 2008.

[6] C. D. Marron, J. Shah, D. J. Mole, and D. Slade, *European Working Time Directive*, Association of Surgeons in Training, 2006, http://www.asit.org/assets/documents/ASiT_EWTD_Final_310506.pdf.

[7] M. J. Tait, G. A. Fellows, S. Pushpananthan, Y. Sergides, M. C. Papadopoulos, and B. A. Bell, "Current neurosurgical trainees' perception of the European Working Time Directive and shift work," *British Journal of Neurosurgery*, vol. 22, no. 1, pp. 28–33, 2008.

[8] K. Grover, M. Gatt, and J. MacFie, "The effect of the EWTD on surgical SpRs: a regional survey," *Annals of the Royal College of Surgeons of England*, vol. 90, pp. 68–70, 2008.

[9] G. J. Morris-Stiff, S. Sarasin, P. Edwards, W. G. Lewis, and M. H. Lewis, "The European working time directive: one for all and all for one?" *Surgery*, vol. 137, no. 3, pp. 293–297, 2005.

[10] G. Morris-Stiff, E. Ball, J. Torkington, M. E. Foster, M. H. Lewis, and T. J. Havard, "Registrar operating experience over a 15-year period: more, less or more or less the same?" *Surgeon*, vol. 2, no. 3, pp. 161–164, 2004.

[11] J. S. Logan, T. Sinnett, and M. Solan, "Surgeon or assistant? Assessing trainee progress from log book activity: a 15-year analysis," *Annals of the Royal College of Surgeons of England*, vol. 94, no. 1, pp. 1–4, 2012.

[12] K. J. Breen, A. M. Hogan, and K. Mealy, "The detrimental impact of the implementation of the European working time directive (EWTD) on surgical senior house officer (SHO) operative experience," *Irish Journal of Medical Science*, vol. 182, no. 3, pp. 383–387, 2013.

[13] C. D. Marron, C. K. Byrnes, and S. J. Kirk, "An EWTD-compliant shift rota decreases training opportunities," *Bulletin of The Royal College of Surgeons of England*, vol. 87, no. 7, pp. 246–248, 2005.

[14] B. A. Parsons, N. S. Blencowe, A. D. Hollowood, and J. R. Grant, "Surgical training: the impact of changes in curriculum and

experience," *Journal of Surgical Education*, vol. 68, no. 1, pp. 44–51, 2011.

[15] *The Working Time Directive 2009: Meeting the Challenge in Surgery*, Royal College of Surgeons of England, London, UK, 2008, https://www.rcseng.ac.uk/surgeons/surgical-standards/docs/WTD%202009%20Meeting%20the%20challenge%20in%20surgery.pdf/view.

[16] M. Eckert, D. Cuadrado, S. Steele, T. Brown, A. Beekley, and M. Martin, "The changing face of the general surgeon: national and local trends in resident operative experience," *American Journal of Surgery*, vol. 199, no. 5, pp. 652–656, 2010.

[17] M. Cullinane, A. J. Gray, C. M. Hargreaves et al., *Who Operates When?* NCEPOD, London, UK, 2003.

[18] Department of Health, "The NHS Improvement Plan: putting people at the heart of public services," June 2004, http://webarchive.nationalarchives.gov.uk/+/www.dh.gov.uk/en/publicationsandstatistics/publications/publicationspolicyandguidance/dh_4084476.

[19] N. S. Blencowe, B. A. Parsons, and A. D. Hollowood, "Effects of changing work patterns on general surgical training over the last decade," *Postgraduate Medical Journal*, vol. 87, no. 1034, pp. 795–799, 2011.

[20] Association of Surgeons of Great Britain and Ireland, *The Impact of EWTD on Delivery of Surgical Services: A Consensus Statement*, Association of Surgeons of Great Britain and Ireland, 2008, http://www.asgbi.org.uk/en/publications/working_time_regulations.cfm.

[21] R. Canter and A. Kelly, "A new curriculum for surgical training within the United Kingdom: the first stages of implementation," *Journal of Surgical Education*, vol. 64, no. 1, pp. 20–26, 2007.

[22] P. Singh and A. Darzi, "Surgical training," *British Journal of Surgery*, vol. 100, no. 3, pp. 307–309, 2013.

[23] J. A. Milburn, G. Khera, S. T. Hornby, P. S. Malone, and J. E. Fitzgerald, "Introduction, availability and role of simulation in surgical education and training: review of current evidence and recommendations from the Association of Surgeons in Training," *International Journal of Surgery*, vol. 10, no. 8, pp. 393–398, 2012.

[24] A. W. Phillips and A. Madhavan, "A critical evaluation of the intercollegiate surgical curriculum and comparison with its predecessor the 'calman' curriculum," *Journal of Surgical Education*, vol. 70, no. 5, pp. 557–562, 2013.

[25] Joint Committee on Surgical Training, *Guidelines for the Award of a CCT in General Surgery*, Joint Committee on Surgical Training, 2014, http://www.jcst.org/quality-assurance/documents/certification-guidelines/general-surgery-certification-guidelines.

[26] W. Allum, S. Hornby, G. Khera et al., "General surgery logbook survey," *Annals of the Royal College of Surgeons of England*, vol. 95, no. 4, pp. 1–6, 2013.

[27] P. J. Bruce, S. D. Helmer, J. S. Osland, and A. D. Ammar, "Operative volume in the new era: a comparison of resident operative volume before and after implementation of 80-hour work week restrictions," *Journal of Surgical Education*, vol. 67, no. 6, pp. 412–416, 2010.

26

Review of Subcutaneous Wound Drainage in Reducing Surgical Site Infections after Laparotomy

B. Manzoor,[1] N. Heywood,[1] and A. Sharma[2]

[1]*Department of Surgery, University Hospital of South Manchester and The University of Manchester, MAHSC, Manchester, UK*
[2]*Wythenshawe Hospital, University Hospital of South Manchester, Southmoor Road, Manchester M23 9LT, UK*

Correspondence should be addressed to A. Sharma; abhiramsharma@nhs.net

Academic Editor: Pramateftakis Manousos-Georgios

Purpose. Surgical site infections (SSIs) remain a significant problem after laparotomies. The aim of this review was to assess the evidence on the efficacy of subcutaneous wound drainage in reducing SSI. *Methods.* MEDLINE database was searched. Studies were identified and screened according to criteria to determine their eligibility for meta-analysis. Meta-analysis was performed using the Mantel-Haenszel method and a fixed effects model. *Results.* Eleven studies were included with two thousand eight hundred and sixty-four patients. One thousand four hundred and fifty patients were in the control group and one thousand four hundred and fourteen patients were in the drain group. Wound drainage in all patients shows no statistically significant benefit in reducing SSI incidence. Use of drainage in high risk patients, contaminated wound types, and obese patients appears beneficial. *Conclusion.* Using subcutaneous wound drainage after laparotomy in all patients is unnecessary as it does not reduce SSI risk. Similarly, there seems to be no benefit in using it in clean and clean contaminated wounds. However, there may be benefit in using drains in patients who are at high risk, including patients who are obese and/or have contaminated wound types. A well designed trial is needed which examines these factors.

1. Introduction

Surgical site infections (SSIs) are defined as wound infection following an invasive surgical procedure [1]. These remain a substantial problem for patients undergoing procedures in spite of advances in surgical techniques and medical care.

SSIs have been shown to contribute up to 20% of nosocomial infections with an overall incidence around 5% across all invasive surgical procedures [1]. Laparotomies carry a higher risk of wound infection and a combined rate of 15% has been reported in upper and lower gastrointestinal surgery, over three times the average risk [2]. Furthermore, in large bowel surgery, an overall infection rate of 17.5% has been identified in the UK [3, 4]. Rates as high as 26% in colorectal procedures [5] and up to 57% in small bowel procedures [6] have also been described.

SSIs lead to increased hospital stay and increased morbidity [7] alongside increasing unnecessary patient suffering and a decreased quality of life (QoL) [8, 9]. A recent study done in Japan identified an increase of mean hospital stay by 17.8 days in patients who developed SSI after colorectal surgery [10] and similarly a 13.2-day length of stay increase following small bowel surgery has also been described [11]. When combining these with the costs of treating the SSIs, in the UK they have been shown to account for up to an extra £700 million of the NHS health budget annually [12, 13].

Numerous risk factors for developing a SSI have been identified. Current smokers are at a 30% increased risk of SSI after major colorectal procedures [14] and smoking cessation reduces SSI [15]. Body Mass Index and obesity have also been linked to increased risk of SSI [16] with studies showing wound complication rates in some procedures rising from 7% up to 23% due to obesity [17]. More specifically, depth of subcutaneous fat has been shown to be a strong risk factor for SSI [18] and has been shown to be a useful predictor for SSI risk [19]. Many other factors including nutrition and diabetes

TABLE 1: Studies detailing the effects of subcutaneous wound drainage in laparotomies and detailing the outcome by infection rates.

Author	Year	Patients	Drain type	Control				Drain				Calculated P value
				Total	SSI	No SSI	% infec.	Total	SSI	No SSI	% infec.	CI 95%
Shaffer et al. [38]	1987	194	Closed suction	92	10	82	**10.9**	102	11	91	**10.8**	0.985
Fujii et al. [35]	2011	79	Open	44	17	27	**38.6**	35	5	30	**14.3**	0.017
Imada et al. [36]	2013	282	Open	131	8	123	**6.1**	151	8	143	**5.3**	0.770
Tochika et al. [39]	2011	100	Closed suction	70	12	58	**17.1**	30	0	30	**0.0**	0.016
Cardosi et al. [33]	2006	144	Closed suction	77	15	62	**17.5**	67	15	52	**22.4**	0.668
Baier et al. [32]	2010	200	Closed suction	100	9	91	**9.0**	100	10	90	**10.0**	0.809
Tsujita et al. [40]	2012	149	Open	88	14	74	**15.9**	61	2	59	**3.3**	0.014
Kozol et al. [37]	1986	98	Suction	45	4	41	**8.9**	53	6	47	**11.3**	0.692
Farnell et al. [34]	1986	1618	Suction	803	41	762	**5.1**	815	45	770	**5.5**	0.709

TABLE 2: Studies in which only the laparotomy data could not be extracted. Nonlaparotomy abdominal incisions were included.

Author	Year	Patients	Drain type	No drain				Drain				Chi-squared 1 DF 2-tailed P Value CI 0.05
				Total	SSI	No SSI	% infec.	Total	SSI	No SSI	% infec.	
Higson and Kettlewell [41]	1978	246	Open	126	11	115	8.7	120	19	101	15.8	0.089
Lubowski and Hunt [42]	1987	349	Closed suction	157	9	148	5.7	192	8	184	4.2	0.499

control, certain comorbidities, ASA class, and operation time have been identified as important factors affecting SSI [19, 20].

Various interventions have been proposed with a view to reducing SSIs. A number of them are used in routine practice. Hand washing, minimising shaving, skin preparation, and preoperative antibiotics have all gained acceptance in the surgical community [21–24]. Use of drains after surgery however has declined in recent times. It has been shown that drains provide no advantage after cholecystectomies, inguinal hernia repairs, and various other types of surgery [25]. Use of drains, however, is still popular after abdominoperineal excision of rectum and repair of incisional hernias due to inconclusive evidence and surgeon preference [26, 27]. They are still used in some major plastic surgery procedures as they are thought to reduce collections in closed spaces [28].

It has been postulated that the presence of haematoma, serous fluid, and dead space in surgical incisional wounds increases the risk of infection as this acts as a culture medium [29, 30]. Subcutaneous drains have been used to reduce the risk of infection [31]. However, the use of postoperative subcutaneous wound drainage is not universally accepted. In addition drains may not be efficacious and cause discomfort and increased hospital stay on their own [32].

The aim of this systematic review is to assimilate and analyse the available evidence regarding the efficacy of subcutaneous wound drainage in reducing s-SSI after laparotomy.

2. Method

A search of the MEDLINE database through PubMed was performed with the aim of identifying articles regarding the primary search criteria, *Superficial abdominal wound drainage and the impact on wound infection*. Articles were considered from any country and any year but articles that did not meet the language criteria (English) were going to be excluded; however no articles were found that did not meet the language criteria at the end of our screening process.

Search was performed using the terms "*subcutaneous wound drainage*" and "*drain AND subcutaneous AND infection*". All the abstracts were considered against the primary search criteria and 48 articles were retrieved. The articles were then screened for duplicates and 19 articles were highlighted and were removed, leaving a total of 29 articles.

An additional 2 articles were retrieved after reviewing references from these bringing the total number of articles after primary screening to 31.

The retrieved articles were then put through the secondary screening. The articles were screened against the criteria "*primary incision must be a true laparotomy*". Gynaecological procedures and Caesarean sections alongside other nonlaparotomy abdominal incisions were excluded. A total of 19 articles were excluded which left 12 articles. One of the 12 articles was a meta-analysis [25] leaving *11 articles* for the review (Figure 1).

The relevant data for the purpose of this systematic review was extracted from each trial. Chi-squared analysis of each individual trial was performed to determine significance. The data was then used to perform a meta-analysis. The Mantel-Haenszel method was used with a fixed effects model to determine risk ratios (RR) and confidence intervals (CI) for each individual trial in addition to an overall RR, CI, and P value for the collated data.

3. Results

Two thousand eight hundred and sixty-four patients undergoing laparotomies in nine different trials were included in this meta-analysis [32–42] (Table 1). Two studies (Table 2) included some nonlaparotomy incisions and were analysed separately. On meta-analysis (Figure 2), the trials were found to be homogenous (P value of 0.12); therefore the data from

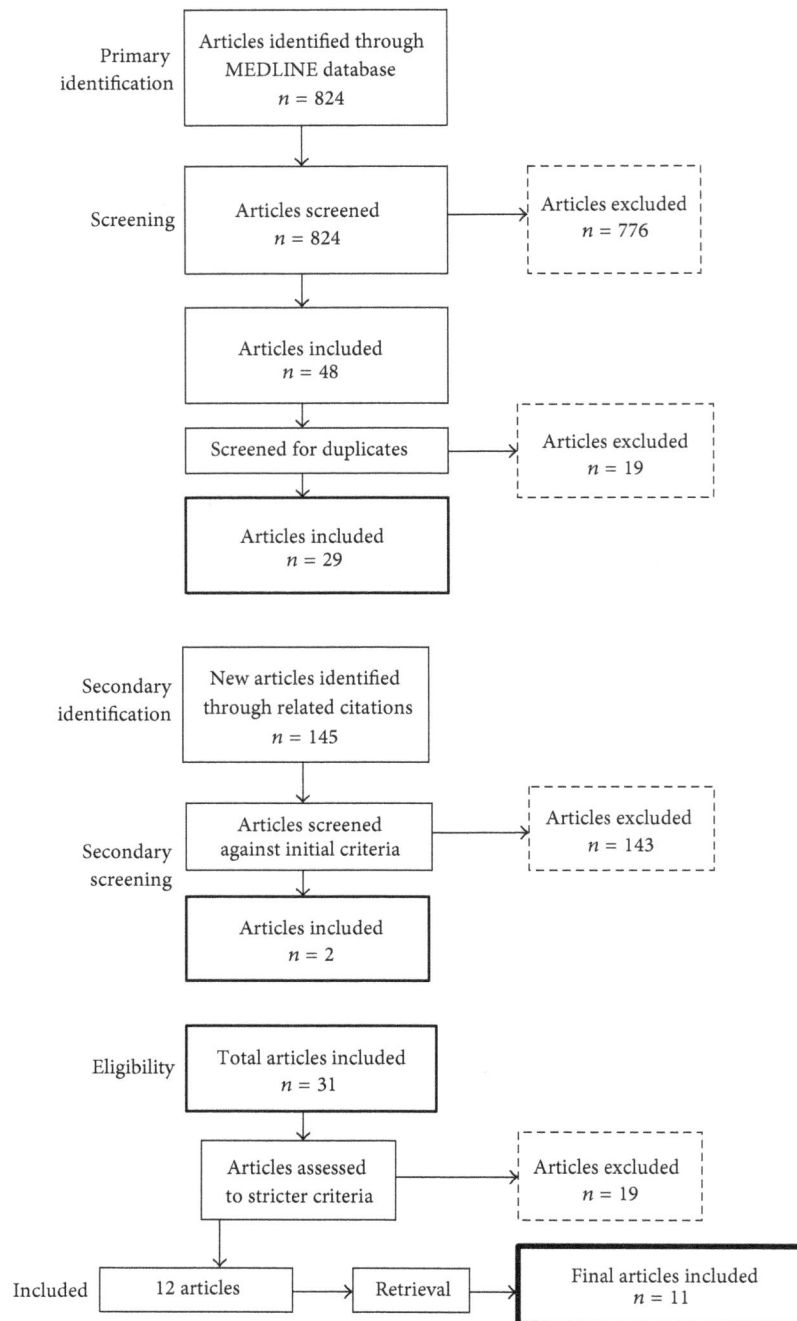

FIGURE 1: Flow chart showing the method of identifying eligible articles for the purpose of our analysis.

the trials was collated and analysed using a fixed effects model.

Chi-squared analysis was used on each of the trials using 95% confidence intervals. Three trials showed a significant reduction in surgical site infections in the drainage group. On assessing the risk ratios and respective confidence intervals, only two showed a significant reduction in SSI in the drain group as opposed to the control group.

Overall no significant difference was found in the SSI rate in the two groups ($P = 0.19$, risk ratio 0.84 (0.66–1.09)).

Two studies with some nonlaparotomy incision were analysed separately. Higson et al. showed a significantly higher infection rate in the drain group compared to the control group. However, on meta-analysis (Figure 3), an overall P value of 0.36 was found [RR 1.29 (0.75–2.23)].

Table 3 shows data extracted from Farnell et al. and Lubowski et al. in which wound type was classified in both the control and drain groups. There was a reduction in both trials of the rate of wound infection in the contaminated wound type when using a drain as opposed to a control group;

TABLE 3: Studies detailing wound type in the control and drain groups.

| Author | Year | Control | | | | | Drain | | | | |
| | | Total patients | Clean | Clean contam. | Contaminated | Dirty | Total patients | Clean | Clean contam. | Contaminated | Dirty |
			Number of (%) infections					Number of (%) infections			
Lubowski and Hunt [42]	1987	157	2 (2.8)	4 (5.1)	2 (33.3)	1 (33.3)	192	2 (2.6)	4 (3.8)	2 (20)	0 (0)
Farnell et al. [34]	1986	803	—	27 (4.1)	7 (7.1)	7 (15.1)	815	—	29 (4.4)	4 (3.9)	12 (22.6)

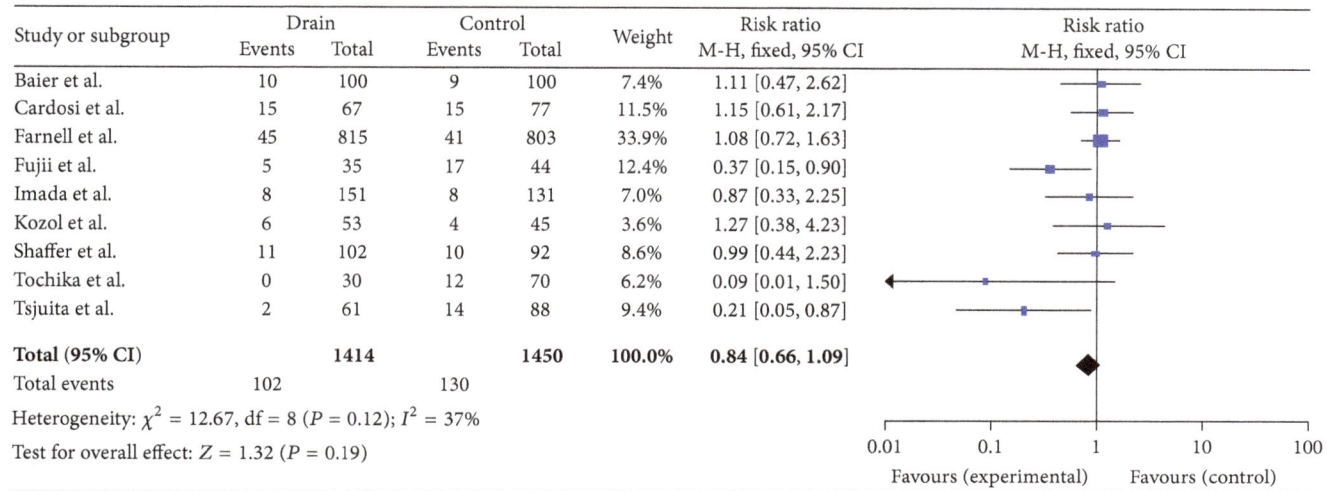

| Study or subgroup | Drain | | Control | | Weight | Risk ratio M-H, fixed, 95% CI | Risk ratio M-H, fixed, 95% CI |
	Events	Total	Events	Total			
Baier et al.	10	100	9	100	7.4%	1.11 [0.47, 2.62]	
Cardosi et al.	15	67	15	77	11.5%	1.15 [0.61, 2.17]	
Farnell et al.	45	815	41	803	33.9%	1.08 [0.72, 1.63]	
Fujii et al.	5	35	17	44	12.4%	0.37 [0.15, 0.90]	
Imada et al.	8	151	8	131	7.0%	0.87 [0.33, 2.25]	
Kozol et al.	6	53	4	45	3.6%	1.27 [0.38, 4.23]	
Shaffer et al.	11	102	10	92	8.6%	0.99 [0.44, 2.23]	
Tochika et al.	0	30	12	70	6.2%	0.09 [0.01, 1.50]	
Tsjuita et al.	2	61	14	88	9.4%	0.21 [0.05, 0.87]	
Total (95% CI)		**1414**		**1450**	**100.0%**	**0.84 [0.66, 1.09]**	
Total events	102		130				

Heterogeneity: $\chi^2 = 12.67$, df = 8 ($P = 0.12$); $I^2 = 37\%$
Test for overall effect: $Z = 1.32$ ($P = 0.19$)

FIGURE 2: Forest plot data comparing ten trials from Table 1.

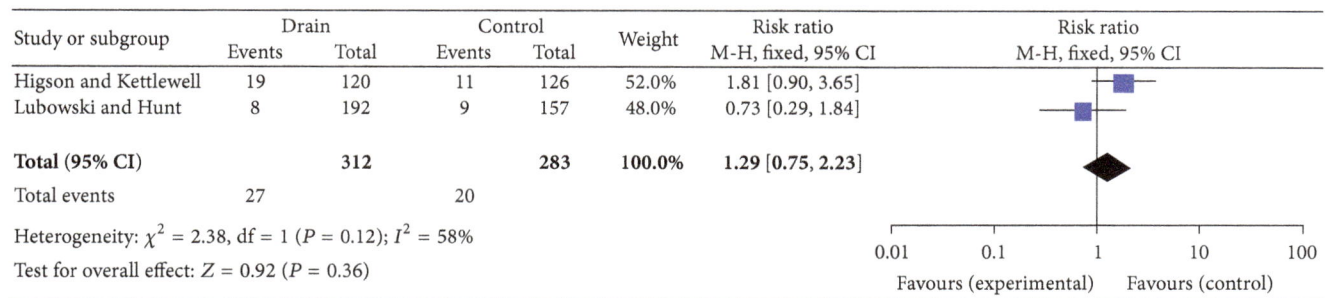

| Study or subgroup | Drain | | Control | | Weight | Risk ratio M-H, fixed, 95% CI | Risk ratio M-H, fixed, 95% CI |
	Events	Total	Events	Total			
Higson and Kettlewell	19	120	11	126	52.0%	1.81 [0.90, 3.65]	
Lubowski and Hunt	8	192	9	157	48.0%	0.73 [0.29, 1.84]	
Total (95% CI)		**312**		**283**	**100.0%**	**1.29 [0.75, 2.23]**	
Total events	27		20				

Heterogeneity: $\chi^2 = 2.38$, df = 1 ($P = 0.12$); $I^2 = 58\%$
Test for overall effect: $Z = 0.92$ ($P = 0.36$)

FIGURE 3: Forest plot data for trials including nonlaparotomy incisions.

however the overall risk ratio was not significant (RR 0.56 (0.21–1.51)).

4. Discussion

The aim of this study was to do a systematic review of the evidence available on the use of subcutaneous wound drainage after laparotomies to determine if there is a reduction in the incidence of surgical site infections (SSIs).

We only included studies with laparotomy incisions in this review. The aim was to include a homogenous group of studies which could be compared and data combined to perform a meta-analysis. Incidence of SSI is higher in laparotomies compared to hernia operations or pfannenstiel incisions and this is accentuated further in emergency laparotomies. A recent systematic review and meta-analyses by Kosin et al. looking at subcutaneous wound drainage for a variety of incisions showed that drains could be omitted in most procedures but there was no specific focus on laparotomies. Two trials analysed the types of surgery (clean, clean contaminated, contaminated, and dirty) separately (Table 3). There was no statistically significant difference in the groups in these trials.

There was no significant reduction in SSI incidence when all the laparotomies were analysed together in our meta-analyses. The risk ratio determined was 0.84 (0.66–1.09) which cannot be taken as a reliable indication about the efficacy of using drains. Two trials were analysed separately.

Higson et al. and Lubowski et al. trials showed no significant difference either in the rate of SSI. Higson et al. showed an almost double infection rate in the drain group as opposed to the control group. However this difference was not statistically significant ($P = 0.089$). Alongside this, both trials consisted of a relatively small sample size; hence reliable conclusions cannot be formed on this alone.

Out of all the trials in the meta-analysis, only two trials showed a significant reduction in SSI incidence in the drain group. Fujii et al. included high risk patients, including emergency laparotomies, and patients with thick subcutaneous fat and the risk ratio showed a reduction in the SSI rate in the drain group (RR 0.37 (0.15–0.9)). Imada et al. showed no significant difference in SSI incidence when using a drain in all patients; however there was a reduction in SSIs in the high risk patient group from 15% to 8%. It has also been reported by Soper et al. [18] that the depth of subcutaneous fat in a patient is an independent risk factor for SSI. It may therefore be possible that subcutaneous drains may be of benefit in high risk and/or obese patients and this is not evident in the meta-analysis due to underpowering. Indeed two trials detailed the wound types in each of the control and the drain groups and in these trials there was an overall reduction of 44% in SSI in the contaminated wound type where a subcutaneous drain was placed.

Various newer potential interventions may be used to reduce SSIs in this group of patients. The recently concluded ROSSINI trial assesses the efficacy of using wound edge protection devices in reducing SSI rates in laparotomies [43]. The trial results have recently been presented (ACPGBI Liverpool 1st–3rd July 2013) and do not show any advantage of using wound protectors. The authors are currently designing a further trial to address some of the shortcomings of the trial. Wound wicks which are removed at 72 hours can be used to prevent subcutaneous collection and may be useful. The National Emergency Laparotomy Audit (NELA) is a new initiative in the United Kingdom to audit and subsequently reduce complication rates after emergency laparotomies [44]. SSIs remain a major problem after emergency laparotomies and would be within the remit of NELA. This would further highlight the significance of interventions that reduce SSI in emergency laparotomies.

We aimed at keeping the studies as homogenous as possible for a reliable systematic review and analysis but despite this, there are still many variables between the trials which may have had an influence on the results. Wound drainage in all patients does not seem to be of significant benefit in reducing SSI and may add up to unnecessary cost, discomfort, and prolonged postoperative stay.

However, there may be potential benefit in higher risk patients, patients with deeper subcutaneous fat, and patients with contaminated or dirty wounds. These individual factors need to be carefully investigated in patients who undergo laparotomy. Other novel devices are also available which utilise suction to reduce the formation of collections under wounds. These have not been evaluated in a controlled trial. Wound wicks may also be used to ensure drainage of wounds in the immediate postoperative period. There is a need for a randomised controlled trial with well defined inclusion/exclusion criteria to evaluate use of such interventions in patients undergoing emergency laparotomies.

Conflict of Interests

No conflict of interests exists for the authors.

Authors' Contribution

A. Sharma contributed to study conception and design and critical revision of the paper. B. Manzoor and A. Sharma contributed to acquisition of data and analysis and interpretation of data and drafting of the paper.

References

[1] NICE, "Clinical Guideline 74—prevention and treatment of surgical site infection," NICE, October 2008, http://www.nice.org.uk/nicemedia/pdf/CG74NICEguideline.pdf.

[2] A. Watanabe, S. Kohnoe, R. Shimabukuro et al., "Risk factors associated with surgical site infection in upper and lower gastrointestinal surgery," Surgery Today, vol. 38, no. 5, pp. 404–412, 2008.

[3] HPS, Surveillance of Surgical Site Infection. Annual Report for Procedures Carried out from: January 2003–December 2011, Health Protection Scotland, Glasgow City, UK, 2012, http://www.documents.hps.scot.nhs.uk/hai/sshaip/publications/ssi/ssi-2011.pdf.

[4] Health Protection Agency, Surveillance of Surgical Site Infections in NHS Hospitals in England, 2010/2011, Health Protection Agency, 2011.

[5] R. L. Smith, J. K. Bohl, S. T. McElearney et al., "Wound infection after elective colorectal resection," Annals of Surgery, vol. 239, no. 5, pp. 599–607, 2004.

[6] V. Satyanarayana, H. V. Prashanth, B. Bhandare, and A. N. Kavyashree, "Study of surgical site infections in abdominal surgeries," Journal of Clinical and Diagnostic Research, vol. 5, no. 5, pp. 935–939, 2011.

[7] P. Astagneau, C. Rioux, F. Golliot, and G. Brücker, "Morbidity and mortality associated with surgical site infections: results from the 1997–1999 INCISO surveillance," The Journal of Hospital Infection, vol. 48, no. 4, pp. 267–274, 2001.

[8] A. Sharma, D. M. Sharp, L. G. Walker, and J. R. T. Monson, "Predictors of early postoperative quality of life after elective resection for colorectal cancer," Annals of Surgical Oncology, vol. 14, no. 12, pp. 3435–3442, 2007.

[9] D. E. Reichman and J. A. Greenberg, "Reducing surgical site infections: a review," Reviews in Obstetrics and Gynecology, vol. 2, no. 4, pp. 212–221, 2009.

[10] N. Kashimura, S. Kusachi, T. Konishi et al., "Impact of surgical site infection after colorectal surgery on hospital stay and medical expenditure in Japan," Surgery Today, vol. 42, no. 7, pp. 639–645, 2012.

[11] R. Coello, A. Charlett, J. Wilson, V. Ward, A. Pearson, and P. Borriello, "Adverse impact of surgical site infections in English hospitals," The Journal of Hospital Infection, vol. 60, no. 2, pp. 93–103, 2005.

[12] Department of Health, Under the Knife Report, Department of Health, 2011.

[13] R. Plowman, N. Graves, M. A. S. Griffin et al., "The rate and cost of hospital-acquired infections occurring in patients admitted to selected specialties of a district general hospital in England and the national burden imposed," *The Journal of Hospital Infection*, vol. 47, no. 3, pp. 198–209, 2001.

[14] A. Sharma, A.-P. Deeb, J. C. Iannuzzi, A. S. Rickles, J. R. T. Monson, and F. J. Fleming, "Tobacco smoking and postoperative outcomes after colorectal surgery," *Annals of Surgery*, vol. 258, no. 2, pp. 296–300, 2013.

[15] L. T. Sørensen, "Wound healing and infection in surgery. The clinical impact of smoking and smoking cessation: a systematic review and meta-analysis," *Archives of Surgery*, vol. 147, no. 4, pp. 373–383, 2012.

[16] M. R. Kwaan, A. M. E. Sirany, D. A. Rothenberger, and R. D. Madoff, "Abdominal wall thickness: is it associated with superficial and deep incisional surgical site infection after colorectal surgery?" *Surgical Infections*, vol. 14, no. 4, pp. 363–368, 2013.

[17] C. van Walraven and R. Musselman, "The Surgical Site Infection Risk Score (SSIRS): a model to predict the risk of surgical site infections," *PLoS ONE*, vol. 8, no. 6, Article ID e67167, 2013.

[18] D. E. Soper, R. C. Bump, and W. G. Hurt, "Wound infection after abdominal hysterectomy: effect of the depth of subcutaneous tissue," *American Journal of Obstetrics and Gynecology*, vol. 173, no. 2, pp. 465–471, 1995.

[19] T. Fujii, S. Tsutsumi, A. Matsumoto et al., "Thickness of subcutaneous fat as a strong risk factor for wound infections in elective colorectal surgery: impact of prediction using preoperative CT," *Digestive Surgery*, vol. 27, no. 4, pp. 331–335, 2010.

[20] W. G. Cheadle, "Risk factors for surgical site infection," *Surgical Infections*, vol. 7, supplement 1, pp. S7–S11, 2006.

[21] M. Diana, M. Hübner, M.-C. Eisenring, G. Zanetti, N. Troillet, and N. Demartines, "Measures to prevent surgical site infections: what surgeons (should) do," *World Journal of Surgery*, vol. 35, no. 2, pp. 280–288, 2011.

[22] R. O. Darouiche, M. J. Wall Jr., K. M. F. Itani et al., "Chlorhexidine-alcohol versus povidone-iodine for surgical-site antisepsis," *The New England Journal of Medicine*, vol. 362, no. 1, pp. 18–26, 2010.

[23] J. W. Alexander, J. E. Fischer, M. Boyajian, J. Palmquist, and M. J. Morris, "The influence of hair-removal methods on wound infections," *Archives of Surgery*, vol. 118, no. 3, pp. 347–352, 1983.

[24] B. W. Murray, S. Huerta, S. Dineen, and T. Anthony, "Surgical site infection in colorectal surgery: a review of the nonpharmacologic tools of prevention," *Journal of the American College of Surgeons*, vol. 211, no. 6, pp. 812–822, 2010.

[25] A. M. Kosins, T. Scholz, M. Cetinkaya, and G. R. D. Evans, "Evidence-based value of subcutaneous surgical wound drainage: the largest systematic review and meta-analysis," *Plastic and Reconstructive Surgery*, vol. 132, no. 2, pp. 443–450, 2013.

[26] J. M. A. Bohnen, "Use of drains," in *Abdominal Wall Hernias: Principles and Management*, R. Bendavid, Ed., p. 328, Springer, New York, NY, USA, 2001.

[27] K. S. Gurusamy and K. Samraj, "Wound drains after incisional hernia repair," *The Cochrane Database of Systematic Reviews*, no. 1, Article ID CD005570, 2007.

[28] X.-D. He, Z.-H. Guo, J.-H. Tian, K.-H. Yang, and X.-D. Xie, "Whether drainage should be used after surgery for breast cancer? A systematic review of randomized controlled trials," *Medical Oncology*, vol. 28, supplement 1, pp. S22–S30, 2011.

[29] D. Chelmow, E. J. Rodriguez, and M. M. Sabatini, "Suture closure of subcutaneous fat and wound disruption after cesarean delivery: a meta-analysis," *Obstetrics and Gynecology*, vol. 103, no. 5, part 1, pp. 974–980, 2004.

[30] Drains, "Dead space management," in *Complications in Surgery*, M. W. Mulholland and G. M. Doherty, Eds., p. 148, Wolters Kluwer, Lippincott Williams & Wilkins Health, Philadelphia, Pa, USA, 2nd edition, 2011.

[31] D. J. Leaper, "Risk factors for surgical infection," *The Journal of Hospital Infection*, vol. 30, supplement, pp. 127–139, 1995.

[32] P. K. Baier, N. C. Glück, U. Baumgartner, U. Adam, A. Fischer, and U. T. Hopt, "Subcutaneous Redon drains do not reduce the incidence of surgical site infections after laparotomy. A randomized controlled trial on 200 patients," *International Journal of Colorectal Disease*, vol. 25, no. 5, pp. 639–643, 2010.

[33] R. J. Cardosi, J. Drake, S. Holmes et al., "Subcutaneous management of vertical incisions with 3 or more centimeters of subcutaneous fat," *American Journal of Obstetrics and Gynecology*, vol. 195, no. 2, pp. 607–614, 2006.

[34] M. B. Farnell, S. Worthington-Self, P. Mucha Jr., D. M. Ilstrup, and D. C. McIlrath, "Closure of abdominal incisions with subcutaneous catheters. A prospective randomized trial," *Archives of Surgery*, vol. 121, no. 6, pp. 641–648, 1986.

[35] T. Fujii, Y. Tabe, R. Yajima et al., "Effects of subcutaneous drain for the prevention of incisional SSI in high-risk patients undergoing colorectal surgery," *International Journal of Colorectal Disease*, vol. 26, no. 9, pp. 1151–1155, 2011.

[36] S. Imada, S. Noura, M. Ohue et al., "Efficacy of subcutaneous penrose drains for surgical site infections in colorectal surgery," *World Journal of Gastrointestinal Surgery*, vol. 5, no. 4, pp. 110–114, 2013.

[37] R. A. Kozol, D. Fromm, N. B. Ackerman, and R. Chung, "Wound closure in obese patients," *Surgery Gynecology & Obstetrics*, vol. 162, no. 5, pp. 442–444, 1986.

[38] D. Shaffer, P. N. Benotti, A. Bothe Jr., R. L. Jenkins, and G. L. Blackburn, "A prospective, randomized trial of abdominal wound drainage in gastric bypass surgery," *Annals of Surgery*, vol. 206, no. 2, pp. 134–137, 1987.

[39] N. Tochika, T. Namikawa, I. Kamiji, M. Kitamura, K. Okamoto, and K. Hanazaki, "Subcutaneous continuous suction drainage for prevention of surgical site infection," *Journal of Hospital Infection*, vol. 78, no. 1, pp. 67–68, 2011.

[40] E. Tsujita, Y.-I. Yamashita, K. Takeishi et al., "Subcuticular absorbable suture with subcutaneous drainage system prevents incisional SSI after hepatectomy for hepatocellular carcinoma," *World Journal of Surgery*, vol. 36, no. 7, pp. 1651–1656, 2012.

[41] R. H. Higson and M. G. W. Kettlewell, "Parietal wound drainage in abdominal surgery," *The British Journal of Surgery*, vol. 65, no. 5, pp. 326–329, 1978.

[42] D. Lubowski and D. R. Hunt, "Abdominal wound drainage—a prospective, randomized trial," *The Medical Journal of Australia*, vol. 146, no. 3, pp. 133–135, 1987.

[43] T. D. Pinkney, M. Calvert, D. C. Bartlett et al., "Impact of wound edge protection devices on surgical site infection after laparotomy: multicentre randomised controlled trial (ROSSINI Trial)," *British Medical Journal*, vol. 347, Article ID f4305, 2013.

[44] D. I. Saunders, D. Murray, A. C. Pichel, S. Varley, and C. J. Peden, "Variations in mortality after emergency laparotomy: the first report of the UK emergency laparotomy network," *British Journal of Anaesthesia*, vol. 109, no. 3, pp. 368–375, 2012.

27

Leakage after Surgery for Rectum Cancer: Inconsistency in Reporting to the Danish Colorectal Cancer Group

L. Borly, M. B. Ellebæk, and N. Qvist

Surgical Department A, Odense University Hospital, Denmark

Correspondence should be addressed to L. Borly; lars.borly@gmail.com

Academic Editor: Gregory Kouraklis

Purpose. Anastomotic leakage accounts for up to 1/3 of all fatalities after rectal cancer surgery. Evidence suggests that anastomotic leakage has a negative prognostic impact on local cancer recurrence and long-term cancer specific survival. The reported leakage rate in 2011 in Denmark varied from 7 to 45 percent. The objective was to clarify if the reporting of anastomotic leakage to the Danish Colorectal Cancer Group was rigorous and unequivocal. *Methods*. An Internet-based questionnaire was e-mailed to all Danish surgical departments, who reported to Danish Colorectal Cancer Group (DCCG) in 2011. There were 23 questions. Four core questions were whether pelvic collection, fecal appearance in a pelvic drain, rectovaginal fistula, and "watchfull" waiting patients were reported as anastomotic leakage. *Results*. Fourteen out of 17 departments, who in 2011 according to DDCG performed rectal cancer surgery, answered the questionnaire. This gave a response rate of 82%. In three of four core questions there was disagreement in what should be reported as anastomotic leakage. *Conclusion*. The reporting of anastomotic leakage to the Danish Colorectal Cancer Group was not rigorous and unequivocal. The reported anastomotic leakage rate in Danish Colorectal Cancer Group should be interpreted with caution.

1. Introduction

A unique international accepted definition of anastomotic leakage (AL) is paramount to gather knowledge about the true incidence of AL and to perform valid comparison between different departments, regions, or countries. Furthermore it is important for the study of risk factors and the consequences of AL on local cancer recurrence and long-term cancer specific survival [1, 2].

Another problem is the different clinical presentation of AL, which includes peroperative demonstrated leakage, air, or intestinal content in drain, pelvic sepsis, or leakage demonstrated by a CT-scan, suture line dehiscence demonstrated by endoscopy, and overt peritonitis.

In Denmark all departments performing colorectal cancer surgery are obliged to report their results to the Danish Colorectal Cancer Group (DCCG) [3]. The DCCG database is a prospective, nationwide database with a patient completeness rate of 99%. One of the quality indicators in the DCCG yearly report is the individual department AL frequency, which must be no more than 10%.

In 2011 seventeen Danish surgical departments reported their results to the DCCG database. Out of 382 patients with rectum cancer who underwent a colorectal or coloanal anastomosis, 51 patients or 13.35% were reported having an AL. The reported department frequency varied from 7 to 45 percent [4]. The Danish national guidelines did not include any strict definitions on anastomotic leakage and there might be a risk of inconsistent reporting of AL.

The aim of the present study was by a structured questionnaire to clarify whether the reporting of AL to the DCCG database could be considered as rigorous and unequivocal.

2. Material and Methods

In March 2013 a self-administrated Internet-based questionnaire was e-mailed to all Danish surgical departments who reported to the DCCG database in 2011. The departments received a reminder after 2 months followed by information on the project by phone in order to maximize response rate.

There were 23 questions, which were a mixture of open format, closed format, and leading questions. The different

TABLE 1: Core question about fluid collection, rectovaginal fistula, drainage, and watchful waiting.

	Question	Yes		No		Always		Some times		Never		
		n	%	n	%	n	%	n	%	n	%	
6	Do you report patients to DCCG with a fluid collection in the small pelvis as a leakage - regardless of the patients has a radiologic or endoscopic proven leakage?	5	39	8	61							
7	Do you report patients to DCCG with rectovaginal fistula as a leakage?	8	62	5	38							
8	Do you use drainage close to the anastomosis?					4	31	5	38	4	31	If always or sometimes the responder was asked to answer question 9
9	Do you report patients with air, pus or faeces in the drain as a leakage if no leakage is shown by reoperation, radiology or endoscopy?	5	56	4	44							
22	Do you occasionally use watchful waiting in patients suspicious of anastomotic leakage?	7	54	6	46							If yes the responder was asked to answer question 23
23	Do you report watchful waiting patients to the DCCG database as a leakage?	6	86	1	14							

formats were used when appropriate. An online survey service (Survey Monkey) was used.

3. Results

Fourteen out of a total of 17 departments answered the questionnaire. This gave a response rate of 82%. One department had not performed surgery for rectum cancer and was excluded. Thus, thirteen responders were available for the per protocol analysis. None of the responders reported having made significant changes in their definition or reporting of AL to the database within the last two years. The 13 departments who answered the questionnaire represented 94% of all rectum resections and 93% of all AL in Denmark in 2011.

Eight out of thirteen departments answered yes to the existence of a department approved guideline for diagnosing AL. Six of these 8 responders described in a few keywords their guideline content or referred to a web-based guideline. CT with contrast enema per rectum, diagnostic laparoscopy, and endoscopy were the methods they described.

Core questions about reporting fluid collection in the pelvis, rectovaginal fistula and air, pus, or feces in drainage and watchful waiting as AL (questions 6 to 9) showed disagreement whether these events should be reported to DCCG as AL (Table 1).

In questions 10 to 13 the responders were asked to describe their perioperative procedures. All of the responders used a leak test with air insufflation. Ten of the responders used a rigid scope and 3 used a flexible scope.

In questions 14 to 20 the responders were asked to describe if they postoperatively used routine laboratory measurements or clinical algorithms for postoperative surveillance (Table 2 and Box 1).

The very last question was if the responders always performed a laparoscopy or a laparotomy if they had a confirmed AL. Two of the thirteen responded yes.

4. Discussion

The study shows that the reporting of AL to DCCG is not rigorous and unequivocal, and therefore the results of that specific parameter in the database should be interpreted with caution.

The response rate on 82% was high compared to most other studies. A systematic review of Internet-based surveys of health professionals found response rates, which ranged from 9% to 94% [5]. The high response rate in the present study could be explained by an e-mail reminder after 2 months followed by information on the project by phone [6–8].

In comparison a survey using the same online service was conducted among colorectal surgeons in UK. As in our study the objective was the definition of AL. A response rate on only 28.4% was achieved [9]. In that study extravasation of contrast on enema and fecal matter seen in pelvic drain or from the wound was accepted as diagnostic for AL.

To elucidate the validity of the questionnaire, ideally the results should have been compared to the patients records and case forms reported to the database for each separate

TABLE 2: Questions about postoperatively used routine measurements or algorithms.

		Yes		No		
		n	%	*n*	%	
14	Do you postoperative on routine and daily basis measure C-reactive protein [CRP]?	10	77	3	23	
15	Do you postoperative on routine- and daily basis measure other biomarkers such as D-dimer, procalcitonin, cytokines or others?	1	8	12	92	The one yes responder measured cytokines as part of a project.
16	Do you postoperative on routine basis use clinical scoring systems or algorithms?	4	31	9	69	If yes the responder was asked to answer question 17
17	Kindly describe the clinical scoring systems or algorithms you use					Four of the responders described their clinical scoring systems or algorithms. They were based on "early warning system" EWS
18	Do you always use the same diagnostics methods in the same order when you have a suspicion of AL?	9	69	4	31	If yes the responder was asked to answer question 19 and If no the responder was asked to answer question 21
19	Kindly describe the diagnostics methods in the same order?	The answer is shown in Box 1				
20	Kindly describe the diagnostics methods in different order?					The 4 responders answered that they on suspicion of AL used different diagnostics methods in different order. Three of the four responders described that the choice of method and order depended on the patients clinical condition and the surgical approach (open versus laparoscopic).

Eight of the nine yes responders in question 19 described their diagnostics methods when they had a suspicion of AL
(i) CT scanning with administration of rectal contrast: endoscopy
(ii) CT scanning with administration of rectal contrast: endoscopy or diagnostic laparoscopy
(iii) CT scanning with administration of rectal contrast
(iv) Divided into early and delayed AL
    (a) Early AL: diagnostic laparoscopy or endoscopy or CT scanning with administration of rectal contrast
    (b) Delayed AL: CT with i.v. and peroral contrast, maybe supplemented with administration of rectal contrast
        or endoscopy, depending on the findings at CT
(v) Rectal exploration followed by CT scanning with administration of rectal contrast
(vi) Rectal exploration performed by colorectal surgeon followed by CT scanning with administration of rectal contrast followed
    by endoscopy depending on the CT findings. If there is a pelvic abscess it is treated with a sponge
(vii) CT scanning with administration of rectal contrast: endoscopy
(viii) CT scanning with administration of both i.v. and rectal contrast: endoscopy and rectal exploration

Box 1

department. Furthermore, it should have been compared to a national gold standard in the definition of AL. However in 2011 this was nonexisting but has been introduced from 2013 and onwards. The aim of this investigation was not to define the true incidence of AL but to investigate any differences in reporting AL to the DCCG database. None of the responders had any remarks concerning the understanding of the questionnaire. The validity of this questionnaire analysis therefore seems to be high.

Drainage of the small pelvis can be considered as indicator of AL [10]. Interestingly only half of the responders in this survey reported patients with air, pus, or feces in the drain as being an AL. Only half of the UK surgeons agreed that radiological collection treated with antibiotics or percutaneous drainage constituted an AL [9]. This is similar to the findings in our study, where only 38% reported a fluid collection in the small pelvis as an AL. It has been found that both patients with and without AL have fluid collection in the small pelvis [11]. Sixty-nine percent of the UK surgeons agreed that intra-abdominal sepsis requiring laparotomy constituted an AL. The precise formulation of their questionnaire was not apparent [9]. An increase in C reactive protein (CRP) may be a predictor of septic complications after elective colorectal surgery [12]. In our study 76.92% of the responders used daily measurements of CRP concentration on routine, and 31% routinely used postoperative clinical scoring systems or algorithms. The use of the postoperative surveillance programs may detect more subclinical AL resulting in a higher frequency of reported AL in these departments.

The international study group of rectal cancer (ISREC) [13] has proposed a definition for AL and suggested grading system for AL according to clinical severity: firstly the AL should be defined as a defect of the intestinal wall integrity at the colorectal or coloanal anastomotic site (including suture and staple lines of neorectal reservoirs) leading to a communication between the intra- and extraluminal compartments. A pelvic abscess close to the anastomosis should also be considered as anastomotic leakage. Grade A is an AL requiring no active therapeutic intervention, grade B is an AL requiring active therapeutic intervention but manageable without relaparotomy, and grade C is an AL requiring relaparotomy.

ISREC validated the definition and severity grading in a cohort of 746 patients [14]. ISREC concluded that their definition and grading system of AL may facilitate comparisons of results from different studies on AL after sphincter-preserving rectal surgery. Only 16% of the patients had a grade A AL. In a recent study from 2014, which included 129 patients with low anterior resection, the ISREC definition and severity-grading system was applied. Of 19 patients with contrast enema proven AL, 61% had grade A, 17% grade B, and 22% grade C [15]. These results show that this new grading system has its own shortcomings. The only way to get precise information on the true incidence and possible consequences for the patient is a routine CT scanning with contras enema at a fixed and generally accepted postoperative day. This approach will also elucidate those AL, which are hidden by a diverting stoma.

After this study was presented in Danish as an abstract to the Danish Surgical Society's annual meeting 2013 changes have been made.

The Danish surgeons are now asked to report if the AL do not demand treatment, demand treatment but not surgery, or demand relaparotomy or relaparoscopy and if the anastomosis is taken down.

5. Conclusion

There is a demand of more precise knowledge on the rate of AL and the possible consequences on disease-free survival, morbidity, and functional outcome. We suggest a multicenter prospective study, where the proposed ISREC definition and severity grading of AL are combined with a CT scan with rectal administration of contrast and measurement at a fixed postoperative day.

Disclosure

This study was presented in Danish as an abstract to the Danish Surgical Society's annual meeting 2013 and as a poster at the 7th European Colorectal Congress (ECC) December 2013 in St. Gallen. The paper does not contain clinical studies or patient data.

Conflict of Interests

The authors declare that they have no conflict of interests.

References

[1] S. W. Bell, K. G. Walker, M. J. F. X. Rickard et al., "Anastomotic leakage after curative anterior resection results in a higher prevalence of local recurrence," *British Journal of Surgery*, vol. 90, no. 10, pp. 1261–1266, 2003.

[2] A. Mirnezami, R. Mirnezami, K. Chandrakumaran, K. Sasapu, P. Sagar, and P. Finan, "Increased local recurrence and reduced survival from colorectal cancer following anastomotic leak: systematic review and meta-analysis," *Annals of Surgery*, vol. 253, no. 5, pp. 890–899, 2011.

[3] DCCG Guidelines, http://www.dccg.dk/03_Publikation/01_ret.html.

[4] DCCG Year report, http://www.dccg.dk/03_Publikation/02_arsraport_pdf/aarsrapport_2011.pdf.

[5] D. Braithwaite, J. Emery, S. de Lusignan, and S. Sutton, "Using the internet to conduct surveys of health professionals: a valid alternative?" *Family Practice*, vol. 20, no. 5, pp. 545–551, 2003.

[6] C. Fischbacher, D. Chappel, R. Edwards, and N. Summerton, "Health surveys via the internet: quick and dirty or rapid and robust?" *Journal of the Royal Society of Medicine*, vol. 93, no. 7, pp. 356–359, 2000.

[7] S. A. McLean and J. A. Feldman, "The impact of changes in HCFA documentation requirements on academic emergency medicine: results of a physician survey," *Academic Emergency Medicine*, vol. 8, no. 9, pp. 880–885, 2001.

[8] A. Gandsas, K. Draper, E. Chekan et al., "Laparoscopy and the internet: a surgeon survey," *Surgical Endoscopy*, vol. 15, no. 9, pp. 1044–1048, 2001.

[9] K. Adams and S. Papagrigoriadis, "Little consensus in either definition or diagnosis of a lower gastro-intestinal anastomotic leak amongst colorectal surgeons," *International Journal of Colorectal Disease*, vol. 28, no. 7, pp. 967–971, 2013.

[10] S. Tsujinaka and F. Konishi, "Drain vs no drain after colorectal surgery," *Indian Journal of Surgical Oncology*, vol. 2, no. 1, pp. 3–8, 2011.

[11] P. Matthiessen, M. Henriksson, O. Hallböök, E. Grunditz, B. Norén, and G. Arbman, "Increase of serum C-reactive protein is an early indicator of subsequent symptomatic anastomotic leakage after anterior resection," *Colorectal Disease*, vol. 10, no. 1, pp. 75–80, 2008.

[12] A. B. Almeida, G. Faria, H. Moreira, J. Pinto-de-Sousa, P. Correia-da-Silva, and J. C. Maia, "Elevated serum C-reactive protein as a predictive factor for anastomotic leakage in colorectal surgery," *International Journal of Surgery*, vol. 10, no. 2, pp. 87–91, 2012.

[13] N. N. Rahbari, J. Weitz, W. Hohenberger et al., "Definition and grading of anastomotic leakage following anterior resection of

the rectum: a proposal by the International Study Group of Rectal Cancer," *Surgery*, vol. 147, no. 3, pp. 339–351, 2010.

[14] Y. Kulu, A. Ulrich, T. Bruckner et al., "Validation of the International Study Group of Rectal Cancer definition and severity grading of anastomotic leakage," *Surgery*, vol. 153, no. 6, pp. 753–761, 2013.

[15] F. Reilly, J. P. Burke, E. Appelmans, T. Manzoor, J. Deasy, and D. A. McNamara, "Incidence, risks and outcome of radiological leak following early contrast enema after anterior resection," *International Journal of Colorectal Disease*, vol. 29, no. 4, pp. 453–458, 2014.

28

Comparing Supervised Exercise Therapy to Invasive Measures in the Management of Symptomatic Peripheral Arterial Disease

Thomas Aherne,[1] **Seamus McHugh,**[1] **Elrasheid A. Kheirelseid,**[1] **Michael J. Lee,**[2] **Noel McCaffrey,**[3] **Daragh Moneley,**[1] **Austin L. Leahy,**[1] **and Peter Naughton**[1]

[1]*Department of Vascular Surgery, Beaumont Hospital, Dublin 9, Ireland*
[2]*Department of Interventional Radiology, Beaumont Hospital, Dublin 9, Ireland*
[3]*Department of Human and Health Performance, Dublin City University, Dublin 9, Ireland*

Correspondence should be addressed to Thomas Aherne; thomasaherne@rcsi.ie

Academic Editor: Miltiadis I. Matsagkas

Peripheral arterial disease (PAD) is associated with considerable morbidity and mortality. Consensus rightly demands the incorporation of supervised exercise training (SET) into PAD treatment protocols. However, the exact role of SET particularly its relationship with intervention requires further clarification. While supervised exercise is undoubtedly an excellent tool in the conservative management of mild PAD its use in more advanced disease as an adjunct to open or endovascular intervention is not clearly defined. Indeed its use in isolation in this cohort is incompletely reported. The aim of this review is to clarify the exact role of SET in the management of symptomatic PAD and in particular to assess its role in comparison with or as an adjunct to invasive intervention. A systematic literature search revealed a total 11 randomised studies inclusive of 969 patients. All studies compared SET and intervention with monotherapy. Study results suggest that exercise is a complication-free treatment. Furthermore, it appears to offer significant improvements in patients walk distances with a combination of both SET and intervention offering a superior walking outcome to monotherapy in those requiring invasive measures.

1. Introduction

Peripheral arterial disease (PAD) affects 12–16% of the population over the age of 60 years with intermittent claudication (IC), its primary symptom, proving detrimental to patient quality of life [1–4]. Typically PAD follows a stable course with management confined to conservative measures; however one in ten PAD patients will develop critical limb ischaemia (CLI) with all-cause mortality in the CLI cohort rising to 50% at 5 years [5–7]. This reduction in life expectancy is due largely to concomitant cardiovascular disease [8, 9].

Therefore, treatment goals should focus not only on the alteration of disease progression and symptomatic relief but also on the improvement of patient long-term survival [10]. Approaches include the modification of risk factors through optimum medical therapy (OMT) and supervised exercise therapy (SET) with endovascular (EVR) and open surgical revascularization reserved for those failing conservative

measures. Further novel therapies including kinesitherapy and electrotherapeutic procedures have also been proposed [11]. While endovascular treatment offers a minimally invasive revascularization option for many patients data supporting its ability to improve long-term survival is lacking. Regular exercise, on the other hand, is associated with a 50% reduction in cardiovascular mortality [12]. Supervised exercise training consists of a prescribed, evidence based exercise program which is performed under the direct observation of a trained practitioner. It is now well established as an initial noninvasive option in all PAD patients with robust supporting data [13–15].

Rationale for Review. Despite its intuitive benefits a wide variation in the use and availability of SET exists and it remains a greatly underutilized resource due to limited patient access [16]. The BASIL study highlights the deficiencies in the current medical optimization with few participants utilizing

TABLE 1: Treatment groups and disease level.

Study	Patient number	EVR	SET	EVR + SET	INV	Surgery	Surgery + SET	Fem-pop	Aortoiliac	Multilevel
Lundgren et al. [30]	75		25			25	25		Not recorded	
Creasy et al./Perkins et al. [19, 20]	56	30	26					28	25	0
Gelin et al. [29]	164		88		66				Not recorded	
Hobbs et al. [21]	23	9	7					23	0	0
Badger et al. [31]	14		6				8	14	0	0
Greenhalgh et al. [26]	127		60	67				93	94	
Kruidenier et al. [27]	70	35		35				5	60	5
Mazari et al. [25]	178	60	60	58					Not recorded	
Spronk et al./Fakhry et al. [22–24]	151	76	75					44	106	—
Murphy et al. [18, 32]	111	46	43					0	111	0
Bø et al. [28]	50	21		29				25	25	0

EVR: endovascular revascularization; SET: supervised exercise therapy; INV: invasive management; Fem-pop: femoropopliteal.

clinically proven best medical therapy [7, 17]. The issue is further clouded by conflicting literature as to the optimal nonsurgical management of these patients [18–32]. Thus while its use is strongly supported by current literature it appears that SET is underutilized in mild-to-moderate PAD while its use in more advanced disease requires further clarification. With this likely in mind the Institute of Medicine has prioritized research into the comparative efficacy of the different treatment modalities for PAD [33]. Furthermore, the role of SET as an adjunct to or substitute for intervention remains unclear.

The aim of this review was to compare the use of supervised exercise therapy to invasive measures in the management of symptomatic peripheral arterial disease thus clarifying an exact role for SET in the management of this patient cohort.

2. Methods

2.1. Study Eligibility. All randomised controlled trials (RT) assessing exercise in conjunction with or in comparison to an endovascular or open intervention in the management of peripheral arterial disease were included for review (Table 1). All observational and review data were excluded from the results. Relevant papers were searched and evaluated independently by two assessors. Outcomes were tabulated where figures were included.

2.2. Literature Search. The online medical literature database PUBMED was systematically searched. All studies and relevant reviews were manually cross-referenced to identify any outstanding articles.

PubMed was last searched on September 18, 2015 (Figure 1). The database was comprehensively searched without date or language restriction using the following search strategy.

[[[[[[[peripheral arterial disease] OR peripheral vascular disease] OR claudication] AND angioplasty] OR revascularization] OR endovascular] OR open surgery] OR bypass] AND exercise. A total of 8544 studies were identified. After

the filter for randomised controlled trials was applied 820 studies were identified. Relevant full articles were reviewed by two reviewers [TA, PN].

3. Results

A total of 15 papers (Table 1) report outcomes of 11 RT. These trials include a total of 969 patients and all directly compare supervised exercise with various invasive interventions. Maximum walking distance (MWD), intermittent claudication distance (ICD), and ankle brachial pressure index (ABPI) measurement form the cornerstones of vascular assessment in each study.

3.1. Quality Assessment of Assessed Data. The risk of bias in each included study is summarised in Table 2. Few papers reported any participant heterogeneity with regard to baseline function, comorbidities, and smoking status. Risk assessment was performed with guidance from the Cochrane Handbook for Systematic Reviews of Interventions [34].

3.2. Supervised Exercise versus Endovascular Intervention. Five trials including 519 patients directly compare the outcomes of EVR and SET in the management of peripheral arterial disease (Table 3).

At six months Murphy et al. reported significant improvements in maximum walk times in those undergoing SET compared to those in the EVR group [18]. However, at 18-month follow-up this benefit was lost with no significant difference in walk times identified [32]. ABPI were consistently higher in the EVR group. Creasy and Perkins noted significant improvements in the functionality of both groups [19, 20]. Again, no significant change in ABPI was noted in any SET cohort. Improvement in mobility was most significant when the disease affected the superficial femoral artery. Hobbs et al. only noted significant improvements in walk distances in those receiving EVR [21]. No improvement was seen with SET alone. Spronk et al. reported a 1-week clinical success rate of 88% following EVR decreasing to 68% at 12 months while the SET group had an early success rate of

TABLE 2: Assessment of bias.

Lundgren et al. [30]	Random sequence generation	Randomised but not described	Unclear risk of bias
	Allocation concealment	Randomised but not described	Unclear risk of bias
	Blinding of participants and personnel	Blinding not possible	Not assessed
	Incomplete outcome data	Follow-up data in each group incomplete	Moderate risk of bias
	Selective reporting	Clear outcomes	Low risk of bias
	Other sources of bias	None	Low risk of bias
Creasy et al./Perkins et al. [19, 20]	Random sequence generation	Randomised but not described	Unclear risk of bias
	Allocation concealment	Randomised but not described	Unclear risk of bias
	Blinding of participants and personnel	Blinding not possible	Not assessed
	Incomplete outcome data	No loss to follow-up reported	Low risk of bias
	Selective reporting	Clear outcomes	Low risk of bias
	Other sources of bias	None	Low risk of bias
Gelin et al. [29]	Random sequence generation	Randomised via computer based algorithm	Low risk of bias
	Allocation concealment	Randomised via computer based system	Low risk of bias
	Blinding of participants and personnel	Blinding not possible	Not assessed
	Incomplete outcome data	Some loss to follow-up	Moderate risk of bias
	Selective reporting	Clear outcomes	Low risk of bias
	Other sources of bias	None	Low risk of bias
Hobbs et al. [21]	Random sequence generation	Randomised with 2 × 2 factorial design	Low risk of bias
	Allocation concealment	Computer generated randomisation	Low risk of bias
	Blinding of participants and personnel	Blinding not possible	Not assessed
	Incomplete outcome data	Four withdrawals	Low risk of bias
	Selective reporting	Clear outcomes	Low risk of bias
	Other sources of bias	None	Low risk of bias
Badger et al. [31]	Random sequence generation	Randomised but not described	Unclear risk of bias
	Allocation concealment	Randomised but not described	Unclear risk of bias
	Blinding of participants and personnel	Blinding not possible	Not assessed
	Incomplete outcome data	All patients lost to 6-month follow-up	High risk of bias
	Selective reporting	Clear outcomes	Low risk of bias
	Other sources of bias	None	Low risk of bias
Greenhalgh et al. [26]	Random sequence generation	Detailed description of Stata generated randomisation	Low risk of bias
	Allocation concealment	Computer generated randomisation	Low risk of bias
	Blinding of participants and personnel	Blinding not possible	Not assessed
	Incomplete outcome data	Moderate loss to follow-up	Moderate risk of bias
	Selective reporting	Clear outcomes	Low risk of bias
	Other sources of bias	None	Low risk of bias
Kruidenier et al. [27]	Random sequence generation	Computer generated block randomisation	Low risk of bias
	Allocation concealment	Computer generated block randomisation	Low risk of bias
	Blinding of participants and personnel	No blinding	High risk of bias
	Incomplete outcome data	Moderate losses to follow-up	Moderate risk of bias
	Selective reporting	Clear outcomes	Low risk of bias
	Other sources of bias	None	Low risk of bias
Mazari et al. [25]	Random sequence generation	Sealed envelope used to randomise	Low risk of bias
	Allocation concealment	Sealed envelope used to randomise	Low risk of bias
	Blinding of participants and personnel	Blinding not described	Unclear risk of bias
	Incomplete outcome data	Moderate loss to follow-up	Moderate risk of bias
	Selective reporting	Clear outcomes	Low risk of bias
	Other sources of bias	None	Low risk of bias

TABLE 2: Continued.

Spronk et al./Fakhry et al. [22–24]	Random sequence generation	Computer generated block randomisation	Low risk of bias
	Allocation concealment	Computer generated block randomisation	Low risk of bias
	Blinding of participants and personnel	Blinding not possible	Not assessed
	Incomplete outcome data	Prolonged study with some loss to follow-up	Moderate risk of bias
	Selective reporting	Clear outcomes	Low risk of bias
	Other sources of bias	None	Low risk of bias
Murphy et al. [18, 32]	Random sequence generation	Web based randomisation	Low risk of bias
	Allocation concealment	Web based randomisation	Low risk of bias
	Blinding of participants and personnel	Observers blinded	Low risk of bias
	Incomplete outcome data	Prolonged study with some loss to follow-up	Moderate risk of bias
	Selective reporting	Clear outcomes	Low risk of bias
	Other sources of bias	None	Low risk of bias
Bø et al. [28]	Random sequence generation	Computer based randomisation	Low risk of bias
	Allocation concealment	Computer based randomisation	Low risk of bias
	Blinding of participants and personnel	Observers blinded	Low risk of bias
	Incomplete outcome data	No loss to follow-up	Low risk of bias
	Selective reporting	Clear outcomes	Low risk of bias
	Other sources of bias	None	Low risk of bias

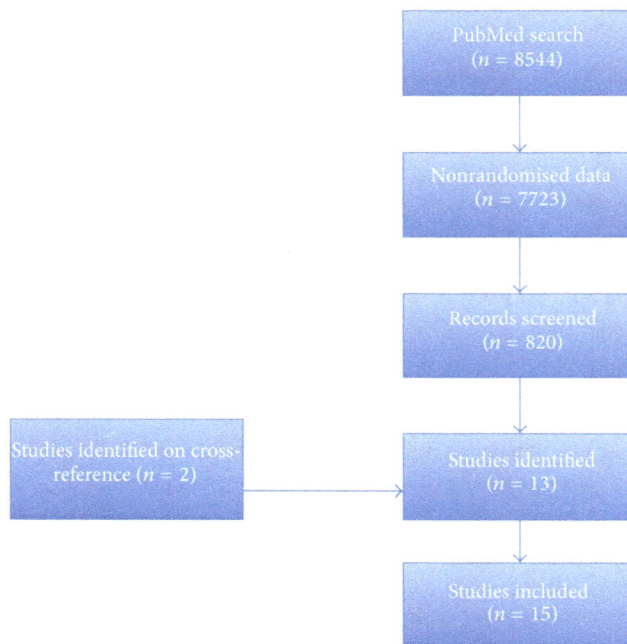

FIGURE 1: Flow diagram depicting study identification.

16% increasing to 65% by 12 months [22, 23]. Clinical success was defined as an improvement in at least one category in the Rutherford scale posttreatment. Long-term outcomes (7 years) from this RT show maintenance of the functional gains achieved at 1 year with no variance in amputation rate 10 between groups [24]. Finally, Mazari et al. identified significant functional improvements in both groups at one year; however no statistically significant difference was identified between cohorts [25]. Again, only EVR was associated with improved ABPI measurements.

3.3. Supervised Exercise Plus Invasive Measures (Open Surgery or EVR) versus Monotherapy.
In total six studies inclusive of 514 patients compare the merits of combination therapy consisting of invasive intervention and SET and single intervention alone (Table 4). Two included studies examine the benefits of a combination of open arterial surgical reconstruction and SET [30, 31] while four articles assess dual therapy including both EVR and SET [25–28].

The earliest work in this area by Lundgren et al. compares open arterial reconstruction and SET with open surgery

TABLE 3: Supervised exercise versus endovascular revascularization.

Study	Follow-up	ABPI		P	MWD		P	ICD		P
		Baseline	Endpoint		Baseline	Endpoint		Baseline	Endpoint	
Hobbs et al. [21]										
EVR	6 months	0.69	0.93	0.013[†]	185	698	0.008[†]	84	698	0.011[†]
SET		0.66	0.70	0.46[†]	111	124	0.35[†]	59	92	0.074[†]
Mazari et al. [25]										
EVR	12 months	0.71	0.90		77	146		31	75	
SET		0.72	0.84	0.093	83	215	0.2	42	97	0.48
Spronk et al./Fakhry et al. [22–24]										
EVR	7 years	0.63	0.84		174	1248		82	1022	
SET		0.62	0.82	0.8	186	1168	0.48	104	804	0.15
Murphy et al. [18, 32]										
EVR	18 months	0.7	0.7		5.2 min	8.4 min		1.8 min	4.8 min	
SET		0.6	0.6	<0.001	5.6 min	10.6 min	0.16	1.8 min	5.1 min	0.77

ABPI: ankle brachial pressure index; MWD: maximal walk distance; ICD: intermittent claudication distance; EVR: endovascular revascularization; SET: supervised exercise therapy. Distances in metres unless otherwise stated. min represents time in minutes, claudication onset time/maximal walk time. P value represents statistical comparison of interventions except in Hobbs et al. [21] where † represents change in measurement over study period.

TABLE 4: Supervised exercise plus invasive measures (open surgery or EVR) versus monotherapy.

Study	Follow-up	ABPI		P	MWD		P	ICD		P
		Baseline	Endpoint		Baseline	Endpoint		Baseline	Endpoint	
Lundgren et al. [30]										
Surgery		0.55	—		209	570		85	405	
SET	13 months	0.59	—		180	654		70	559	
Surgery + SET		0.59	—	<0.001	183	459	0.05	67	187	0.006
Badger et al. [31]										
Surgery	6 months	—	—		—	—		—	—	—
Surgery + SET		—	—	0.02*	—	—	0.001*	—	—	—
Greenhalgh et al. [26] (Aortoiliac)										
SET	24 months	0.66	0.74		126	168		—	—	—
EVR + SET		0.68	0.90	0.02	114	354	0.05	—	—	—
Greenhalgh et al. [26] (Femoropopliteal)										
SET	24 months	0.69	0.72		126	155		—	—	—
EVR + SET		0.66	0.83	0.01	133	245	0.4	—	—	—
Kruidenier et al. [27]										
EVR	6 months	0.71	0.93		282	685		343	547	
EVR + SET		0.69	0.88	0.755	186	956	0.001	293	842	0.001
Mazari et al. [25]										
EVR		0.71	0.9		77	146		31	75	
SET	12 months	0.72	0.84		83	215		42	97	
EVR + SET		0.64	0.92	0.93	85	187	0.259	43	99	0.484
Bø et al. [28]										
EVR	3 months	—	—		213	427		94	267	
EVR + SET		—	—	<0.001*	385	584	NS	101	456	NS

ABPI: ankle brachial pressure index; MWD: maximal walk distance; ICD: intermittent claudication distance; EVR: endovascular revascularization; SET: supervised exercise therapy. Distances in metres unless otherwise stated. * represents significant improvement favouring combined treatment. P value represents statistical comparison of interventions. — represents nonreported figures.

TABLE 5: Invasive (EVR or surgery) management versus supervised exercise.

Study	Follow-up	ABPI		P	MWD		P	ICD		P
		Baseline	Endpoint		Baseline	Endpoint		Baseline	Endpoint	
Gelin et al. [29]										
INV	12 months	0.55	0.71	<0.01[†]	274	344	<0.01[†]	—	—	—
SET		0.56	0.54	—	258	247	—	—	—	—

ABPI: ankle brachial pressure index; MWD: maximal walk distance; ICD: intermittent claudication distance; EVR: endovascular revascularization; SET: supervised exercise therapy. Distances in metres unless otherwise stated. P value represents statistical comparison of interventions. † represents change in measurement over study period.

alone [30]. This study identified improvements in walk distances in both groups; however, those undergoing combination therapy experienced significantly improved walking performance at 13 months. Similarly, Badger et al. identified significant improvements in MWD in patients undergoing peripheral arterial bypass in conjunction with SET compared to those undergoing bypass in isolation [31].

More recently, studies have focused on the use of SET as an adjunct to EVR. Mazari et al. identified that a combined treatment group achieved the greatest (but not statistically significant) improvement in MWD and ICD with a lower incidence of reintervention compared to the monotherapy groups [25]. This benefit was further supported by randomised data from Greenhalgh et al. [26–28]. At six months Kruidenier et al. identified significantly lengthened walk distances when SET was used as an adjunct to EVR. Furthermore, both Greenhalgh and Bø et al. examined patients with both aortoiliac and infrainguinal disease in separate trial limbs. While Greenhalgh compared combination therapy with SET alone Bø et al. contrasted dual therapy with EVR alone. Both studies identified improvements in walk distances in both trial limbs for patients undergoing combination therapy versus monotherapy; however only Greenhalgh identified significantly better ABPI in the dual intervention group.

3.4. Invasive (EVR or Surgery) Management versus Supervised Exercise. Gelin alone compared invasive intervention (either EVR or open surgery based on preoperative angiography) and supervised exercise [29] (Table 5). At one year only those randomised to invasive measures experienced any improvement in walk distance or lower limb arterial pressures.

3.5. Open Surgery versus Supervised Exercise. Lundgren et al. included a comparison of open revascularisation and SET in the previously discussed RT (Table 4) [30]. At 13 months those undergoing open surgery had better functional performance than those undergoing SET alone. In addition, those undergoing surgery experienced a significantly higher ABPI to those in the exercise group.

4. Discussion

Peripheral arterial disease is a widespread phenomenon in the elderly population [35]. The optimum management of claudication continues to raise debate. Exercise is a straightforward and effective conservative treatment option. Meta-analysis

has shown a 122% increase in walking distances in patients undergoing exercise therapy [15]. This has been reinforced by the more recent Cochrane review examining exercise for IC [36]. However, despite its success intensive programs continue to be associated with high dropout rates [37].

The exact physiological mechanism by which exercise improves performance is incompletely understood. Multiple physiological adaptions have been proposed as contributing factors. Arterial collateralization has the potential to improve peripheral blood flow in the ischaemic limb with the exercised muscle displaying increased levels of the proangiogenic vascular endothelial growth factor [38]. However, improved functional performance in the trained limb is not reflective of improved ABPI measurements as seen in endovascular revascularization [18, 39]. Increased arterial shear stress in exercise is associated with nitric oxide (NO) release, a powerful vasoactive agent [40]. This endothelial-mediated response is impaired in patients with PAD [41]. The concept of "hemorheologic fitness" suggests that a proven reduction in blood viscosity in the trained individual may result in improved peripheral metabolic efficiency [42]. In addition, gait proficiency, reversal of acquired metabolic myopathies, and modified inflammatory responses all have the potential to improve exercise related function [43–46].

This review suggests a number of roles for supervised exercise therapy in the symptomatic PAD patient (Figure 2). Significantly, no study reported exercise related complications.

(i) Direct comparison of SET and endovascular measures revealed similar functional outcomes for both interventions in the medium term across a number of studies with long-term data from one study identifying comparable limb salvage between groups. However, only EVR alone resulted in significant improvements in lower limb perfusion as measured by ABPI. These data have significant applicability to symptomatic patients whose comorbidities allow them to exercise to an adequate level for SET. Supervised exercise offers this group an acceptable, effective initial step in those capable and motivated to take part.

(ii) In those requiring intervention a combination of surgical intervention and SET offered superior outcomes to monotherapy across multiple studies. Two trials assessed open surgery with adjunctive SET with both suggesting significant benefits in walk distances

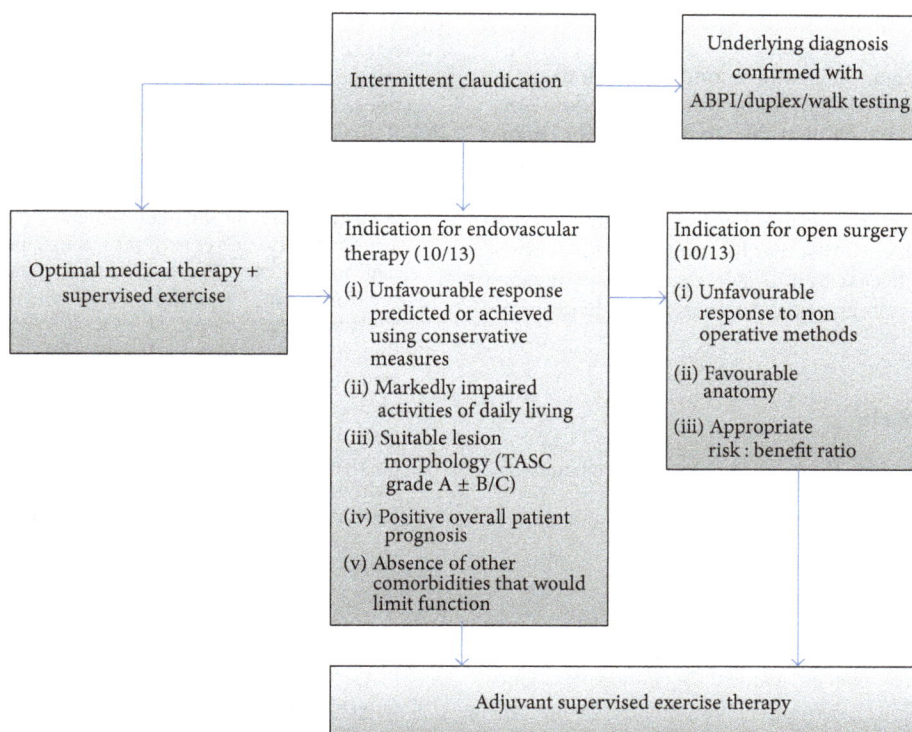

FIGURE 2: Management of intermittent claudication incorporating supervised exercise therapy.

in the dual therapy group. Similarly, all four trials assessing endovascular intervention in conjunction with SET compared to monotherapy found greater improvements in the walking distances of those undergoing dual therapy. These data would strongly support the use of SET as an adjunct to any operative intervention in the management of symptomatic PAD.

(iii) Only one study directly compared open surgery and SET. This strongly supported the surgical approach in terms of both function and perfusion outcomes.

Multiple exercise modalities including treadmill walking, resistance training, and upper limb ergometry have proven benefit in PAD [12, 36, 47, 48]. Unfortunately, the success of SET is reliant on excellent compliance and availability. Supervised exercise training has been shown to consistently result in improved functionality with superior outcomes to a "go home and walk" approach [49–51]. Compliance can further be augmented by regular exercise reminders, patient specific exercise prescriptions, target setting, and the incorporation of exercise into daily activities [52]. Gains in walk time and claudication onset occur rapidly over the initial 2 months and can be maintained with good compliance [53]. An exercise prescription of at least two 30-minute sessions per week offers optimal walking outcomes [54].

In those failing or unable to partake in an initial exercise program endovascular revascularization offers low rates of periprocedural morbidity and mortality with excellent initial success rates [55–57]. However the two main shortcomings

of endovascular intervention include long-term durability and overall poor survival rates associated with concomitant cardiovascular disease. Supervised exercise addresses some of these concerns. By stimulating collateralization and the release of vasodilators such as nitric oxide exercise therapy should confer superior functional results in the longer-term. This is supported by a number of studies [58, 59]. Thus, for this patient group SET offers not only functional improvement but also significant benefits to the cardiovascular health of these patients [12].

4.1. Strengths and Limitations. This review is strengthened by the fact that all incorporated data are from well-designed randomised controlled studies. Follow-up ranged from 6 months to 12 years. Cumulatively these trials incorporate a significant number of claudicants. Individually papers provide strong data that exercise results in significant gains in walk distance. In addition, a number of studies have found that a combination of SET and intervention provides a superior outcome to monotherapy.

This review is however subject to a number of limitations. Firstly, while all patients had significant arterial symptoms a degree of heterogeneity exists in this cohort. Each included study describes slight variations in the level of disease, the symptomatic presentation, and the intervention received rendering definitive conclusion difficult. Secondly, many studies included small numbers of participants with a number reporting moderate losses to follow-up. Finally, due to the heterogeneity of outcome data meta-analysis was not performed as part of this review.

5. Conclusion

Exercise is an effective, safe, and economical method of treating symptomatic PAD [23]. Some randomised data now suggests that it may be comparable to EVR in the management of symptomatic noncritical ischaemia. Furthermore there is emerging evidence that combining endovascular intervention following by supervised exercise achieves better long-term results than endovascular intervention alone; however greater surgeon access to and awareness of this important adjuvant therapy is essential to maximize therapeutic outcomes.

Conflict of Interests

The authors declare that there is no conflict of interests regarding the publication of this paper.

References

[1] M. H. Criqui, A. Fronek, E. Barrett-Connor, M. R. Klauber, S. Gabriel, and D. Goodman, "The prevalence of peripheral arterial disease in a defined population," *Circulation*, vol. 71, no. 3, pp. 510–515, 1985.

[2] M. Schroll and O. Munck, "Estimation of peripheral arteriosclerotic disease by ankle blood pressure measurements in a population study of 60-year-old men and women," *Journal of Chronic Diseases*, vol. 34, no. 6, pp. 261–269, 1981.

[3] E. Selvin and T. P. Erlinger, "Prevalence of and risk factors for peripheral arterial disease in the United States: results from the National Health and Nutrition Examination Survey, 1999-2000," *Circulation*, vol. 110, no. 6, pp. 738–743, 2004.

[4] I. C. Chetter, P. Dolan, J. I. Spark, D. J. A. Scott, and R. C. Kester, "Correlating clinical indicators of lower-limb ischaemia with quality of life," *Cardiovascular Surgery*, vol. 5, no. 4, pp. 361–366, 1997.

[5] K. Bloor, "Natural history of arteriosclerosis of the lower extremities—hunterian lecture delivered at the Royal College of Surgeons of England on 22nd April 1960," *Annals of the Royal College of Surgeons of England*, vol. 28, no. 1, pp. 36–52, 1961.

[6] J. A. Dormandy, L. Heeck, and S. Vig, "The fate of patients with critical leg ischemia," *Seminars in Vascular Surgery*, vol. 12, no. 2, pp. 142–147, 1999.

[7] A. W. Bradbury, D. J. Adam, J. D. Beard et al., "Bypass versus angioplasty in severe ischaemia of the leg (BASIL): multicentre, randomised controlled trial," *The Lancet*, vol. 366, no. 9501, pp. 1925–1934, 2005.

[8] M. H. Criqui, R. D. Langer, A. Fronek et al., "Mortality over a period of 10 years in patients with peripheral arterial disease," *The New England Journal of Medicine*, vol. 326, no. 6, pp. 381–386, 1992.

[9] F. G. R. Fowkes, "Epidemiology of atherosclerotic arterial disease in the lower limbs," *European Journal of Vascular Surgery*, vol. 2, no. 5, pp. 283–291, 1988.

[10] J. A. Dormandy and R. B. Rutherford, "Management of peripheral arterial disease (PAD). TASC Working Group. TransAtlantic Inter-Society Consensus (TASC)," *Journal of Vascular Surgery*, vol. 31, no. 1, part 2, pp. S1–S296, 2000.

[11] M. D. Markovic, D. M. Markovic, M. V. Dragas et al., "The role of kinesitherapy and electrotherapeutic procedures in nonoperative management of patients with intermittent claudications," *Vascular*, 2015.

[12] K. E. Powell and M. Pratt, "Physical activity and health," *British Medical Journal*, vol. 313, no. 7050, pp. 126–127, 1996.

[13] A. T. Hirsch, Z. J. Haskal, N. R. Hertzer et al., "ACC/AHA 2005 guidelines for the management of patients with peripheral arterial disease (lower extremity, renal, mesenteric, and abdominal aortic): executive summary a collaborative report from the American Association for Vascular Surgery/Society for Vascular Surgery, Society for Cardiovascular Angiography and Interventions, Society for Vascular Medicine and Biology, Society of Interventional Radiology, and the ACC/AHA Task Force on practice guidelines (writing committee to develop guidelines for the management of patients with peripheral arterial disease): endorsed by the American Association of Cardiovascular and Pulmonary Rehabilitation; National Heart, Lung, and Blood Institute; Society for Vascular Nursing; TransAtlantic Inter-Society Consensus; and Vascular Disease Foundation," *Journal of the American College of Cardiology*, vol. 47, no. 6, pp. 1239–1312, 2006.

[14] L. Norgren, W. R. Hiatt, and J. A. Dormandy, "Inter-society consensus for the management of peripheral arterial disease (TASC II)," *European Journal of Vascular and Endovascular Surgery*, vol. 33, supplement 1, pp. S1–S75, 2007.

[15] A. W. Gardner and E. T. Poehlman, "Exercise rehabilitation programs for the treatment of claudication pain. A meta-analysis," *The Journal of the American Medical Association*, vol. 274, no. 12, pp. 975–980, 1995.

[16] A. H. Stewart and P. M. Lamont, "Exercise for intermittent claudication. Supervised programmes should be universally available," *The British Medical Journal*, vol. 323, no. 7315, pp. 703–704, 2001.

[17] P. Burns, S. Gough, and A. W. Bradbury, "Management of peripheral arterial disease in primary care," *British Medical Journal*, vol. 326, no. 7389, pp. 584–588, 2003.

[18] T. P. Murphy, D. E. Cutlip, J. G. Regensteiner et al., "Supervised exercise versus primary stenting for claudication resulting from aortoiliac peripheral artery disease: six-month outcomes from the claudication: exercise versus endoluminal revascularization (CLEVER) study," *Circulation*, vol. 125, no. 1, pp. 130–139, 2012.

[19] T. S. Creasy, P. J. McMillan, E. W. L. Fletcher, J. Collin, and P. J. Morris, "Is percutaneous transluminal angioplasty better than exercise for claudication? Preliminary results from a prospective randomised trial," *European Journal of Vascular Surgery*, vol. 4, no. 2, pp. 135–140, 1990.

[20] J. M. T. Perkins, J. Collin, T. S. Creasy, E. W. L. Fletcher, and P. J. Morris, "Exercise training versus angioplasty for stable claudication. Long and medium term results of a prospective, randomised trial," *European Journal of Vascular and Endovascular Surgery*, vol. 11, no. 4, pp. 409–413, 1996.

[21] S. D. Hobbs, T. Marshall, C. Fegan, D. J. Adam, and A. W. Bradbury, "The constitutive procoagulant and hypofibrinolytic state in patients with intermittent claudication due to infrainguinal disease significantly improves with percutaneous transluminal balloon angioplasty," *Journal of Vascular Surgery*, vol. 43, no. 1, pp. 40–46, 2006.

[22] S. Spronk, J. L. Bosch, P. T. den Hoed, H. F. Veen, P. M. T. Pattynama, and M. G. M. Hunink, "Intermittent claudication: clinical effectiveness of endovascular revascularization versus supervised hospital-based exercise training—randomized controlled trial," *Radiology*, vol. 250, no. 2, pp. 586–595, 2009.

[23] S. Spronk, J. L. Bosch, P. T. den Hoed, H. F. Veen, P. M. T. Pattynama, and M. G. M. Hunink, "Cost-effectiveness of endovascular revascularization compared to supervised hospital-based exercise training in patients with intermittent claudication: a randomized controlled trial," *Journal of Vascular Surgery*, vol. 48, no. 6, pp. 1472–1480, 2008.

[24] F. Fakhry, E. V. Rouwet, P. T. Den Hoed, M. G. M. Hunink, and S. Spronk, "Long-term clinical effectiveness of supervised exercise therapy versus endovascular revascularization for intermittent claudication from a randomized clinical trial," *British Journal of Surgery*, vol. 100, no. 9, pp. 1164–1171, 2013.

[25] F. A. K. Mazari, J. A. Khan, D. Carradice et al., "Randomized clinical trial of percutaneous transluminal angioplasty, supervised exercise and combined treatment for intermittent claudication due to femoropopliteal arterial disease," *British Journal of Surgery*, vol. 99, no. 1, pp. 39–48, 2012.

[26] R. M. Greenhalgh, J. J. Belch, L. C. Brown, P. A. Gaines, L. Gao, and J. A. Reise, "The adjuvant benefit of angioplasty in patients with mild to moderate intermittent claudication (MIMIC) managed by supervised exercise, smoking cessation advice and best medical therapy: results from two randomised trials for stenoticfemoropopliteal and aortoiliac arterial disease," *European Journal of Vascular and Endovascular Surgery*, vol. 36, no. 6, pp. 680–688, 2008.

[27] L. M. Kruidenier, S. P. Nicolaï, E. V. Rouwet, R. J. Peters, M. H. Prins, and J. A. W. Teijink, "Additional supervised exercise therapy after a percutaneous vascular intervention for peripheral arterial disease: a randomized clinical trial," *Journal of Vascular and Interventional Radiology*, vol. 22, no. 7, pp. 961–968, 2011.

[28] E. Bø, J. Hisdal, M. Cvancarova et al., "Twelve-months follow-up of supervised exercise after percutaneous transluminal angioplasty for intermittent claudication: a randomised clinical trial," *International Journal of Environmental Research and Public Health*, vol. 10, no. 11, pp. 5998–6014, 2013.

[29] J. Gelin, L. Jivegård, C. Taft et al., "Treatment efficacy of intermittent claudication by surgical intervention, supervised physical exercise training compared to no treatment in unselected randomised patients I: one year results of functional and physiological improvements," *European Journal of Vascular and Endovascular Surgery*, vol. 22, no. 2, pp. 107–113, 2001.

[30] F. Lundgren, A.-G. Dahllof, K. Lundholm, T. Schersten, and R. Volkmann, "Intermittent claudication—surgical reconstruction or physical training? A prospective randomized trial of treatment efficiency," *Annals of Surgery*, vol. 209, no. 3, pp. 346–355, 1989.

[31] S. A. Badger, C. V. Soong, M. E. O'Donnell, C. A. G. Boreham, and K. E. McGuigan, "Benefits of a supervised exercise program after lower limb bypass surgery," *Vascular and Endovascular Surgery*, vol. 41, no. 1, pp. 27–32, 2007.

[32] T. P. Murphy, D. E. Cutlip, J. G. Regensteiner et al., "Supervised exercise, stent revascularization, or medical therapy for claudication due to aortoiliac peripheral artery disease: the CLEVER study," *Journal of the American College of Cardiology*, vol. 65, no. 10, pp. 999–1009, 2015.

[33] 100 initial topics for comparative effectiveness research, 2009, http://www.iom.edu/Reports/2009/ComparativeEffectiveness-ResearchPriorities.aspx.

[34] J. A. C. Sterne, M. Egger, and D. Moher, "Addressing reporting biases," in *Cochrane Handbook for Systematic Reviews of Interventions Version 5.1.0*, J. P. T. Higgins and S. Green, Eds., The Cochrane Collaboration, 2011.

[35] G. C. Leng, O. Papacosta, P. Whincup et al., "Femoral atherosclerosis in an older British population: prevalence and risk factors," *Atherosclerosis*, vol. 152, no. 1, pp. 167–174, 2000.

[36] L. Watson, B. Ellis, and G. C. Leng, "Exercise for intermittent claudication," *The Cochrane Database of Systematic Reviews*, no. 4, Article ID CD000990, 2008.

[37] B. L. Bendermacher, E. M. Willigendael, S. P. Nicolaï et al., "Supervised exercise therapy for intermittent claudication in a community-based setting is as effective as clinic-based," *Journal of Vascular Surgery*, vol. 45, no. 6, pp. 1192–1196, 2007.

[38] T. Gustafsson, A. Puntschart, L. Kaijser, E. Jansson, and C. J. Sundberg, "Exercise-induced expression of angiogenesis-related transcription and growth factors in human skeletal muscle," *American Journal of Physiology: Heart and Circulatory Physiology*, vol. 276, no. 2, pp. H679–H685, 1999.

[39] R. Ekroth, A.-G. Dahllöf, B. Gundevall, J. Holm, and T. Scherstén, "Physical training of patients with intermittent claudication: indications, methods, and results," *Surgery*, vol. 84, no. 5, pp. 640–643, 1978.

[40] M. Noris, M. Morigi, R. Donadelli et al., "Nitric oxide synthesis by cultured endothelial cells is modulated by flow conditions," *Circulation Research*, vol. 76, no. 4, pp. 536–543, 1995.

[41] A. R. Yataco, M. C. Corretti, A. W. Gardner, C. J. Womack, and L. I. Katzel, "Endothelial reactivity and cardiac risk factors in older patients with peripheral arterial disease," *American Journal of Cardiology*, vol. 83, no. 5, pp. 754–758, 1999.

[42] E. Ernst, "Influence of regular physical activity on blood rheology," *European Heart Journal*, vol. 8, pp. 59–62, 1987.

[43] C. J. Womack, D. J. Sieminski, L. I. Katzel, A. Yataco, and A. W. Gardner, "Improved walking economy in patients with peripheral arterial occlusive disease," *Medicine & Science in Sports & Exercise*, vol. 29, no. 10, pp. 1286–1290, 1997.

[44] T. A. Beckitt, J. Day, M. Morgan, and P. M. Lamont, "Calf muscle oxygen saturation and the effects of supervised exercise training for intermittent claudication," *Journal of Vascular Surgery*, vol. 56, no. 2, pp. 470–475, 2012.

[45] P. V. Tisi, M. Hulse, A. Chulakadabba, P. Gosling, and C. P. Shearman, "Exercise training for intermittent claudication: does it adversely affect biochemical markers of the exercise-induced inflammatory response?" *European Journal of Vascular and Endovascular Surgery*, vol. 14, no. 5, pp. 344–350, 1997.

[46] K. J. Stewart, W. R. Hiatt, J. G. Regensteiner, and A. T. Hirsch, "Exercise training for claudication," *The New England Journal of Medicine*, vol. 347, no. 24, pp. 1941–1951, 2002.

[47] M. M. McDermott, P. Ades, J. M. Guralnik et al., "Treadmill exercise and resistance training in patients with peripheral arterial disease with and without intermittent claudication: a randomized controlled trial," *The Journal of the American Medical Association*, vol. 301, no. 2, pp. 165–174, 2009.

[48] I. Zwierska, R. D. Walker, S. A. Choksy, J. S. Male, A. G. Pockley, and J. M. Saxton, "Upper—vs lower-limb aerobic exercise rehabilitation in patients with symptomatic peripheral arterial disease: a randomized controlled trial," *Journal of Vascular Surgery*, vol. 42, no. 6, pp. 1122–1130, 2005.

[49] F. A. Frans, S. Bipat, J. A. Reekers, D. A. Legemate, and M. J. W. Koelemay, "Systematic review of exercise training or percutaneous transluminal angioplasty for intermittent claudication," *British Journal of Surgery*, vol. 99, no. 1, pp. 16–28, 2012.

[50] A. A. Ahimastos, E. P. Pappas, P. G. Buttner, P. J. Walker, B. A. Kingwell, and J. Golledge, "A meta-analysis of the outcome of endovascular and noninvasive therapies in the treatment of

intermittent claudication," *Journal of Vascular Surgery*, vol. 54, no. 5, pp. 1511–1521, 2011.

[51] B. L. Bendermacher, E. M. Willigendael, J. A. Teijink, and M. H. Prins, "Supervised exercise therapy versus non-supervised exercise therapy for intermittent claudication," *Cochrane Database of Systematic Reviews*, no. 2, Article ID CD005263, 2006.

[52] L. Bourke, K. E. Homer, M. A. Thaha et al., "Interventions for promoting habitual exercise in people living with and beyond cancer," *The Cochrane Database of Systematic Reviews*, vol. 9, Article ID CD010192, 2013.

[53] A. W. Gardner, P. S. Montgomery, and D. E. Parker, "Optimal exercise program length for patients with claudication," *Journal of Vascular Surgery*, vol. 55, no. 5, pp. 1346–1354, 2012.

[54] S. P. A. Nicolaï, E. J. M. Hendriks, M. H. Prins, and J. A. W. Teijink, "Optimizing supervised exercise therapy for patients with intermittent claudication," *Journal of Vascular Surgery*, vol. 52, no. 5, pp. 1226–1233, 2010.

[55] V. G. Papavassiliou, S. R. Walker, A. Bolia, G. Fishwick, and N. J. M. London, "Techniques for the endovascular management of complications following lower limb percutaneous transluminal angioplasty," *European Journal of Vascular and Endovascular Surgery*, vol. 25, no. 2, pp. 125–130, 2003.

[56] V. S. Kashyap, M. L. Pavkov, J. F. Bena et al., "The management of severe aortoiliac occlusive disease: endovascular therapy rivals open reconstruction," *Journal of Vascular Surgery*, vol. 48, no. 6, pp. 1451.e3–1457.e3, 2008.

[57] G. S. R. Muradin, J. L. Bosch, T. Stijnen, and M. G. M. Hunink, "Balloon dilation and stent implantation for treatment of femoropopliteal arterial disease: meta-analysis," *Radiology*, vol. 221, no. 1, pp. 137–145, 2001.

[58] M. M. McDermott, T. J. Carroll, M. Kibbe et al., "Proximal superficial femoral artery occlusion, collateral vessels, and walking performance in peripheral artery disease," *JACC: Cardiovascular Imaging*, vol. 6, no. 6, pp. 687–694, 2013.

[59] J. D. Allen, T. Stabler, A. Kenjale et al., "Plasma nitrite flux predicts exercise performance in peripheral arterial disease after 3 months of exercise training," *Free Radical Biology and Medicine*, vol. 49, no. 6, pp. 1138–1144, 2010.

Delorme's Procedure for Complete Rectal Prolapse: A Study of Recurrence Patterns in the Long Term

Carlos Placer, Jose M. Enriquez-Navascués, Ander Timoteo, Garazi Elorza, Nerea Borda, Lander Gallego, and Yolanda Saralegui

Department of Colorectal Surgery, Division of General and Gastrointestinal Surgery, Donostia University Hospital, 20014 San Sebastián, Spain

Correspondence should be addressed to Jose M. Enriquez-Navascués; josemaria.enriqueznavascues@osakidetza.net

Academic Editor: Erdinc Kamer

Introduction. The objective of this study was to determine the recurrence rate and associated risk factors of full-thickness rectal prolapse in the long term after Delorme's procedure. *Patients and Methods.* The study involved adult patients with rectal prolapse treated with Delorme's surgery between 2000 and 2012 and followed up prospectively in an outpatient unit. We assessed epidemiological data, Wexner constipation and incontinence score, recurrence patterns, and risk factors. Data were analyzed by univariate and multivariate studies and follow-up was performed according to Kaplan-Meier technique. The primary outcome was recurrence. *Results.* A total of 42 patients, where 71.4% (n = 30) were women, with a median age of 76 years (IQR 66 to 86), underwent Delorme's surgery. The median follow-up was 85 months (IQR 28 to 132). There was no mortality, and morbidity was 9.5%. Recurrence occurred in five patients (12%) within 14 months after surgery. Actuarial recurrence at five years was 9.9%. According to the univariate analysis, constipation and concomitant pelvic floor repair were the only factors found to be associated with recurrence. Multivariate analysis showed no statistically significant differences among variables studied. Kaplan-Meier estimate revealed that constipation was associated with a higher risk of recurrence (log-rank test, p = 0.006). *Conclusions.* Delorme's procedure is a safe technique with an actuarial recurrence at five years of 9.9%. The outcomes obtained in this study support the performance of concomitant postanal repair and levatorplasty to reduce recurrences. Also, severe constipation is associated with a higher recurrence rate.

1. Introduction

Rectal prolapse is a condition with a substantial impact on patient's quality of life. The main clinical symptoms requiring treatment include fecal incontinence, constipation, rectal bleeding, mucous discharge, or the presence of the bulge itself. The goals of surgical treatment are to correct the prolapse and resolve or improve functional disorders (incontinence and constipation), with low morbi-mortality [1].

While a variety of abdominal and perineal procedures have been described to treat rectal prolapse, these are divided into abdominal and perineal approaches. It is considered that abdominal procedures carry a lower rate of recurrence and better functional outcomes but may entail an undesirable risk in young patients: fertility disorders in women and sexual function in men. In addition, the performance of abdominal surgery is technically more difficult in case of recurrence. Conversely, perineal approaches such as Delorme's or Altemeier;s procedure limit these risks at the expense of higher recurrence rates.

At present, laparoscopic surgery has become the treatment of choice for rectal prolapse in many Colorectal Units [2, 3]. However, perineal procedures are still performed in high-risk patients or in case of recurrence following abdominal surgery. A high BMI or the risk for nerve injury involved in abdominal surgery in young males may also lead to an indication of perineal surgery [4].

Although there is a range of ongoing randomized clinical trials (e.g., DeLoRes, Deliver, and Danish trial) whose results have not been published yet, at present there is not strong evidence of the superiority of a treatment over the others [5, 6].

The goal of this study was to assess recurrence rates in the long term following Delorme's procedure and identify the risk factors that might discourage this procedure.

2. Patients and Methods

This is an observational cohort study of patients undergoing Delorme's procedure for complete rectal prolapse at a tertiary hospital between January 2000 and December 2012. Patients' clinical records, physical examination data, and preoperative studies were prospectively collected. Imaging tests were occasionally performed (barium enema, transit time study, endorectal ultrasound, defecography, or pelvic magnetic resonance), as well as a colonoscopy and anorectal manometry. Patients were invited to take a picture of their prolapse when physical examination did not reveal the prolapse itself or there were doubts on the type of prolapse (complete or mucous) reported by the patient.

All patients received a preoperative enema and the administration of prophylactic antibiotic therapy with Metronidazole, Ciprofloxacin, or third-generation cephalosporins, as well as thromboembolic prophylaxis. Surgery was performed either under general or spinal hyperbaric anaesthesia in the lithotomy position. A urinary catheter was inserted. Surgery was performed as described in the literature [7, 8]. A dilution of adrenaline (1:200,000) was injected into the submucosal plane and a mucosectomy twice the length of the prolapse was performed. Reabsorbable suture was used for muscle plication and mucomucous anastomosis 1 cm above the anopectinate line. Park's posterior puborectal plicature or an anterior and posterior levatorplasty were selectively performed in patients with a patulous anus at the physical exploration, through the same incision by developing the intersphincteric plane and using nonreabsorbable monofilament suture. A fiber-supplemented diet was progressively introduced at 24 h following surgery. The urinary catheter was removed within the first day when the patient had no previous prostate disorders. Patients were discharged when they showed tolerance to oral diet, no/mild pain, and normal defecation.

Follow-up was performed in an outpatient clinic setting during the first two years following surgery; then, we contacted the patients or their GP during the first semester of 2013. Patient's baseline characteristics, postoperative complications, or recurrences were recorded. Incontinence and constipation were reassessed using a defecatory diary and Jorge and Wexner score [9].

Categorical variables were analyzed using either Chi-squared test or Fisher's test, as appropriate. Quantitative variables were analyzed by Mann-Whitney U test. Recurrences were assessed with Kaplan-Meier analysis. Risk factors for recurrence were identified by binary logistic regression and the Cox model. Statistical analysis was performed using SPSS 21.0 (SPSS Inc., Chicago, IL) software.

3. Results

A total of 30 women (71.4%) and 12 men (28.6%), with a median age of 76 years (IR 66 to 86), were included in the study. Two patients had undergone surgery for prolapse previously (a posterior rectopexy and a Frykman-Goldberg procedure). At baseline seven patients (16.6%) reported constipation and 15 had severe incontinence (35.7%). Fourteen women (46.6%) had undergone a hysterectomy and eight (26.6%) had some level of associated genital prolapse. As many as 29 patients (69.1%) had an ASA score III and 13 had an ASA score II (30.9%).

During surgery, hyperbaric spinal anaesthesia was used in 31 patients (75.8%) whereas general anaesthesia was used in 11 (26.2%). A levatorplasty was performed in seven patients (16.6%) (four postanal repairs and three anterior and posterior levatorplasty procedures). There was no mortality. Four patients (9.5%) experienced complications: two partial anastomotic dehiscences, a case of urinary retention, and a perineal haematoma. A patient (2.3%) required reintervention (resuture) for partial suture dehiscence. The average hospital stay was five days (IR 4 to 6). Sexual or urinary dysfunctions were not observed in any patient.

The median follow-up was 85 months (IR 28 to 132). Five recurrences (12%) were detected. All recurrences were diagnosed within the first 14 postoperative months: at 3 (one patient), 6 (one patient), 13 (two patients), 14 (one patient) months. Rerecurrence was not observed in any of the five patients who required reintervention after original Delorme's (3 re-Delorme, 1 Altemeier, and 1 laparoscopic ventral rectopexy). Neither de novo incontinence nor de novo constipation was observed during the follow-up.

According to the univariate analysis, none of the main variables (i.e., age, sex, ASA score, previous hysterectomy, and postoperative complications) was found to be associated with recurrence (Table 1). However, significant differences were observed according to the type of anaesthesia ($p = 0.013$), constipation ($p = 0.026$), and performance of concomitant pelvic floor repair ($p = 0.010$). Recurrence was not observed in any patient aged <65 years (9/42), although differences were not statistically significant ($p = 0.567$). Also, of the five recurrences observed, four occurred in patients with a >5 cm prolapse, although differences were not statistically significant ($p = 0.138$). Multivariate analysis showed no statistically significant differences among variables. Kaplan-Meier estimate revealed that constipation was associated with a higher risk of recurrence (log-rank test, $p = 0.006$) (Figures 1, 2, and 3 and Table 2).

Outcomes for functional symptoms are shown in Table 3; as can be seen, during postoperative follow-up of patients, a tendency, to improvement in the degree of constipation, was observed, although it was not statistically significant. However a greater degree of constipation was observed in patients who had a later recurrence of the rectal prolapse. With respect to anal incontinence, no significant improvements were observed after the completion of the procedure Delorme.

4. Discussion

This study demonstrates that Delorme's operation is a safe procedure with very low mortality (0% in our series), a 9.5% morbidity, and an acceptable overall recurrence of 12% after

TABLE 1: Baseline characteristics of rectal prolapse patients.

	Total ($n = 42$)	No recurrence ($n = 37$)	Recurrence ($n = 5$)	p value
Median age (years)	76	72	86	0.180[£]
Sex (men/women)	12/30	10/27	2/3	0.613[¥]
ASA (%)				
I	2 (4.8)	2 (5.5)	0 (0)	
II	12 (28.5)	11 (29.7)	1 (25)	
III	28 (66.7)	24 (64.8)	4 (75)	0.753[¥]
Hysterectomy* (yes/no)	14/16	11/16	3/0	0.090[¥]
Genital prolapse* (Y/N)	8/22	7/20	1/2	0.954[¥]
Incontinence (yes/no)	15/27	13/24	2/3	0.831[¥]
Constipation (yes/no)	7/35	4/33	3/2	0.026[¥]
Prolapse size				
<5 cms (%)	24 (57)	23 (61)	1 (20)	
>5 cms (%)	18 (43)	14 (39)	4 (80)	0.138[¥]
Anaesthesia (spinal/gral.)	31/11	30/7	1/4	0.013[¥]
Levatorplasty (yes/no)*	7/23	7/20	0/3	0.010[¥]
Median hospital stay (days)	5	5	5	0.269[£]
Median follow-up (months)	85	104	43	0.144[£]
Complications (yes/no)	4/38	3/34	1/4	0.410[¥]

*Data for 30 women; [£]Mann-Whitney; [¥]Chi^2.

TABLE 2: Multivariate analysis.

	Total ($n = 42$)	No recurrence ($n = 37$)	Recurrence ($n = 5$)	p value	OR (IC 95%)
Anaesthesia (spinal/general)	31/11	30/7	1/4	0.047[¥]	0.07 (0.005–0.949)
Constipation (yes/no)	7/35	4/33	3/2	0.228[¥]	0.21 (0.017–2.656)
Prolapse size					
<5 cms (%)	24 (57)	23 (61)	1 (20)		
>5 cms (%)	18 (43)	14 (39)	4 (80)	0.483[¥]	0.414 (0.035–4.858)
Levatorplasty (yes/no)*	7/23	7/20	0/3	1[¥]	0.464 (0–)
Hysterectomy* (yes/no)	14/16	11/16	3/0	1[¥]	0.730 (0–)

*Data for 30 women; [£]Mann-Whitney; [¥]Chi^2.

a long median follow-up of seven years. Actuarial recurrence at five years was 9.9%. According to the univariate analysis, constipation and concomitant pelvic floor repair were the only factors found to be associated with recurrence, the former increasing the risk for recurrence and the latter reducing it. However, when multivariate analysis was performed these factors lost their individual influence.

The main limitation of this study is that it is a retrospective and observational study and some final controls were performed by the patient's general practitioner. On the other hand, the main strengths of this study are the long follow-up period, with a median follow-up above seven years, and the low levels of censored data during the study period. This is of special note since the recurrence rates reported in the literature are 47% lower as compared to those reported in an independent review [10].

Different factors have been reported to be associated with recurrence. Early recurrence seems to be clearly related to the execution of the technique and case selection. Two patients had recurrence within six months following surgery, may be due to defects of the technique or to underestimation of the prolapse. Partial resection of the prolapsed mucosa or a large prolapse requiring long muscle repair surgery may play a role in early recurrence.

Late recurrence is usually constant over the years. Variability of recurrence rates may be due to different size of the prolapses, associated pelvic disorders, follow-up periods, reinterventions, constipation, and case-mix [11, 12].

The two pathogenic factors associated with the development of complete rectal prolapse are recto-rectal invagination and a perineal herniation through a deep cul-de-sac of Douglas. It should be elucidated if the modification of these

TABLE 3: Functional outcomes of Delorme's procedure.

	Total (n = 42)	No recurrence (n = 37)	Recurrence (n = 5)	p value
Constipation (Wexner)	7/35	4/33	3/2	0.026[¥]
Baseline (median, IR)	16.28 (8–21)	14.82 (6–19)	14.40 (8–19)	
Postoperative (median, IR)	12.82 (8–18)	13.82 (6–19)	11.33 (5–18)	
Incontinence (Wexner)	15/27	13/24	2/3	0.831[£]
Baseline (median, IR)	7.9 (4–12)	7.8 (4–12)	7.9 (4–12)	
Postoperative (median, IR)	7.4 (4–11)	7.6 (4–12)	7.4 (4–11)	

[£]Mann-Whitney; [¥]Chi^2.

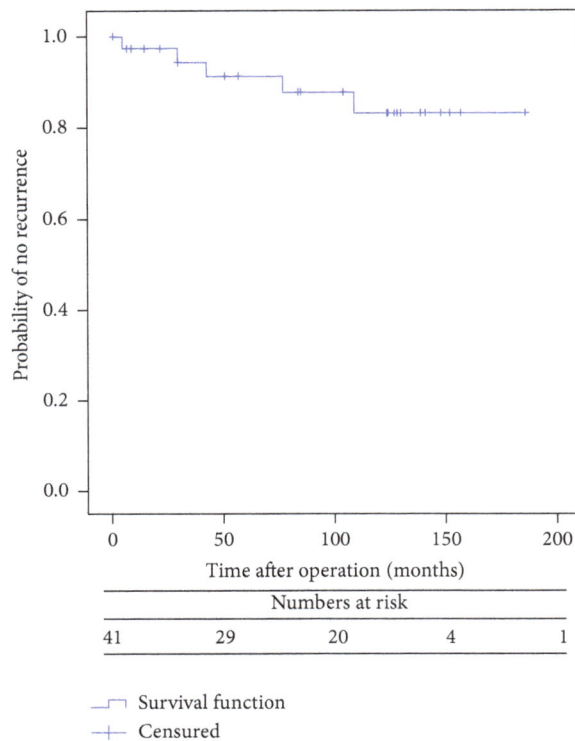

Numbers at risk				
41	29	20	4	1

⊓ Survival function
+ Censored

FIGURE 1: Probability of no recurrence after Delorme procedure (Global series).

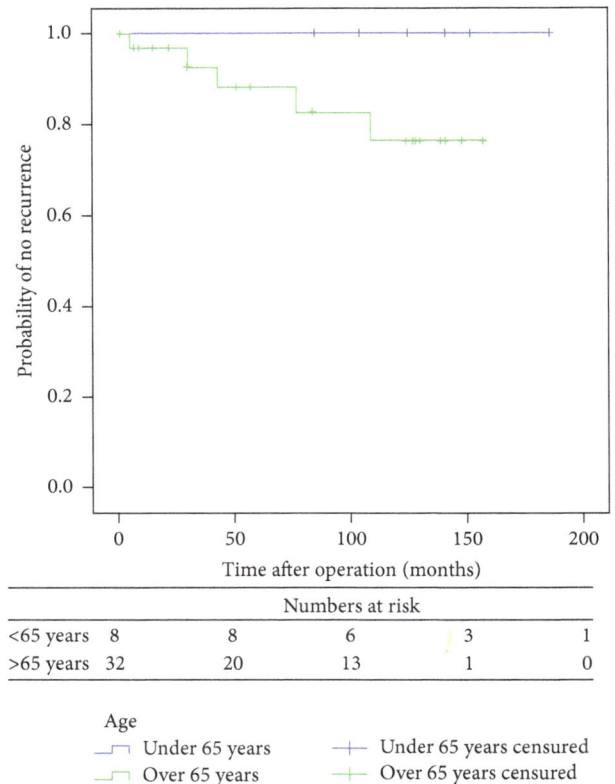

Numbers at risk				
<65 years	8	8	6	3	1
>65 years	32	20	13	1	0

Age
⊓ Under 65 years   + Under 65 years censored
⊓ Over 65 years   + Over 65 years censored

FIGURE 2: Comparison of probability of no recurrence with time for patients according to age (Kaplan-Meier method).

pathogenic factors through perineal surgery may have an influence on long-term outcomes.

Recurrence was not observed in any of the seven women who underwent concomitant posterior or total levatorplasty (7/30). Although differences were not statistically significant probably due to the small sample size, these results are consistent with those reported in the literature [8, 12, 13]. Youssef et al. conducted the only controlled randomized trial performed with 82 patients and found that complete anterior and posterior levatorplasty reduced recurrence from 14.28% to 2.43% [14]. Pelvic floor repair does not seem to influence invagination as a pathogenic mechanism. However, myorrhaphy and elevation of levator ani muscles may delay or prevent the formation of a new peritoneocele and hinder the descent of the longitudinal plication in Delorme's procedure.

To avoid the protrusion of the apex of prolapses repaired by Delorme's procedure, Williams et al. designed the so-called express procedure by which rectal suspension is achieved using collagen strips [15]. The same conclusions can be drawn from other series treated with modified Altemeier's procedure combined with levatorplasty, although this technique can also avoid the "cul-de-sac of Douglas as a pathogenic factor" [16].

Many authors agree that the low recurrence rates among younger patients undergoing Delorme's procedure are due to the good state of their pelvic floor musculature as compared to elderly patients, who have a weak pelvic floor [17]. None of our patients aged <65 years had recurrence, but statistically significant differences were not observed

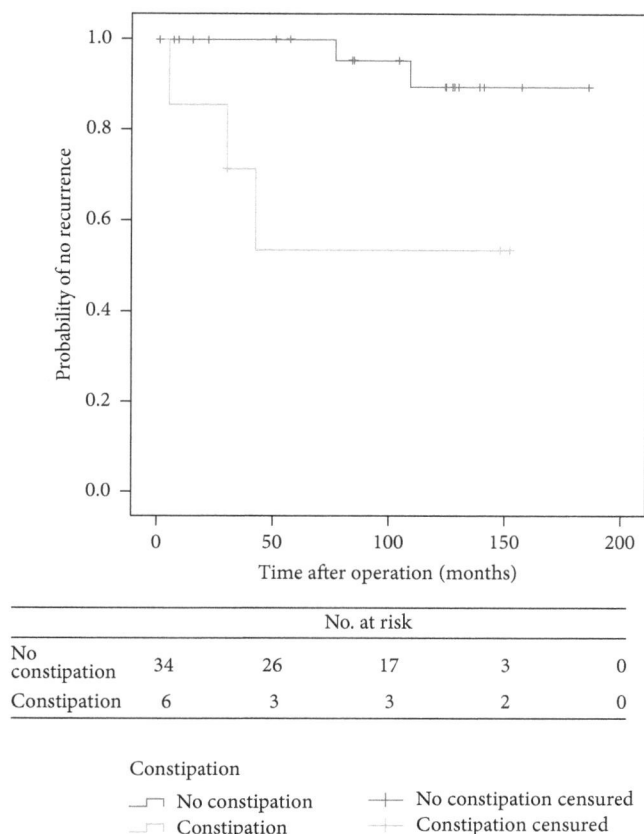

			No. at risk		
No constipation	34	26	17	3	0
Constipation	6	3	3	2	0

Constipation

⊓ No constipation   + No constipation censured
⊓ Constipation   + Constipation censured

FIGURE 3: Comparison of probability of no recurrence with time for patients according to constipation (Kaplan-Meier method).

due to the small sample size. As in our study, persistent constipation is considered a risk factor for recurrence in the literature. Although constipation improved in most patients as evidenced by a lower Wexner score, patients with persistent constipation are at a higher risk of early recurrence. Delorme's procedure improves constipation, as it reduces compliance and improves rectal sensation [18, 19].

Delorme's procedure can be performed for both primary and recurrent prolapse with good outcomes and low technical complexity [20]. No recurrences were observed in the long term in the three patients who underwent reintervention with Delorme's procedure due to recurrence.

Despite its methodological limitations, the recent multicenter controlled study Prosper has rekindled the debate about the effectiveness of the perineal approach [21]. However, this study shows that outcomes seem to depend more on the ability of the surgeon who performs the operation compared to the approach selected.

Although the preferred procedure for rectal prolapse in our Unit is laparoscopic ventral rectopexy, we consider perineal approach useful for particular cases of reintervention, high BMI, small prolapse, and absence of bowel dysfunction. In our opinion, age or surgical risk should not discourage an abdominal approach. A recent survey performed on the American College of Surgeons National Surgical Quality Improvement Program (NSQIP) revealed that the morbidity

and mortality of laparoscopic surgery were similar to those of perineal surgery in elderly patients [22].

On the other hand, anterior and posterior repair of the pelvic floor should be systematically performed in all women requiring surgery for rectal prolapse in order to reduce recurrence rates in these patients. Patients with severe constipation are not ideal candidates for this technique unless abdominal surgery is not indicated for particular reasons. Young males undergoing surgery for rectal prolapse should be informed that abdominal surgery might cause pelvic nerve damage.

Conflict of Interests

The authors declare that there is no conflict of interests regarding the publication of this paper.

References

[1] T. E. Madiba, S. D. Wexner, and M. K. Baig, "Surgical management of rectal prolapse," *Archives of Surgery*, vol. 140, no. 1, pp. 63–73, 2005.

[2] C. B. Samaranayake, C. Luo, A. W. Plank, A. E. Merrie, L. D. Plank, and I. P. Bissett, "Systematic review on ventral rectopexy for rectal prolapse and intussusception," *Colorectal Disease*, vol. 12, no. 6, pp. 504–512, 2010.

[3] A. D'Hoore, R. Cadoni, and F. Penninckx, "Long-term outcome of laparoscopic ventral rectopexy for total rectal prolapse," *British Journal of Surgery*, vol. 91, no. 11, pp. 1500–1505, 2004.

[4] S. R. Brown, "The evidence base for rectal prolapse surgery: is resection rectopexy worth the risk?" *Techniques in Coloproctology*, vol. 18, no. 3, pp. 221–222, 2014.

[5] S. Lee, B.-H. Kye, H.-J. Kim, H.-M. Cho, and J.-G. Kim, "Delorme's procedure for complete rectal prolapse: does it still have it's own role?" *Journal of the Korean Society of Coloproctology*, vol. 28, no. 1, pp. 13–18, 2012.

[6] S. Tou, S. R. Brown, A. I. Malik, and R. L. Nelson, "Surgery for complete rectal prolapse in adults," *Cochrane Database of Systematic Reviews*, no. 4, Article ID CD001758, 2008.

[7] E. Delorme, "Sur le traitement des prolapsus du rectum totaux, par l'excision de la muqueuse rectale ou rectocolique," *Bulletin et Mémoires de la Société des Chirurgiens de Paris*, vol. 26, pp. 499–518, 1900.

[8] J. P. Lechaux, D. Lechaux, and M. Perez, "Results of Delorme's procedure for rectal prolapse: advantages of a modified technique," *Diseases of the Colon & Rectum*, vol. 38, no. 3, pp. 301–307, 1995.

[9] J. M. N. Jorge and S. D. Wexner, "Etiology and management of fecal incontinence," *Diseases of the Colon & Rectum*, vol. 36, no. 1, pp. 77–97, 1993.

[10] G. DiGiuro, D. Ignjatovic, J. Brogger, and R. Bergamaschi, "How accurate are published recurrence rates after rectal prolapse surgery? A meta-analysis of individual patient data," *American Journal of Surgery*, vol. 191, no. 6, pp. 773–778, 2006.

[11] A. M. I. Watts and M. R. Thompson, "Evaluation of Delorme's procedure as a treatment for full-thickness rectal prolapse," *British Journal of Surgery*, vol. 87, no. 2, pp. 218–222, 2000.

[12] B. P. Watkins, J. Landercasper, G. E. Belzer et al., "Long-term follow-up of the modified Delorme procedure for rectal prolapse," *Archives of Surgery*, vol. 138, no. 5, pp. 498–503, 2003.

[13] A. H. ElGadaa, N. Hamrah, and Y. AlAshry, "Complete rectal prolapse in adults: clinical and functional results of Delorme procedure combined with postanal repair," *Indian Journal of Surgery*, vol. 72, no. 6, pp. 443–447, 2010.

[14] M. Youssef, W. Thabet, A. El Nakeeb et al., "Comparative study between Delorme operation with or without postanal repair and levateroplasty in treatment of complete rectal prolapse," *International Journal of Surgery*, vol. 11, no. 1, pp. 52–58, 2013.

[15] N. S. Williams, P. Giordano, L. S. Dvorkin, A. Huang, F. H. Hetzer, and S. M. Scott, "External pelvic rectal suspension (the express procedure) for full-thickness rectal prolapse: evolution of a new technique," *Diseases of the Colon & Rectum*, vol. 48, no. 2, pp. 307–316, 2005.

[16] S. W. Chun, A. J. Pikarsky, S. Y. You et al., "Perineal rectosigmoidectomy for rectal prolapse: role of levatorplasty," *Techniques in Coloproctology*, vol. 8, no. 1, pp. 3–9, 2004.

[17] Y. H. Hwang, "Role of the Delorme procedure for rectal prolapse in young patients," *Annals of Coloproctology*, vol. 29, article 41, 2013.

[18] A. Tsunoda, N. Yasuda, N. Yokoyama, G. Kamiyama, and M. Kusano, "Delorme's procedure for rectal prolapse: clinical and physiological analysis," *Diseases of the Colon and Rectum*, vol. 46, no. 9, pp. 1260–1265, 2003.

[19] M. Lieberth, L. A. Kondylis, J. C. Reilly, and P. D. Kondylis, "The Delorme repair for full-thickness rectal prolapse: a retrospective review," *The American Journal of Surgery*, vol. 197, no. 3, pp. 418–423, 2009.

[20] A. J. Pikarsky, J. S. Joo, S. D. Wexner et al., "Recurrent rectal prolapse. What is the next good option?" *Diseases of the Colon and Rectum*, vol. 43, no. 9, pp. 1273–1276, 2000.

[21] A. Senapati, R. G. Gray, L. J. Middleton et al., "PROSPER: a randomised comparison of surgical treatments for rectal prolapse," *Colorectal Disease*, vol. 15, no. 7, pp. 858–868, 2013.

[22] M. T. Young, M. D. Jafari, M. J. Phelan et al., "Surgical treatments for rectal prolapse: how does a perineal approach compare in the laparoscopic era?" *Surgical Endoscopy*, vol. 29, no. 3, pp. 607–613, 2015.

Surgical Management of Endometrial Polyps in Infertile Women: A Comprehensive Review

Nigel Pereira,[1] **Allison C. Petrini,**[2] **Jovana P. Lekovich,**[1] **Rony T. Elias,**[1] **and Steven D. Spandorfer**[1]

[1]*The Ronald O. Perelman and Claudia Cohen Center for Reproductive Medicine, Weill Cornell Medical College, 1305 York Avenue, 6th Floor, New York, NY 10021, USA*
[2]*Department of Obstetrics and Gynecology, Weill Cornell Medical College, 1305 York Avenue, 6th Floor, New York, NY 10021, USA*

Correspondence should be addressed to Steven D. Spandorfer; sdspando@med.cornell.edu

Academic Editor: Giampiero Capobianco

Endometrial polyps are benign localized lesions of the endometrium, which are commonly seen in women of reproductive age. Observational studies have suggested a detrimental effect of endometrial polyps on fertility. The natural course of endometrial polyps remains unclear. Expectant management of small and asymptomatic polyps is reasonable in many cases. However, surgical resection of endometrial polyps is recommended in infertile patients prior to treatment in order to increase natural conception or assisted reproductive pregnancy rates. There is mixed evidence regarding the resection of newly diagnosed endometrial polyps during ovarian stimulation to improve the outcomes of fresh in vitro fertilization cycles. Hysteroscopy polypectomy remains the gold standard for surgical treatment. Evidence regarding the cost and efficacy of different methods for hysteroscopic resection of endometrial polyps in the office and outpatient surgical settings has begun to emerge.

1. Introduction

The interaction between an embryo and a receptive endometrium forms a critical part of early implantation subsequently allowing for placentation and continuation of a healthy pregnancy [1, 2]. It is believed that intrauterine abnormalities, such as polyps, leiomyomata, or synechiae, may perturb this important event [2, 3]. Although isolated uterine-associated infertility can be found in 2-3% of infertile women [4], intrauterine lesions may be found in approximately 40–50% of subfertile or infertile women [4–6]. Lesions such as endometrial polyps have previously been implicated in the pathogenesis of subfertility and early pregnancy loss, though this association is sometimes debated [5, 6]. Previous observational studies have suggested that resection of endometrial polyps can help increase natural conception rates as well as increase pregnancy rates with assisted reproduction [4]. In this paper, we review the epidemiology, pathogenesis, diagnosis and management of endometrial polyps in infertile women. We also critically evaluate the current evidence related to resection of endometrial polyps and its impact on natural conception and assisted reproductive pregnancy rates.

2. Epidemiology

Endometrial polyps are benign localized outgrowths of the endometrium that contain glands and stroma [5, 7]. They may occur as single or multiple lesions, can be sessile or pedunculated, and may range in size from millimeters to centimeters [2, 7]. Occasionally, endometrial polyps may contain smooth muscle fibers in addition to glands and stroma and are called adenomyomatous polyps [8]. The true incidence of endometrial polyps remains unknown incidence due to its asymptomatic nature [9]. However, depending on the type of population studied, the prevalence of endometrial polyps can vary from 7.8% to 34.9% [10, 11]. Some studies have reported that endometrial polyps can be found in up to 24% of symptomatic women [12, 13]. The prevalence of endometrial polyps is thought to be higher in infertile women [9]. In a prospective study of 1000 patients undergoing hysteroscopic evaluation of the uterine cavity prior to in vitro fertilization (IVF), the prevalence of endometrial polyps was found to be 32% [14]. While this may suggest a causal association between polyps and infertility, this association has been confirmed in only one randomized control trial so far [15].

3. Pathogenesis

Endometrial polyps are rarely diagnosed before menarche [16] suggesting that estrogenic stimulation of the endometrium plays a crucial role in the pathogenesis of endometrial polyps [17]. As these polyps contain immature or functional endometrium, they can develop in conditions associated with increased or unopposed estradiol levels, as in the case of ovarian stimulation during IVF [18]. Age, hypertension, obesity, and diabetes are well known risk factors for the development of endometrial polyps [19, 20]. Of these risk factors, age is perhaps the most well-known risk factor [9]. The prevalence of endometrial polyps increases with age, though it is unclear whether this trend continues past menopause [9]. There also appears to be an association between endometrial polyps and other benign gynecologic conditions such as cervical polyps and endometriosis [21, 22]. Women using tamoxifen are also known to have a higher risk of developing endometrial polyps, and the prevalence of polyps in this patient population is estimated to be between 30 and 60% [23]. Molecular mechanisms such as the overexpression of estrogen and progesterone receptors [24], endometrial aromatase [25, 26], increased B-cell lymphoma 2 protein expression [27], and mutations in the *HMGIC* and *HMGI[Y]* genes [28, 29] have also been implicated in the development of endometrial polyps. Atypical hyperplasia and endometrial cancer may arise in up to 6.7% and 2.2% of endometrial polyps, respectively [30–33]. The risk of malignancy increases with age [9], polyp size [34], and concomitant use of tamoxifen [35].

4. Diagnosis

Patients with symptomatic endometrial polyps usually present with abnormal uterine bleeding [36]. However, a large majority of polyps are asymptomatic and are incidentally discovered [2, 9]. The diagnostic modalities that are commonly utilized to diagnose endometrial polyps include 2-dimensional transvaginal sonography (2D TVUS), 3-dimensional transvaginal sonography (3D TVUS), saline infusion sonography (SIS), hysterosalpingography (HSG), and hysteroscopy [37].

4.1. 2-Dimensional Transvaginal Sonography. An endometrial polyp usually appears as a hyperechoic endometrial mass with regular contours occupying the uterine cavity either partially or fully [15]. Occasionally, cystic spaces may appear within the polyp [38]. Performing sonography in the proliferative phase of the menstrual cycle often provides the most reliable results [39]. 2D TVUS, in experienced hands, can detect endometrial polyps accurately [40]. In a large study of 793 women, the sensitivity, specificity, positive predictive value (PPV), and negative predictive value (NPV) of 2D TVUS in detecting endometrial polyps were found to be 86%, 94%, 91%, and 90%, respectively [41]. The addition of color-flow Doppler can improve the diagnostic capability of 2D TVUS by allowing visualization of the single feeding vessel present in endometrial polyps [9]. Color-flow Doppler, in some studies, has shown to increase the sensitivity of 2D TVUS from 91% to 97% [42].

4.2. 3-Dimensional Transvaginal Sonography. Compared to 2D sonography, 3D TVUS with color-flow Doppler allows for the measurement of endometrial volume, as well as endometrial and subendometrial vascularization indices [43, 44]. Some studies have suggested that using a combination of endometrial echogenicity, thickness, and volume with 3D TVUS may be better than single measurements with 2D TVUS for detecting endometrial polyps [43]. In contrast, others have shown that noncontrast 3D TVUS does not necessarily increase detection of endometrial polyps compared to 2D TVUS [45].

4.3. Saline Infusion Sonography. The addition of intrauterine contrast (saline or gel) increases the diagnostic accuracy of 2D TVUS and 3D TVUS [9]. Additional advantages of SIS include assessment of other uterine cavity abnormalities such as leiomyomata or adhesions and assessment of Müllerian anomalies, if needed [37, 46, 47]. Disadvantages of SIS are related to its learning curve [48] and patient discomfort caused by fluid instillation or leakage [49], as well as the theoretical risk of infection [50]. In a recent systematic review and meta-analysis of 20 studies comparing the diagnostic accuracy of SIS to hysteroscopy, the pooled sensitivity and specificity of SIS in the detection of all intrauterine abnormalities were 88% (95% confidence interval [CI]: 85%–90%) and 94% (95% CI 93%–96%), respectively [37]. Overall, most studies reveal no significant difference between SIS and diagnostic hysteroscopy in diagnosing endometrial polyps [37]. Comparisons between 2D SIS and 3D SIS have also been made [51, 52]. In one such study [51], the sensitivity, specificity, PPV, and NPV for 2D SIS in detecting intrauterine lesions were found to be 71.2%, 94.1%, 90.2%, and 81.0%, respectively. The overall accuracy was 84.2%. For 3D SIS, the sensitivity was 94.2%, specificity 98.5%, positive predictive value 98.0%, negative predictive value 95.7%, and overall accuracy 96.7%. The investigators concluded that 3D SIS was superior to 2D SIS and was comparable to hysteroscopy in diagnosing intrauterine lesions.

4.4. Hysterosalpingography. HSG allows imaging of the cervical canal, uterine cavity, and fallopian tubes with injection of contrast media using fluoroscopic visualization [53]. In general, the cervical canal or endometrial cavity is accessed using aseptic technique [53]. A small volume (10–30 mL) of contrast agent is administered under intermittent fluoroscopy to visualize the structures to be imaged [53]. Occasionally, postdrainage images can be obtained when endometrial pathology is suspected [53]. HSG has high sensitivity (98%) but low specificity (34.6%) and PPV (28.6%) compared with hysteroscopy for endometrial polyps [54, 55].

4.5. Hysteroscopy. Hysteroscopy with guided biopsy is considered the gold standard for diagnosing endometrial polyps [9, 56]. Hysteroscopy also facilitates assessment of size, number, and vascular characteristics of endometrial polyps [9]. Prior to the routine use of hysteroscopy, blind dilation and curettage were used for the diagnosis of endometrial polyps [57]. This technique, however, caused polyp fragmentation making histopathologic diagnosis difficult [58]. The low sensitivity of 8% to 46% and NPV of 7% to 58% of blind endometrial sampling compared to hysteroscopy with guided biopsy [59] suggests that the former technique should not be used for diagnosing endometrial polyps.

5. Treatment Options

5.1. Expectant Management. The natural course of endometrial polyps is not well understood [13, 60]. Given that most polyps are benign, expectant management is a reasonable option in asymptomatic premenopausal women [9]. Small endometrial polyps (<10 mm) are thought to regress spontaneously in about 25% of cases [61, 62].

5.2. Medical Management. There is limited role of medical management for endometrial polyps [9, 62]. Levonorgestrel containing intrauterine devices have been used to reduce the incidence of tamoxifen-related endometrial polyps in some research settings [63]. Gonadotropin releasing hormone agonists have also been used as an adjunctive treatment before hysteroscopic resection [64]. However, there is little-to-no data supporting its utility as a first-line agent for treating endometrial polyps [62, 64].

5.3. Surgical Management. While endometrial polyps may resolve spontaneously and could possibly be amenable to hormonal therapy, definitive treatment options are largely surgical. Blind dilation and curettage can remove endometrial polyps in up to 8% of patients [9]. Addition of polyp forceps increases complete extraction of polyps in approximately 41% of patients [9]. In general, blind dilation and curettage can miss endometrial pathology in approximately 50% of cases and should therefore be avoided when hysteroscopy is available [57–59].

Hysteroscopic polypectomy remains the gold standard for both the diagnosis and treatment of endometrial polyps [9]. The choice of performing hysteroscopy in the office or outpatient surgical setting is generally dependent on patient preference, physician skill, and instrument availability [9, 65]. While equivalent success rates have been reported in both settings, some data indicate that failure to remove a polyp is more likely in the office setting [65]. In contrast, other data suggest that office-based hysteroscopic polypectomy is safe and feasible in patients with endometrial or isthmic polyps

< or = 20 mm, independent of menopausal status or previous vaginal delivery [66].

Several hysteroscopic systems to resect endometrial polyps are currently available, monopolar loop cautery [9], bipolar systems [67], microscissors or graspers [9], and hysteroscopic morcellators [68, 69]. Of these, the monopolar loop is more commonly available and of lower cost [9]. Comparative studies about the aforementioned methods with regard to costs and efficacy have recently begun to emerge. For example, in a prospective, randomized study of 100 patients comparing monopolar to bipolar electrode excision of endometrial polyps, the former technique was found to be better for nonfundal polyps or those >20 mm compared to the latter technique, which was better for small, fundal polyps [70]. In another randomized study of 121 patients, removal of polyps using a hysteroscopic morcellator was found to be significantly quicker, less painful, more acceptable to women, and more likely to completely remove endometrial polyps compared to electrosurgical resection [71]. It is important to note that none of these studies were performed in infertile patients. The overall method of hysteroscopy polypectomy is generally the one which the clinician is trained with and most familiar with [9]. The risk of intrauterine adhesions after hysteroscopy polypectomy is low as the myometrium is generally not incised [72]. Other procedural risks associated with hysteroscopy polypectomy include infection, surgical bleeding, uterine perforation, fluid overload, or anesthesia-related complications.

6. Impact on Fertility

The putative mechanisms by which endometrial polyps adversely impact fertility may be related to mechanical interference with sperm transportation or as space occupying lesions interfering with embryo implantation [5]. The glands and stroma in endometrial polyps are unresponsive to progesterone stimulation, leading to defective implantation at the site of the polyp [8]. Endometrial polyps may also induce local inflammatory changes, which can interfere with normal implantation and embryonic development [6, 73]. These inflammatory changes are mediated by increased number of mast cells in the endometrial cavity [74], as well as increased levels of matrix metalloproteinase-2 and metalloproteinase-9 [75]. Endometrial polyps can produce glycodelin, a glycoprotein that has been shown to inhibit natural killer cell activity, rendering the endometrium less receptive to implantation [2, 76]. It is also speculated that endometrial polyps decrease messenger RNA levels of *HOXA10* and *HOXA11*, which are known molecular markers of endometrial receptivity [7].

6.1. Natural Conception. Previous observational studies have shown that resection of endometrial polyps can improve natural conception rates, particularly in patients with unexplained infertility [3, 5]. In one retrospective study of 78 patients, a pregnancy rate of 78.3% was noted after polypectomy compared to a pregnancy rate 42.1% in patients with normal uterine cavities [77]. Similarly, natural conception rates of 76% [73] and 50% [78] were reported after resection of endometrial polyps. In subfertile women, hysteroscopic polypectomy can improve fertility, with pregnancy rates ranging from 43% to 80% [73, 79].

6.2. Intrauterine Insemination. Studies have shown that pregnancy rates are improved in patients undergoing polypectomy before undergoing intrauterine insemination (IUI) [2]. In one prospective randomized study involving 215 patients, patients who underwent polypectomy prior to IUI had an increased pregnancy rate (51.4%) compared to patients who did not (25.4%) [15]. These findings were similar to another independent study, which reported pregnancy rates of 40.7% and 22.3% in patients who did and did not undergo polypectomy before IUI, respectively [80]. Hysteroscopic resection of endometrial polyps (~16 mm) prior to IUI for unexplained male or female factor has also been shown to increase the odds of clinical pregnancy (odds ratio 4.4, 95% CI 2.5–8.0) for at least 2 years, compared to diagnostic hysteroscopy and polyp biopsy alone [81].

6.3. In Vitro Fertilization. Current evidence supports the resection of endometrial polyps diagnosed prior to commencement of IVF cycles [6]. The time interval between hysteroscopic resection of polyps and the subsequent IVF cycle does not seem to impact the success rates of the IVF cycle [82]. However, the management of newly diagnosed endometrial polyps during ovarian stimulation still remains controversial [2, 5]. Some studies have shown that resection of newly diagnosed endometrial polyps during COH can decrease rates of pregnancy loss [18] and increase clinical pregnancy [83, 84] and live birth rates [77], while others have shown no such benefits [85, 86]. In one of the earliest studies, 83 patients with polyps <20 mm diagnosed during ovarian stimulation were divided into two groups [18]. The first group (49 patients) underwent IVF with fresh embryo transfer (ET), while the second group (34 patients) underwent hysteroscopic polypectomy immediately after oocyte retrieval. The cryopreserved embryos were thawed and transferred in a subsequent cycle. No difference in pregnancy rates was noted between the two groups. At least 2 other studies have confirmed the aforementioned findings [85, 86]. These findings suggest that endometrial polyps <20 mm during fresh IVF-ET cycles can be managed expectantly without compromising clinical pregnancy or live birth rates [2]. This was further confirmed by a retrospective study that showed no difference in the implantation, clinical pregnancy, or live birth rates after fresh IVF-ET cycles when patients with newly diagnosed endometrial polyps were compared to those with normal endometrial stripes [87]. Most recently, our group [2] reported that newly diagnosed endometrial polyps (<20 mm) during ovarian stimulation are associated with an increased biochemical pregnancy rate, without adversely impacting clinical pregnancy or live birth rates after fresh IVF cycles. Thus, one may hypothesize that small endometrial polyps can create a hostile environment for early embryo development; however, if the embryo does overcome this initial insult, the risk of future miscarriage is primarily related to embryonic aneuploidy or other endometrial factors [2].

7. Conclusions

Endometrial polyps are commonly seen in infertile women [6]. The overall evidence suggests a detrimental effect of polyps on fertility [6]. Conservative management of small and asymptomatic polyps is reasonable in most cases [9]. However, surgical resection of endometrial polyps is recommended in infertile patients to possibly increase natural conception and assisted reproductive pregnancy rates [9]. Hysteroscopic polypectomy remains the gold standard for surgical treatment, though evidence regarding the cost and efficacy of different methods for hysteroscopic resection of polyps in the inpatient and outpatient settings has begun to emerge. Management of newly diagnosed endometrial polyps during IVF should be individualized according to the patient's reproductive history, polyp size and location, ovarian stimulation response, the number of good quality embryos, and the individual clinic's success rate with cryopreserved embryo transfer [2, 6].

Conflict of Interests

The authors declare that there is no conflict of interests regarding the publication of this paper.

References

[1] E. R. Norwitz, D. J. Schust, and S. J. Fisher, "Implantation and the survival of early pregnancy," *The New England Journal of Medicine*, vol. 345, no. 19, pp. 1400–1408, 2001.

[2] R. T. Elias, N. Pereira, F. S. Karipcin, Z. Rosenwaks, and S. D. Spandorfer, "Impact of newly diagnosed endometrial polyps during controlled ovarian hyperstimulation on in vitro fertilization outcomes," *Journal of Minimally Invasive Gynecology*, vol. 22, no. 4, pp. 590–594, 2015.

[3] J. Bosteels, J. Kasius, S. Weyers, F. J. Broekmans, B. W. J. Mol, and T. M. D'Hooghe, "Hysteroscopy for treating subfertility associated with suspected major uterine cavity abnormalities," *Cochrane Database of Systematic Reviews*, no. 2, Article ID CD009461, 2015.

[4] M. M. Carneiro, "What is the role of hysteroscopic surgery in the management of female infertility? A review of the literature," *Surgery Research and Practice*, vol. 2014, Article ID 105412, 6 pages, 2014.

[5] E. Taylor and V. Gomel, "The uterus and fertility," *Fertility and Sterility*, vol. 89, no. 1, pp. 1–16, 2008.

[6] K. Afifi, S. Anand, S. Nallapeta, and T. A. Gelbaya, "Management of endometrial polyps in subfertile women: a systematic review," *European Journal of Obstetrics & Gynecology and Reproductive Biology*, vol. 151, no. 2, pp. 117–121, 2010.

[7] B. W. Rackow, E. Jorgensen, and H. S. Taylor, "Endometrial polyps affect uterine receptivity," *Fertility and Sterility*, vol. 95, no. 8, pp. 2690–2692, 2011.

[8] K. Mittal, L. Schwartz, S. Goswami, and R. Demopoulos, "Estrogen and progesterone receptor expression in endometrial polyps," *International Journal of Gynecological Pathology*, vol. 15, no. 4, pp. 345–348, 1996.

[9] American Association of Gynecologic Laparoscopists, "AAGL practice report: practice guidelines for the diagnosis and management of endometrial polyps," *Journal of Minimally Invasive Gynecology*, vol. 19, no. 1, pp. 3–10, 2012.

[10] G. Silló-Seidl, "The analysis of the endometrium of 1,000 sterile women," *Hormones*, vol. 2, no. 2, pp. 70–75, 1971.

[11] M. Lieng, O. Istre, L. Sandvik, and E. Qvigstad, "Prevalence, 1-year regression rate, and clinical significance of asymptomatic endometrial polyps: cross-sectional study," *Journal of Minimally Invasive Gynecology*, vol. 16, no. 4, pp. 465–471, 2009.

[12] L.-J. Van Bogaert, "Clinicopathologic findings in endometrial polyps," *Obstetrics and Gynecology*, vol. 71, no. 5, pp. 771–773, 1988.

[13] R. Haimov-Kochman, R. Deri-Hasid, Y. Hamani, and E. Voss, "The natural course of endometrial polyps: could they vanish when left untreated?" *Fertility and Sterility*, vol. 92, no. 2, pp. 828.e11–828.e12, 2009.

[14] M. D. Hinckley and A. A. Milki, "1000 office-based hysteroscopies prior to *in vitro* fertilization: feasibility and findings," *Journal of the Society of Laparoendoscopic Surgeons*, vol. 8, no. 2, pp. 103–107, 2004.

[15] T. Pérez-Medina, J. Bajo-Arenas, F. Salazar et al., "Endometrial polyps and their implication in the pregnancy rates of patients undergoing intrauterine insemination: a prospective, randomized study," *Human Reproduction*, vol. 20, no. 6, pp. 1632–1635, 2005.

[16] E. Dreisler, S. Stampe Sorensen, P. H. Ibsen, and G. Lose, "Prevalence of endometrial polyps and abnormal uterine bleeding in a Danish population aged 20–74 years," *Ultrasound in Obstetrics and Gynecology*, vol. 33, no. 1, pp. 102–108, 2009.

[17] S. C. Lee, A. M. Kaunitz, L. Sanchez-Ramos, and R. M. Rhatigan, "The oncogenic potential of endometrial polyps: a systematic review and meta-analysis," *Obstetrics & Gynecology*, vol. 116, no. 5, pp. 1197–1205, 2010.

[18] A. Lass, G. Williams, N. Abusheikha, and P. Brinsden, "The effect of endometrial polyps on outcomes of in vitro fertilization (IVF) cycles," *Journal of Assisted Reproduction and Genetics*, vol. 16, no. 8, pp. 410–415, 1999.

[19] R. Onalan, G. Onalan, E. Tonguc, T. Ozdener, M. Dogan, and L. Mollamahmutoglu, "Body mass index is an independent risk factor for the development of endometrial polyps in patients undergoing in vitro fertilization," *Fertility and Sterility*, vol. 91, no. 4, pp. 1056–1060, 2009.

[20] L. Nappi, U. Indraccolo, A. D. S. Sardo et al., "Are diabetes, hypertension, and obesity independent risk factors for endometrial polyps?" *Journal of Minimally Invasive Gynecology*, vol. 16, no. 2, pp. 157–162, 2009.

[21] L.-C. F. Vilodre, R. Bertat, R. Petters, and F. M. Reis, "Cervical polyp as risk factor for hysteroscopically diagnosed endometrial polyps," *Gynecologic and Obstetric Investigation*, vol. 44, no. 3, pp. 191–195, 1997.

[22] J. H. McBean, M. Gibson, and J. R. Brumsted, "The association of intrauterine filling defects on hysterosalpingogram with endometriosis," *Fertility and Sterility*, vol. 66, no. 4, pp. 522–526, 1996.

[23] C. Exacoustos, E. Zupi, B. Cangi, M. Chiaretti, D. Arduini, and C. Romanini, "Endometrial evaluation in postmenopausal breast cancer patients receiving tamoxifen: an ultrasound, color flow Doppler, hysteroscopic and histological study," *Ultrasound in Obstetrics & Gynecology*, vol. 6, no. 6, pp. 435–442, 1995.

[24] C. Saccardi, S. Gizzo, K. Ludwig et al., "Endometrial polyps in women affected by levothyroxine-treated hypothyroidism—histological features, immunohistochemical findings, and possible explanation of etiopathogenic mechanism: a pilot study," *BioMed Research International*, vol. 2013, Article ID 503419, 5 pages, 2013.

[25] L. Pal, A. L. Niklaus, M. Kim, S. Pollack, and N. Santoro, "Heterogeneity in endometrial expression of aromatase in polyp-bearing uteri," *Human Reproduction*, vol. 23, no. 1, pp. 80–84, 2008.

[26] H. Maia Jr., K. Pimentel, T. M. Correia Silva et al., "Aromatase and cyclooxygenase-2 expression in endometrial polyps during the menstrual cycle," *Gynecological Endocrinology*, vol. 22, no. 4, pp. 219–224, 2006.

[27] A. Pinheiro, A. Antunes Jr., L. Andrade, L. De Brot, A. M. Pinto-Neto, and L. Costa-Paiva, "Expression of hormone receptors, Bcl-2, Cox-2 and Ki67 in benign endometrial polyps and their association with obesity," *Molecular Medicine Reports*, vol. 9, no. 6, pp. 2335–2341, 2014.

[28] P. dal Cin, S. Wanschura, B. Kazmierczak et al., "Amplification and expression of the HMGIC gene in a benign endometrial polyp," *Genes Chromosomes and Cancer*, vol. 22, no. 2, pp. 95–99, 1998.

[29] P. dal Cin, R. Vanni, S. Marras et al., "Four cytogenetic subgroups can be identified in endometrial polyps," *Cancer Research*, vol. 55, no. 7, pp. 1565–1568, 1995.

[30] A. Ben-Arie, C. Goldchmit, Y. Laviv et al., "The malignant potential of endometrial polyps," *European Journal of Obstetrics Gynecology and Reproductive Biology*, vol. 115, no. 2, pp. 206–210, 2004.

[31] A. Shushan, A. Revel, and N. Rojansky, "How often are endometrial polyps malignant?" *Gynecologic and Obstetric Investigation*, vol. 58, no. 4, pp. 212–215, 2004.

[32] S. H. Bakour, K. S. Khan, and J. K. Gupta, "The risk of premalignant and malignant pathology in endometrial polyps," *Acta Obstetricia et Gynecologica Scandinavica*, vol. 79, no. 4, pp. 317–320, 2000.

[33] E. Ferrazzi, E. Zupi, F. P. Leone et al., "How often are endometrial polyps malignant in asymptomatic postmenopausal women? A multicenter study," *American Journal of Obstetrics and Gynecology*, vol. 200, no. 3, pp. 235.e1–235.e6, 2009.

[34] A. Papadia, D. Gerbaldo, E. Fulcheri et al., "The risk of premalignant and malignant pathology in endometrial polyps: should every polyp be resected?" *Minerva Ginecologica*, vol. 59, no. 2, pp. 117–124, 2007.

[35] L. Bernstein, D. Deapen, J. R. Cerhan et al., "Tamoxifen therapy for breast cancer and endometrial cancer risk," *Journal of the National Cancer Institute*, vol. 91, no. 19, pp. 1654–1662, 1999.

[36] M. G. Munro, H. O. D. Critchley, M. S. Broder, and I. S. Fraser, "FIGO classification system (PALM-COEIN) for causes of abnormal uterine bleeding in nongravid women of reproductive age," *International Journal of Gynecology and Obstetrics*, vol. 113, no. 1, pp. 3–13, 2011.

[37] S. Seshadri, T. El-Toukhy, A. Douiri, K. Jayaprakasan, and Y. Khalaf, "Diagnostic accuracy of saline infusion sonography in the evaluation of uterine cavity abnormalities prior to assisted reproductive techniques: a systematic review and meta-analyses," *Human Reproduction Update*, vol. 21, no. 2, pp. 262–274, 2015.

[38] C. A. Hulka, D. A. Hall, K. McCarthy, and J. F. Simeone, "Endometrial polyps, hyperplasia, and carcinoma in postmenopausal women: differentiation with endovaginal sonography," *Radiology*, vol. 191, no. 3, pp. 755–758, 1994.

[39] K. M. Nalaboff, J. S. Pellerito, and E. Ben-Levi, "Imaging the endometrium: disease and normal variants," *Radiographics*, vol. 21, no. 6, pp. 1409–1424, 2001.

[40] J. Shalev, I. Meizner, I. Bar-Hava, D. Dicker, R. Mashiach, and Z. Ben-Rafael, "Predictive value of transvaginal sonography performed before routine diagnostic hysteroscopy for evaluation of infertility," *Fertility and Sterility*, vol. 73, no. 2, pp. 412–417, 2000.

[41] P. Vercellini, I. Cortesi, S. Oldani, M. Moschetta, O. De Giorgi, and P. G. Crosignani, "The role of transvaginal ultrasonography and outpatient diagnostic hysteroscopy in the evaluation of patients with menorrhagia," *Human Reproduction*, vol. 12, no. 8, pp. 1768–1771, 1997.

[42] A. Jakab, L. Óvári, B. Juhász, L. Birinyi, G. Bacskó, and Z. Tóth, "Detection of feeding artery improves the ultrasound diagnosis of endometrial polyps in asymptomatic patients," *European Journal of Obstetrics Gynecology and Reproductive Biology*, vol. 119, no. 1, pp. 103–107, 2005.

[43] L. Fang, Y. Su, Y. Guo, and Y. Sun, "Value of 3-dimensional and power Doppler sonography for diagnosis of endometrial polyps," *Journal of Ultrasound in Medicine*, vol. 32, no. 2, pp. 247–255, 2013.

[44] F. Ahmadi, F. Zafarani, H. Haghighi, M. Niknejadi, and A. V. T. Dizaj, "Application of 3D ultrasonography in detection of uterine abnormalities," *International Journal of Fertility and Sterility*, vol. 4, no. 4, pp. 144–147, 2011.

[45] R. La Torre, C. De Felice, C. De Angelis, F. Coacci, M. Mastrone, and E. V. Cosmi, "Transvaginal sonographic evaluation of endometrial polyps: a comparison with two dimensional and three dimensional contrast sonography," *Clinical and Experimental Obstetrics and Gynecology*, vol. 26, no. 3-4, pp. 171–173, 1999.

[46] N. Makris, N. Skartados, K. Kalmantis, G. Mantzaris, A. Papadimitriou, and A. Antsaklis, "Evaluation of abnormal uterine bleeding by transvaginal 3-D hysterosonography and diagnostic hysteroscopy," *European Journal of Gynaecological Oncology*, vol. 28, no. 1, pp. 39–42, 2007.

[47] F. W. Jansen, C. D. de Kroon, H. van Dongen, C. Grooters, L. Louwé, and T. Trimbos-Kemper, "Diagnostic hysteroscopy and saline infusion sonography: prediction of intrauterine polyps and myomas," *The Journal of Minimally Invasive Gynecology*, vol. 13, no. 4, pp. 320–324, 2006.

[48] N. Exalto, C. Stappers, L. A. M. van Raamsdonk, and M. H. Emanuel, "Gel instillation sonohysterography: first experience with a new technique," *Fertility and Sterility*, vol. 87, no. 1, pp. 152–155, 2007.

[49] C. H. Syrop and V. Sahakian, "Transvaginal sonographic detection of endometrial polyps with fluid contrast augmentation," *Obstetrics and Gynecology*, vol. 79, no. 6, pp. 1041–1043, 1992.

[50] V. I. Shavell, I. P. Le, and F. D. Yelian, "Tuboovarian abscess after saline infusion sonohysterography: an unusual complication," *Journal of Minimally Invasive Gynecology*, vol. 16, no. 5, pp. 652–654, 2009.

[51] W. El-Sherbiny, A. El-Mazny, N. Abou-Salem, and W. S. Mostafa, "The diagnostic accuracy of two- vs three-dimensional sonohysterography for evaluation of the uterine cavity in the reproductive age," *Journal of Minimally Invasive Gynecology*, vol. 22, no. 1, pp. 127–131, 2015.

[52] N. Abou-Salem, A. Elmazny, and W. El-Sherbiny, "Value of 3-dimensional sonohysterography for detection of intrauterine lesions in women with abnormal uterine bleeding," *The Journal of Minimally Invasive Gynecology*, vol. 17, no. 2, pp. 200–204, 2010.

[53] ACR Practice Parameter for the Performance of Hysterosalpingography Res. 50-2011, Amended 2014 (Res. 39), 2015, http://www.acr.org/Quality-Safety/Standards-Guidelines/Practice-Guidelines-by-Modality/Radiography.

[54] S. Preutthipan and V. Linasmita, "A prospective comparative study between hysterosalpingography and hysteroscopy in the detection of intrauterine pathology in patients with infertility," *Journal of Obstetrics and Gynaecology Research*, vol. 29, no. 1, pp. 33–37, 2003.

[55] S. R. Soares, M. M. B. B. Dos Reis, and A. F. Camargos, "Diagnostic accuracy of sonohysterography, transvaginal sonography, and hysterosalpingography in patients with uterine cavity diseases," *Fertility and Sterility*, vol. 73, no. 2, pp. 406–411, 2000.

[56] K. W. K. Lo and P. M. Yuen, "The role of outpatient diagnostic hysteroscopy in identifying anatomic pathology and histopathology in the endometrial cavity," *Journal of the American Association of Gynecologic Laparoscopists*, vol. 7, no. 3, pp. 381–385, 2000.

[57] R. J. Gimpelson and H. O. Rappold, "A comparative study between panoramic hysteroscopy with directed biopsies and dilatation and curettage. A review of 276 cases," *American Journal of Obstetrics and Gynecology*, vol. 158, no. 3, pp. 489–492, 1988.

[58] R. Svirsky, N. Smorgick, U. Rozowski et al., "Can we rely on blind endometrial biopsy for detection of focal intrauterine pathology?" *The American Journal of Obstetrics and Gynecology*, vol. 199, no. 2, pp. 115.e1–115.e3, 2008.

[59] S. Bettocchi, O. Ceci, M. Vicino, F. Marello, L. Impedovo, and L. Selvaggi, "Diagnostic inadequacy of dilatation and curettage," *Fertility and Sterility*, vol. 75, no. 4, pp. 803–805, 2001.

[60] D. J. DeWaay, C. H. Syrop, I. E. Nygaard, W. A. Davis, and B. J. Van Voorhis, "Natural history of uterine polyps and leiomyomata," *Obstetrics and Gynecology*, vol. 100, no. 1, pp. 3–7, 2002.

[61] Y. Hamani, I. Eldar, H. Y. Sela, E. Voss, and R. Haimov-Kochman, "The clinical significance of small endometrial polyps," *European Journal of Obstetrics Gynecology and Reproductive Biology*, vol. 170, no. 2, pp. 497–500, 2013.

[62] M. Lieng, O. Istre, and E. Qvigstad, "Treatment of endometrial polyps: a systematic review," *Acta Obstetricia et Gynecologica Scandinavica*, vol. 89, no. 8, pp. 992–1002, 2010.

[63] F. J. E. Gardner, J. C. Konje, S. C. Bell et al., "Prevention of tamoxifen induced endometrial polyps using a levonorgestrel releasing intrauterine system. Long-term follow-up of a randomised control trial," *Gynecologic Oncology*, vol. 114, no. 3, pp. 452–456, 2009.

[64] P. Vercellini, L. Trespidi, T. Bramante, S. Panazza, F. Mauro, and P. G. Crosignani, "Gonadotropin releasing hormone agonist treatment before hysteroscopic endometrial resection," *International Journal of Gynecology & Obstetrics*, vol. 45, no. 3, pp. 235–239, 1994.

[65] N. A. Cooper, T. J. Clark, L. Middleton et al., "Outpatient versus inpatient uterine polyp treatment for abnormal uterine bleeding: randomised controlled non-inferiority study," *British Medical Journal*, vol. 350, article h1398, 2015.

[66] P. Litta, E. Cosmi, C. Saccardi, C. Esposito, R. Rui, and G. Ambrosini, "Outpatient operative polypectomy using a 5 mm-hysteroscope without anaesthesia and/or analgesia: advantages and limits," *European Journal of Obstetrics Gynecology and Reproductive Biology*, vol. 139, no. 2, pp. 210–214, 2008.

[67] A. Golan, R. Sagiv, M. Berar, S. Ginath, and M. Glezerman, "Bipolar electrical energy in physiologic solution—a revolution in operative hysteroscopy," *Journal of the American Association of Gynecologic Laparoscopists*, vol. 8, no. 2, pp. 252–258, 2001.

[68] M. H. Emanuel and K. Wamsteker, "The Intra Uterine Morcellator: a new hysteroscopic operating technique to remove intrauterine polyps and myomas," *The Journal of Minimally Invasive Gynecology*, vol. 12, no. 1, pp. 62–66, 2005.

[69] H. van Dongen, M. H. Emanuel, R. Wolterbeek, J. B. Trimbos, and F. W. Jansen, "Hysteroscopic morcellator for removal of intrauterine polyps and myomas: a randomized controlled pilot study among residents in training," *The Journal of Minimally Invasive Gynecology*, vol. 15, no. 4, pp. 466–471, 2008.

[70] L. Muzii, F. Bellati, M. Pernice, N. Manci, R. Angioli, and P. B. Panici, "Resectoscopic versus bipolar electrode excision of endometrial polyps: a randomized study," *Fertility and Sterility*, vol. 87, no. 4, pp. 909–917, 2007.

[71] P. P. Smith, L. J. Middleton, M. Connor, and T. J. Clark, "Hysteroscopic morcellation compared with electrical resection of endometrial polyps: a randomized controlled trial," *Obstetrics and Gynecology*, vol. 123, no. 4, pp. 745–751, 2014.

[72] R. Deans and J. Abbott, "Review of intrauterine adhesions," *Journal of Minimally Invasive Gynecology*, vol. 17, no. 5, pp. 555–569, 2010.

[73] B. Śpiewankiewicz, J. Stelmachów, W. Sawicki, K. Cendrowski, P. Wypych, and K. Świderska, "The effectiveness of hysteroscopic polypectomy in cases of female infertility," *Clinical and Experimental Obstetrics & Gynecology*, vol. 30, no. 1, pp. 23–25, 2003.

[74] M. Al-Jefout, K. Black, L. Schulke et al., "Novel finding of high density of activated mast cells in endometrial polyps," *Fertility and Sterility*, vol. 92, no. 3, pp. 1104–1106, 2009.

[75] N. Inagaki, L. Ung, T. Otani, D. Wilkinson, and A. Lopata, "Uterine cavity matrix metalloproteinases and cytokines in patients with leiomyoma, adenomyosis or endometrial polyp," *European Journal of Obstetrics Gynecology and Reproductive Biology*, vol. 111, no. 2, pp. 197–203, 2003.

[76] S. S. Richlin, S. Ramachandran, A. Shanti, A. A. Murphy, and S. Parthasarathy, "Glycodelin levels in uterine flushings and in plasma of patients with leiomyomas and polyps: implications for implantation," *Human Reproduction*, vol. 17, no. 10, pp. 2742–2747, 2002.

[77] N. N. Varasteh, R. S. Neuwirth, B. Levin, and M. D. Keltz, "Pregnancy rates after hysteroscopic polypectomy and myomectomy in infertile women," *Obstetrics and Gynecology*, vol. 94, no. 2, pp. 168–171, 1999.

[78] T. A. Shokeir, H. M. Shalan, and M. M. El-Shafei, "Significance of endometrial polyps detected hysteroscopically in eumenorrheic infertile women," *Journal of Obstetrics and Gynaecology Research*, vol. 30, no. 2, pp. 84–89, 2004.

[79] R. F. Valle, "Therapeutic hysteroscopy in infertility," *International Journal of Fertility*, vol. 29, no. 3, pp. 143–148, 1984.

[80] T. Kalampokas, D. Tzanakaki, S. Konidaris, C. Iavazzo, E. Kalampokas, and O. Gregoriou, "Endometrial polyps and their relationship in the pregnancy rates of patients undergoing intrauterine insemination," *Clinical and Experimental Obstetrics and Gynecology*, vol. 39, no. 3, pp. 299–302, 2012.

[81] J. Bosteels, J. Kasius, S. Weyers, F. J. Broekmans, B. W. J. Mol, and T. M. D'Hooghe, "Treating suspected uterine cavity abnormalities by hysteroscopy to improve reproductive outcome in women with unexplained infertility or prior to IUI, IVF, or ICSI," *Gynecological Surgery*, vol. 10, no. 3, pp. 165–167, 2013.

[82] O. G. Eryilmaz, C. Gulerman, E. Sarikaya, H. Yesilyurt, F. Karsli, and N. Cicek, "Appropriate interval between endometrial polyp resection and the proceeding IVF start," *Archives of Gynecology and Obstetrics*, vol. 285, no. 6, pp. 1753–1757, 2012.

[83] I. Stamatellos, A. Apostolides, P. Stamatopoulos, and J. Bontis, "Pregnancy rates after hysteroscopic polypectomy depending on the size or number of the polyps," *Archives of Gynecology and Obstetrics*, vol. 277, no. 5, pp. 395–399, 2008.

[84] A. Yanaihara, T. Yorimitsu, H. Motoyama, S. Iwasaki, and T. Kawamura, "Location of endometrial polyp and pregnancy rate in infertility patients," *Fertility and Sterility*, vol. 90, no. 1, pp. 180–182, 2008.

[85] M. Isikoglu, Z. Berkkanoglu, Z. Senturk, K. Coetzee, and K. Ozgur, "Endomerial polyps smaller than 1.5 cm do not affect ICSI outcome," *Reproductive BioMedicine Online*, vol. 12, no. 2, pp. 199–204, 2006.

[86] B. Tiras, U. Korucuoglu, M. Polat, H. B. Zeyneloglu, A. Saltik, and H. Yarali, "Management of endometrial polyps diagnosed before or during ICSI cycles," *Reproductive BioMedicine Online*, vol. 24, no. 1, pp. 123–128, 2012.

[87] J. H. Check, C. A. Bostick-Smith, J. K. Choe, J. Amui, and D. Brasile, "Matched controlled study to evaluate the effect of endometrial polyps on pregnancy and implantation rates following in vitro fertilization-embryo transfer (IVF-ET)," *Clinical and Experimental Obstetrics and Gynecology*, vol. 38, no. 3, pp. 206–208, 2011.

Permissions

List of Contributors

Pınar Solmaz Hasdemir, Tevfik Guvenal, Hasan Tayfun Ozcakir, Faik Mumtaz Koyuncu, Mustafa Erkan and Semra Oruc Koltan
Department of Obstetrics and Gynecology, Celal Bayar University Medical School, 45000 Manisa, Turkey

Gonul Dinc Horasan
Department of Statistics, Celal Bayar University Medical School, Manisa, Turkey

Jan H. Koetje, Karsten D. Ottink, Iris Feenstra and Wilbert M. Fritschy
Department of Vascular Surgery, Isala Zwolle, 8025 AB Zwolle, Netherlands

Rati Agrawal, K. C. Sood and Bhupender Agarwal
DNB (General Surgery), Department of General Surgery, Maharaja Agrasen Hospital (MAH), New Delhi 110026, India

Sivakumar Sudhakaran
Texas A&M Health Science Center, 8447 State Highway 47, Bryan, TX 77807, USA

Salim R. Surani
Division of Pulmonary, Critical Care & Sleep Medicine, Texas A&M Health Science Center, Corpus Christi, 1177 West Wheeler Avenue, Suite 1, Aransas Pass, TX 78336, USA

Matthew Richardson, Jonathan Hayes, J. Randall Jordan and Matthew Fort
University of Mississippi Medical Center, Department of Otolaryngology and Communicative Sciences, 2500 N. State Street, Jackson, MS 39216, USA

Aaron Puckett
University of Mississippi Medical Center, Department of Biomedical Materials Science, 2500 N. State Street, Jackson, MS 39216, USA

Neelima Gupta, P. P. Singh and Rahul Kumar Bagla
Department of Otorhinolaryngology, University College of Medical Sciences and GTB Hospital, Delhi 110095, India

Mahmut Deniz, Zafer Ciftci and Erdogan Gultekin
Department of Otorhinolaryngology, School of Medicine, Namik Kemal University, 59100 Tekirdag, Turkey

Hemkant Verma, Siddharth Pandey, Kapil Dev Sheoran and Sanjay Marwah
Department of Surgery, Pt. B.D. Sharma, PGIMS, Rohtak 124001, India

M. Ezzedien Rabie, Abdullah Saad Al Qahtani, Sherif B. M. Taha and Ismail El Hakeem
Department of Surgery, Armed Forces Hospital, Southern Region, Khamis Mushait, Saudi Arabia

Olajide Ogunbiyi and Ahmad El Hadad
Department of Radiology, Armed Forces Hospital, Southern Region, Khamis Mushait, Saudi Arabia

Ming-Ho Wu and Han-Yun Wu
Department of Surgery, Tainan Municipal Hospital, 670 Chung-Te Road, Tainan 701, Taiwan

William D. Harrison, Deborah Lees, Jamie A'Court, Thomas Ankers, Ian Harper, Dominic Inman and Mike R. Reed
Orthopaedic Department, Wansbeck General Hospital, Northumbria Healthcare Trust, Woodhorn Lane, Ashington, Northumberland NE63 9JJ, UK

Siripong Sirikurnpiboon and Suparat Amornpornchareon
Department of Surgery, Rajavithi Hospital, College of Medicine, Rangsit University, Phayathai Road, Rajathewee, Bangkok 10400, Thailand

S. Roy
Global Health Economics and Market Access, Ethicon, Somerville, NJ 08876, USA

S. Ghosh
Global Health Economics and Market Access, Ethicon, Cincinnati, OH 45242, USA

A. Yoo
Medical Devices Epidemiology, Johnson & Johnson, New Brunswick, NJ 08901, USA

Freahiywot Aklew Teshager
Gondar University Referral Hospital, University of Gondar, P.O. Box 196, Gondar, Ethiopia

Eshetu Haileselassie Engeda and Workie ZemeneWorku
Department of Nursing, College of Medicine and Health Sciences, University of Gondar, P.O. Box 196, Gondar, Ethiopia

Fionn Coughlan, Prasad Ellanti, Cliodhna Ní Fhoghlu, Andrew Moriarity and Niall Hogan
St. James's Hospital, Dublin, Ireland

Vincenzo Colabianchi and Marika Langella
1Plastic SurgeryUnit, Casa di Cura Villa Alba, Bologna Medical Center, 40136 Bologna, Italy

Giancarlo de Bernardinis
General Surgery Unit, Presidio Ospedaliero Villa Letizia, 67100 L'Aquila, Italy

Matteo Giovannini
General Surgery Unit, Casa di Cura Villa Alba, Bologna Medical Center, 40136 Bologna, Italy

Danilo Dodero
Divisione di Ostetricia e Ginecologia, ASL 4 Chiavarese, Ospedale Rivoli, 16033 Lavagna, Italy

Luca Bernardini
Dipartimento Materno Infantile, Ostetricia e Ginecologia, ASL 5 Spezzino, 19100 La Spezia, Italy

Ehsan Yıldız and Yavuz Savas Koca
Department of General Surgery, School of Medicine, Suleyman Demirel University, Isparta, Turkey

Rangsan Niramis, Maitree Anuntkosol, Veera Buranakitjaroen, Achariya Tongsin, Varaporn Mahatharadol, Wannisa Poocharoen, Suranetr La-orwong and Kulsiri Tiansri
Department of Surgery, Queen Sirikit National Institute of Child Health, Bangkok 10400, Thailand
College of Medicine, Rangsit University, Bangkok 10400, Thailand

Darpanarayan Hazra, Indrani Sen, Edwin Stephen and Sunil Agarwal
Department of Vascular Surgery, The Christian Medical College, Vellore 632004, India

Sukesh Chandran Nair and Joy Mammen
Department of Transfusion Medicine and Immunohaematology, The Christian Medical College, Vellore 632004, India

Daniel Kinyuru Ojuka
Department of Surgery, University of Nairobi, P.O. Box 19969-00202, Nairobi, Kenya

Jana Macleod
Department of Surgery, Kenyatta University, Kenya

Catherine Kwamboka Nyabuto
Spinal Injury Hospital, Nairobi, Kenya

Rajith Mendis
Westmead Hospital, Sydney, NSW2145, Australia

Caran Cheung
University of Sydney, Sydney, NSW2006, Australia

David Martin
Department of Upper GI Surgery, Concord Hospital, Sydney, NSW 2139, Australia
Department of Upper GI Surgery, Royal Prince Alfred Hospital, Sydney, NSW 2050, Australia
Department of Upper GI Surgery, Strathfield Private Hospital, Sydney, NSW 2135, Australia

George Whittaker
School of Medical Education, King's College London, London SE1 1UL, UK

Hamid Abboudi, Muhammed Shamim Khan, Prokar Dasgupta and Kamran Ahmed
Department of Urology, Guy's and St.Thomas' NHS Foundation Trust, London SE1 9RT, UK
MRC Centre for Transplantation, King's College London, London SE1 9RT, UK

Rossella Sgarzani, Luca Negosanti, Paolo Giovanni Morselli, Veronica Vietti Michelina and Riccardo Cipriani
Plastic Surgery Department, Sant'Orsola-Malpighi Hospital, University of Bologna, Via Massarenti 9, 40138 Bologna, Italy

Luigi Maria Lapalorcia
Plastic Surgery Department, Asl 1 of Umbria, Citta di Castello, Località Chioccolo, 06012 Perugia, Italy

Andrew Emmanuel, Ezzat Chohda, Carolyn Sands, Joseph Ellul and Hamid Khawaja
Department of General Surgery, Princess Royal University Hospital, Kings College NHS Foundation Trust, Farnborough Common, Orpington, Kent BR6 8ND, UK

B. Manzoor and N. Heywood
Department of Surgery, University Hospital of South Manchester and The University of Manchester, MAHSC, Manchester, UK

A. Sharma
Wythenshawe Hospital, University Hospital of South Manchester, Southmoor Road, Manchester M23 9LT, UK

L. Borly, M. B. Ellebæk and N. Qvist
Surgical Department A, Odense University Hospital, Denmark

Thomas Aherne, Seamus McHugh, Elrasheid A. Kheirelseid, Daragh Moneley, Austin L. Leahy and Peter Naughton
Department of Vascular Surgery, Beaumont Hospital, Dublin 9, Ireland

Michael J. Lee
Department of Interventional Radiology, Beaumont Hospital, Dublin 9, Ireland

Noel McCaffrey
Department of Human and Health Performance, Dublin City University, Dublin 9, Ireland

Carlos Placer, JoseM. Enriquez-Navascués, Ander Timoteo, Garazi Elorza, Nerea Borda, Lander Gallego and Yolanda Saralegui
Department of Colorectal Surgery, Division of General and Gastrointestinal Surgery, Donostia University Hospital, 20014 San Sebastián, Spain

Nigel Pereira, Jovana P. Lekovich, Rony T. Elias and Steven D. Spandorfer
The Ronald O. Perelman and Claudia Cohen Center for Reproductive Medicine, Weill Cornell Medical College, 1305 York Avenue, 6th Floor, New York, NY 10021, USA

Allison C. Petrini
Department of Obstetrics and Gynecology, Weill Cornell Medical College, 1305 York Avenue, 6th Floor, New York, NY 10021, USA

9 781632 413840